# A Pocket Guide to
Long-Term Care Medicine

# CURRENT CLINICAL PRACTICE

Neil S. Skolnik, MD, Series Editor

For other titles published in this series, go to
www.springer.com/series/7633

# Long-Term Care Medicine
# A Pocket Guide

## *Pamela Ann Fenstemacher*

*Abington Memorial Hospital,
Family Medicine Residency Program Associate Director of Geriatric
Education Abington, PA, USA*

*and*

## *Peter Winn*

*University of Oklahoma,
Department of Family and Preventive Medicine,
Professor and Head of Geriatric Program, Oklahoma City, OK, USA*

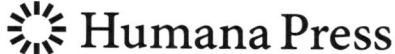

*Editors*

Pamela Ann Fenstemacher
Associate Director of Geriatric
Education of the Family
Medicine Residency Program
Abington Memorial Hospital
Suite 108
500 Old York Road
Jenkintown, Pennsylvania
19046 USA
pfenstemacher@gmail.com

Peter Winn
Professor and
Head of Geriatric Program,
University of Oklahoma,
Department of Family and
Preventive Medicine,
NE. 10th St. 900
73104 Oklahoma City Oklahoma
USA
peter-winn@ouhsc.edu

ISBN 978-1-60761-141-7          e-ISBN 978-1-60761-142-4
DOI 10.1007/978-1-60761-142-4
Springer New York Dordrecht Heidelberg London

© Springer Science+Business Media, LLC 2011
All rights reserved. This work may not be translated or copied in whole or in part without the written permission of the publisher (Humana Press, c/o Springer Science+Business Media, LLC, 233 Spring Street, New York, NY 10013, USA), except for brief excerpts in connection with reviews or scholarly analysis. Use in connection with any form of information storage and retrieval, electronic adaptation, computer software, or by similar or dissimilar methodology now known or hereafter developed is forbidden.
The use in this publication of trade names, trademarks, service marks, and similar terms, even if they are not identified as such, is not to be taken as an expression of opinion as to whether or not they are subject to proprietary rights.
While the advice and information in this book are believed to be true and accurate at the date of going to press, neither the authors nor the editors nor the publisher can accept any legal responsibility for any errors or omissions that may be made. The publisher makes no warranty, express or implied, with respect to the material contained herein.

Printed on acid-free paper

Humana Press is part of Springer Science+Business Media (www.springer.com)

Individuals over 65 represent the fasted growing portion of the population in the United States, consume the highest proportion of the country's healthcare dollars, and often live in a long-term care facility for the latter portion of their lives. The care in long-term care facilities is provided for by primary care physicians who may or may not be board certified in geriatrics and who more likely than not have never had a directed learning experience in long-term care. It is to this group of physicians, who provide to bulk of care to the most vulnerable portion of our population that this needed book is directed.

The editors, Drs. Fenstemacher and Winn, have extensive academic and practical experience in long-term care and have been involved in leadership positions with the American Medical Directors Association, which is the professional association for long-term care physicians. From this vantage point they have selected authors who have given both an academic and practical perspective on the issues most relevant to the patients we take care of in long-term care facilities. The book's emphasis is on giving the practicing physician a digestible guide to understand and better manage many of the issue that come up in long-term care facilities.

The book is readable, practical, interesting, and increasingly relevant. For this the editors and authors are owed our thanks.

>   -Neil Skolnik, M.D.
>   Professor of Family and Community Medicine
>   Temple University School of Medicine
>   Associate Director
>   Family Medicine Residency Program
>   Abington Memorial Hospital

Practical, interesting, relevant

# Preface

Whether practitioners are still in training, recently graduated, or deciding to change the direction or focus of their career paths, either by choice or necessity, they can find themselves immersed in the long-term care (LTC) arena. Any practitioner of LTC can be overwhelmed when confronted by a LTC system that is both complex and highly regulated, let alone taking care of patients who are challenging even to the most experienced among us. These patients are challenging not only because they have numerous chronic medical conditions and extensive and complicated medication regimens, but also advanced age and frailty. As experienced clinicians, educators, and medical directors in LTC, we have written this guide for practitioners in hopes of continuing to improve the quality of care provided throughout the LTC continuum by imparting to practitioners the current knowledge in this field as well as the experience our chapter authors have acquired over many years working in LTC.

Even the most experienced practitioners who have taken AMDA's course on medical direction have commented on how much of the information on LTC care presented in the course is not readily available or frequently taught. The content of this guide for practitioners is aimed at filling this void. Both the American Medical Directors Association (AMDA) and its state chapters continue to work tirelessly to meet the LTC practitioner's needs.

The chapters of this guide address the varied components of the LTC system as well as how to take care of the patients and residents living within it. The contributors to this guide are passionate about LTC and many have worked within AMDA to create and disseminate a knowledge base for practitioners through varied means such as AMDA's clinical practice guidelines, conferences, and white papers, all of which have served as resources to this guide.

We hope that you find The Pocket Guide to Long-Term Care an invaluable resource to complement your quest to optimize the care and living experience of your patients in LTC that supports patient-centered care as well as patient choice, well-being, dignity, and an improved quality of life.

This guide is dedicated to the AMDA staff, especially Lorraine Tarnove, and all our AMDA colleagues who have mentored both of us over the years.

Jenkintown, PA  Pamela Ann Fenstemacher
Oklahoma City, OK  Peter Winn

# Contents

Part 1  An Introduction to Long-Term Care

1  Home Care ............................................................................. 3

2  Assisted Living and Residential Care ................................... 15

3  Nursing Facilities .................................................................. 37

4  The Role of Practitioners and the Medical Director ........... 55

Part 2  Common Clinical Conditions in Long-Term Care

5  Common Clinical Conditions in Long-Term Care .............. 75

6  Acute Change in Condition .................................................. 123

7  Health Maintenance and Prevention ................................... 145

8  Integrating Palliative Care into Practice .............................. 159

9  Weight and Nutrition ............................................................ 187

10  Wound Care .......................................................................... 205

Part 3  Psychosocial Aspects of Long-Term Care

11  Dementia, Delirium, and Depression ................................... 225

12  Ethical and Legal Issues ....................................................... 247

13  Caring for Families ............................................................... 269

## Part 4  Special Issues in Long-Term Care

14  Documentation and Coding ................................................. 285

15  Medication Management in Long-Term Care ..................... 299

16  Rehabilitation and Maximizing Function .......................... 323

Erratum .................................................................................... E1

Index ......................................................................................... 337

# Contributors

**Ross H. Albert MD, PhD**
Hospitalist, Connecticut Multispecialty Group,
Hartford Hospital, Hartford, CT 06107

**Alva Baker MD, CMD**
Former AMDA President, 2811 Carlisle Drive New Windsor MD,
21776, USA

**David Brechtelsbauer MD, CMD**
Department of Family Medicine, Sanford School of Medicine at the
University of South Dakota, 1115 East 20th Street Sioux Falls SD,
57105-1013, USA

**J. Kenneth Brubaker MD, CMD**
Chief Medical Director, Pennsylvania Office of Long Term Living,
Director of Senior Services, Lancaster General Health, Department
of Geriatrics Specialists, Lancaster General Hospital, 2110 Harrisburg Pike, Ste. 300 Lancaster PA, 17604, USA

**Leonard Gelman MD, CMD**
Medical Director, Capital Care Ballston Spa, 20 Prospect Street,
Suite 106 Ballston Spa NY, 12020, USA

**Todd H. Goldberg MD, CMD, FACP**
Associate Professor, Director of Geriatric Medicine, WVU Health
Sciences Center, Internal Medicine, Geriatrics Section, Charleston
Area Medical Center, Charleston WV, 25304, USA

**Daniel Haimowitz MD, FACP, CMD**
Geriatrician and Multi-facility Medical Director, 1 Gardenia Road
Levittown PA, 19057, USA

**Randall D. Huss MD, CMD**
President, St. John's Clinic – Rolla Division, Administration,
1605 Martin Springs Drive, Suite 360b Rolla MO, 65401, USA

**Thomas Lawrence MD**
Multi-Facility Medical Director for Long-Term Care and Geriatrician, Main Line Health System, Main Line Geriatrics, Bryn Mawr Hospital Health Center, 3855 West Chester Pike, Suite 300 Newtown Square PA, 19073, USA

**Steven A. Levenson MD, CMD**
Multi-Facility Medical Director for Long-Term Care, 7801 Ruxwood Road Baltimore MD, 21204, USA

**Joel A. Levine MD, FACP, FACG**
Chief of Gastroenterology and Associate Professor, WVU Health Sciences Center, Internal Medicine, GI Section, Charleston Area Medical Center, Charleston WV, 25304, USA

**Susan T. Marcolina MD**
Geriatrician for Overlake Medical Clinics, Downtown Bellevue, 400 108th Avenue, Suite 100, Bellevue, WA 98004, USA

**Naushira Pandya MD, CMD**
Associate Professor and Chair Director, Geriatrics Education Center, Department of Geriatrics, Nova Southeastern University College of Osteopathic Medicine, 3200 S University Dr Ft. Lauderdale FL, 33328, USA

**Andrew Rosenzweig MD, FACP**
Associate Fellowship Director, Division of Geriatrics, Abington Memorial Hospital, Clinical Assistant Professor of Medicine, Drexel University College of Medicine, 1200 Old York Rd, Elkins Building Suite 2B Abington PA, 19001, USA

**Robert Salinas MD, CAQ (G, HPM)**
Associate Professor, Director Community Medicine, Department of Family and Preventative Medicine, The University of Oklahoma, 900 NE 10th Street Oklahoma City OK, 73104, USA

**David A. Smith MD, FAAFP, CMD**
Professor of Family & Community Medicine, Texas A&M, President, Geriatric Consultants of Central Texas, PA, Family Medicine Department, Texas A&M University College of Medicine, 901 North Fisk #224 Brownwood TX, 76801, USA

**Richard G. Stefanacci DO, MGH, MBA, AGSF, CMD**
CMS Health Policy Scholar 2003–04, The Institute for Geriatric Studies, Center for Medicare Medication Management (cm$^3$), Mayes College of Healthcare Business & Policy, University of the Sciences in Philadelphia, Mayes College of Healthcare Business & Policy, 600 South 43rd Street Philadelphia PA, 19104-4495, USA

**Keith Swanson Pharm. D., CGP**
Associate Professor, Department of Pharmacy: Clinical and Administrative Sciences, University of Oklahoma Health Sciences Center, PO Box 26901, 1110 N. Stonewall, College of Pharmacy Oklahoma City OK, 73126-0901, USA

**Deborah Way MD**
Geriatrician and Palliative Care Specialist, LIFE – Living Independently for Elders, 4508 Chestnut Street Philadelphia PA, 19139, USA

**Peter Winn MD, CMD**
Professor and Head of Geriatrics Program, Department of Family and Preventive Medicine, University of Oklahoma, 900 NE 10th Street Oklahoma City OK, 73104, USA

# Part I
An Introduction to Long-Term Care

# Chapter 1
# Home Care

Robert Salinas

**Keywords:** Home care • House call • Agency home health care • Skilled care • Reimbursement

## INTRODUCTION

It is estimated that by the year 2020, the number of people aged 65 and over in the United States will increase from 36 to 50 million, the fastest growing segment of our population. Although this age group still represents approximately 13% of the current population, they account for roughly 36% of all health care-related expenditures in the United States [1]. As this demographic enlarges with Americans aging well into their golden years, a groundswell of home care needs will be created. Baby boomers have a strong desire to remain in their homes and age in place, which will increase this need for home care even further.

The continued growth in the number of older Americans afflicted with multiple chronic conditions will also cause an increased need for home care. Currently, many of these elderly persons remain homebound and experience great difficulty in accessing timely and needed health care services, including regular visits to a physician's office. As a result, many of these frail elderly remain isolated with their medical care fragmented.

Recent trends suggest that the number of frail elderly requiring emergency room evaluation and hospital admission are on the rise. Often, these emergency room visitations are driven by exacerbation of symptoms from chronic conditions such as congestive heart failure, chronic obstructive pulmonary disease, and diabetes [2]. In addition, for those patients who are admitted to the hospital, many are also now experiencing shorter lengths of hospital stays [3]. This increase in chronically ill elderly and the changing reimbursement of hospital-based care are shifting health care from the acute hospital to community-based care. A dramatic paradigm shift is not only occurring in the way health care is being delivered, but also developed for this vulnerable segment of the population [4]. With the aid of technology and more strategies to support the prevention of acute care hospitalization, home care has emerged as a viable delivery of care model that will help meet the needs of both an overworked health care system and those homebound patients who experience difficulties accessing medical care [5].

This chapter reviews the important components of the delivery of medical care in the home, including physician house calls and the services provided by home health care agencies.

## HOME CARE

Home care is defined as the provision of health care-related services and equipment to patients in the home for the purpose of restoring and maintaining his or her maximal level of comfort, function, and health [6]. The term also implies the use of any therapeutic, diagnostic, or social support services provided in the individual's home. Generally, the goals of care or the stated care plan help determine the level of home care interventions. This may include a series of house calls by a physician, nurse practitioner, or physician assistant and the services of a home health care agency. The term also encompasses an interdisciplinary team approach to the delivery of care in the home that includes individually tailored therapeutic, diagnostic, and/or social support services aimed at restoring or maintaining independent functional status [6].

The services of home health are generally available to patients who have a need for services in the home when acutely ill, declining in function, or when transitioning back to home or an assisted living facility, after being discharged from an acute care hospital or rehabilitation setting [5].

## THE PHYSICIAN HOUSE CALL

The traditional place called "home" has changed as older adults have opted to leave their community dwelling and move to an assisted living or independent living facility. There are many reasons why a practitioner might decide to visit a patient in their home. It may be for either an acute care visit in which the patient is unable to come to the outpatient clinic setting or for ongoing management of a progressive chronic condition. A home visit is also justified when the clinician attempts to gather more information about the environmental conditions of a patient who continues to experience recurrent falls and injuries. At other times, a home visit might be necessary to explore end-of-life care preferences in a patient with advanced illness who is transitioning to hospice care [7]. Some physicians perform episodic home visits on a group of selected frail patients, while others have been able to establish a practice exclusively in home care.

Contrary to a common belief, patients are not required to be homebound in order for a physician to submit billing for medical services rendered during a house call. The requirements are different for those patients who require agency-delivered home health care services (to be discussed later in this chapter).

**Preparing for the House Call**

When making a home visit, it is important to determine the purpose and goals of the visit. This may require advance notice to both family members and members of the home health care team. At times, this might include the hospice team or community-based case worker involved with coordination of patient care. Planning ahead will help determine what procedural instruments may be required for a particular patient such as toe nail clippers or supplies for injection of medication. Table 1.1 lists some of the common items found in the modern house call doctor's bag.

During the home visit, clinicians should not only assess the patient's medical conditions but also assess the patient's functional status, cognitive ability, and level of independence. This includes evaluation of basic activities of daily living (ADLs) such as ambulation, transfers, feeding, bathing, and toileting. For those patients with severe physical and mental limitations, assessment of functional status will identify the need for adaptive equipment that may delay institutionalization. Many assistive devices and durable

TABLE 1.1. The doctor's bag

Stethoscope
Blood pressure cuff
Thermometer
Pen light
Prescription pad
Pharmacopeia
Toe nail clippers
Examination gloves
Syringes and needles
Sharp containing box
Scissors
Street map or GPS

TABLE 1.2. Assessment in the home

Patient assessment
    Functional assessment
    Mental/cognitive assessment
    Nutritional assessment
    Medication use and compliance
    Advance care planning
Caregiver assessment
    Assessment of burden of caregiving
    Assessment of caregiver
Environmental assessment
    Safety in the home
    Needs for special durable medical equipment (DME)
Community assessment
    Safety of neighborhood for patient care
    Use of community resources

medical equipment (DME) such as a walker or bedside commode can aide a person in remaining independent in the home.

Often, a decline in ADLs is preceded by a decline in instrumental activities of daily living (IADL'S) and identifying a deficit in the latter might help assess a person's ability to safely live alone as well as to identify strategies to maximize safety measures and promote independence. As opposed to an office visit, a house call might identify the need for home remodeling and retrofitting that will allow better access and facilitate mobility.

Formal or informal caregiver assessment is also important in determining whether a plan of care can be successfully implemented in the home. Often, the caregiver might be a spouse or immediate family member who is involved with day in and day out continual care of the patient and therefore is at risk for burn out. Table 1.2. lists some important aspects of a home assessment.

### Billing for House Call Services

Under current Medicare rules, any licensed physician, nurse practitioner, or physician assistant is allowed to make a house call and bill appropriately for those services that are rendered. Physicians are allowed to bill the patient or a third-party payer using the appropriate CPT codes for the level of service provided [6]. Most third-party payers follow the rates and guidelines for billing set forth by Medicare and state Medicaid offices. Physicians are also allowed, as they are in other health care settings, to bill based on the amount of time directly spent with or in counseling the patient. It is important that each component of the encounter be appropriately documented for the level of services provided. Currently, physicians are not allowed to bill for travel time associated with making a house call (Table 1.3).

TABLE 1.3. Medicare part B reimbursement 2009

| New patients | | Established patients | |
|---|---|---|---|
| Code | Reimbursement | Code | Reimbursement |
| 99341 | $54.10 | 99347 | $52.66 |
| 99342 | $78.63 | 99348 | $79.35 |
| 99343 | $129.48 | 99349 | $115.41 |
| 99344 | $199.09 | 99359 | $160 |

## AGENCY HOME HEALTH CARE

Under the current Medicare guidelines, beneficiaries who require episodic care in the home may be eligible for home health care. The purpose of home health care is to assemble a team of qualified caregivers (Table 1.4) that can provide assistance in the home of a person who requires skilled nursing care, physical therapy, speech therapy, and other services. Often the referral is made when the physician notes a decline in the patient's level of functional independence, which has been shown to place the elderly at risk for hospitalization or institutionalization [5].

TABLE 1.4. Members of the home health care team

Skilled nurse
Physical therapist
Speech therapist
Occupational therapist
Home health care aide
Social worker
Case manager

### Requirements for Agency Home Health Care

Two important requirements that must be met before a physician can prescribe agency home health care for a Medicare beneficiary are worthy of review. First, a physician must deem that the patient meets the requirement for "homebound" status and has demonstrated a need for episodic skilled nursing care, physical therapy, or speech therapy [6]. The interpretation of homebound status often leads to confusion. Its definition is fully explained in Figure. 1.1.

A patient is considered homebound if "leaving the home would require a considerable and taxing effort" and if the patient "has a condition due to illness or injury which restricts ability to leave the residence except with the aid of supportive devices, the use of special transportation, or the assistance of another person, or if the patient has a condition such that leaving the home is medically contraindicated." Homebound patients may leave the home "if absences are infrequent or for periods of relatively short duration…or for the purpose of receiving medical treatment."

FIGURE. 1.1. Definition of homebound status (Revised from the publication "Medicare and Home Health Care," Baltimore, MD: Centers for Medicaid and Medicare, U.S. Department of Health and Human Services, 2007).

At times, the home setting may not be the best venue to execute a complex care plan, especially for those very frail patients with multiple health care needs. In such cases, other options to deliver episodic care may be more realistic and consistent with the patients needs, and therefore should be explored. Such options might include admission to a rehabilitation hospital or a skilled nursing facility after an acute hospitalization.

When a patient is deemed appropriate for home health care, any physician may order home health and begin a care plan. More recently with the new delivery of hospital-based home care, many patients are leaving the hospital setting with prescribed home health care services that facilitate transition back to their homes [8]. Often multiple medical providers are involved with patient care as they go from one to another health care setting. Communication among providers during an episode of care transition is of paramount importance in making sure that all team members are aware of changes in patient's needs and the individual care plan [9, 10].

A physician can either write a prescription or give a verbal order to a representative of an agency to begin services. The initiation of the care plan needs to include information on the patient's overall functional status as well as why the patient was referred to home health care, while keeping goals and purposes in mind. Background information regarding caregivers in the home or other concerns related to frailty should be shared with the home health care team as well. This information will help ensure that the correct care plan can be carried out in the home and identify potential barriers that could prevent successful implementation. The approach to delivering good home health care is based on the team approach for which each member of the team provides a valuable skill set that is aimed at restoring health or rehabilitating a patient with individualized needs [11].

## MEMBERS OF THE TEAM

The approach to delivering good home health care services is based on the premise of negotiating individual health care goals with the patient and family and then developing a plan of care that can sustain the efforts in reaching these goals. Similar to the skilled nursing facility or rehabilitation setting, each team member provides valuable shared information and skills that are used in collaboration for maximizing patient outcomes. Many of the home health care team members might have regular contact with the patient's family and thus be in a better position to ascertain whether a plan of care can be successfully instituted in the home.

### Skilled Nursing Care

Homebound patients often require licensed practical nurse (LPN) or registered nurses (RN) to provide skilled level of care for patients in the home that includes educating patients and caregivers on acute or chronic medical conditions and administration of medication, obtaining laboratory specimens, infusing IV therapy, and/or providing local wound care. Upon admission to home health, each patient is assessed in terms of functional status, memory, and cognitive status, and a reconciliation of all prescribed and over-the-counter medications is performed [12–15]. Most home health care agencies are now capable of using computer-based programs to look for potential drug interactions.

Once the care plan has been determined, skilled care nurses will generally provide services two to three times a week. However, they can be authorized by the physician to see patients more frequently at the beginning of care (front-loaded visits) to ensure an appropriate care plan based on the needs of the patient. Skilled nurses may either identify another medical problem that has not been listed in the physician's medical record or aid in identifying barriers to the delivery of good care in the home like caregiver stress or financial burdens.

Nurses are also poised to gather beneficial information for the physician, including end-of-life care preferences. The function of community-based nurses continues to expand and their role in caring for the homebound chronically ill continues to emerge [16]. Community-based nurses are involved in the promotion, monitoring, and maintenance of health, especially in homebound persons afflicted with chronic illness.

### Physical Therapist

Physical therapists are members of the home health care team who provide therapy to improve or maximize lower extremity strength and conditioning of patients. Many times these patients have a history of recurrent falls or have become deconditioned following an acute illness or hospitalization. Referrals for physical therapy in the home frequently involve patients who have suffered an acute cerebral vascular accident (CVA) or had major lower extremity orthopedic surgery [17, 18].

Physical therapists also participate in the overall care plan, as well as assisting in educating the patient's caregivers on how to improve the patient's function, safety, and independence. Physicians may also receive recommendations from the physical therapist about assisted devices or other forms of DME that the patient may benefit from such as canes, walkers, shower chairs, or bathroom grab bars.

### Speech Therapist

Under the current Medicare home health care guidelines, a physician can request a referral for home health care solely for the purpose of providing speech therapy in the home. Speech therapy is frequently sought in a patient who has suffered a recent stroke with subsequent speaking and swallowing difficulties or has had repeated episodes of aspiration pneumonia. A recommended change in dietary consistency may also be necessary in patients who demonstrate swallowing difficulties due to illnesses such as progressive dementia or Parkinson's disease.

### Occupational Therapist

Occupational therapists often work in tandem with other members of the home health care team to promote functional independence with more focus on improving ADLs. Homebound patients often experience a decline in level of independence during or following an acute illness. The occupational therapist may also recommend special adaptive equipment or DME that they feel will assist the patient's independence.

### Aide in Attendance

Based on eligibility and medical necessity, home health care agencies can provide nursing aides to assist patients in ADLs as well as light housework if a patient is still too weak to function independently. They are important members of the team and supplement the care provided by family members or other caregivers in the home.

## PHYSICIAN REIMBURSEMENT FOR HOME HEALTH CARE SERVICES

Physicians who order home health care from a qualified Medicare agency are eligible to receive payment for reviewing the home health care agency plan of care. Once a referral to home health has been made, the physician will receive an initial certification form (Form 485) which the physician will review, agree with the plan of care, and return the form to the home health care agency after signing it. Once this has been done, the physician is allowed to bill for the initial certification period/initial plan of care (G01800), if they are in agreement with the need for home health care services.

If the patient continues to require home health care services, the physician must sign a recertification (G0179) and once again the physician can submit billing for this review. Licensed physicians are the only ones who can sign these forms and bill for certification or recertification of home health care services. Mid-level providers cannot sign these certification forms. If the physician spends a minimum of 30 min in a 30-day period providing oversight and directing services during the episode of home health, he or she is also allowed to bill for Care Plan Oversight (CPO) as well (G0181). This oversight and direction of services should be documented. In contrast to billing requirements for certification and recertification, nurse practitioners or physician assistants *are* allowed to bill for CPO. One important caveat is that surgeons are not allowed to bill for CPO if the oversight is related to a surgical procedure that they performed, because their services are bundled into postoperative care fees. Table 1.5 lists the G codes for billing for agency home health care.

TABLE 1.5. Care plan oversight (CPO)

| Certification and recertification | |
|---|---|
| HCPCS code | Description |
| G0180-Certifcation | Initial home health certification, also known as reviewing and signing the initial plan of care |
| G0179-Recertification | Recertification of the plan of care-if the patient's care continues for an additional 60 days, the physician must review and sign recertification plan of care |
| G0181-Care plan oversight | Indicated for the supervision of a patient under the care of a Medicare-certified home health care agency (patient not present) |
| | Oversight is indicated for the patient whose care is complex and involves multiple disciplines, therapy requiring regular physician contact |

## THE FUTURE OF HOME HEALTH CARE

Due to the sustained growth in the number of people living with chronic illnesses that are associated with escalating medical expenditures, the provision of medical care in the home continues to evolve as a viable means of curtailing costs. It is alarming that approximately two million people, or 5% of the Medicare population, account for nearly half on the Medicare budget in the United States [4]. Medical technology breakthroughs and the expected increase in the number of older and chronically ill Americans are predicted to push medical costs up even higher. Currently, the government is exploring innovative cost-effective alternative health care delivery models because it will be crucial to contain future cost increases.

New technological advances being studied allow monitoring of vital signs in the home of heart failure patients in order to catch exacerbations early and prevent costly hospitalizations [19-21]. This telemedicine technology not only allows home health care nurses to monitor a patient's blood pressure, pulse rate, and daily weight from a distance, but also to share vital signs with the patient's physician [22-24]. In the future, other models of care such as the "hospital at home" program can serve to reduce the high costs associated with hospitalization while obtaining good health outcomes for those patients who opt for treatment in the home [25-26].

## PEARLS FOR THE PRACTITIONER

- Many frail elderly are homebound and experience great difficulty in accessing timely and needed health care services, including regular visits to a physician's office.
- Home care is defined as the provision of health care-related services and equipment to patients in the home for the purpose of restoring and maintaining his or her maximal level of comfort, function, and health.
- Home health care assembles an interdisciplinary team of qualified collaborating caregivers that maximizes outcomes by sharing information and skills in the patient's home.
- Home health care services are best delivered by negotiating individual health care goals with the patient and family and then developing a plan of care that can sustain the efforts in reaching those goals.
- Only licensed physicians working with a qualified Medicare agency are eligible to receive payment for reviewing the home health care agency plan of care. But, physicians and mid-level providers are allowed to bill for CPO.

- During a home visit, clinicians should not only assess the patient's medical conditions but also assess the patient's functional status, cognitive ability, and level of independence.
- Patients are not required to be homebound in order for a physician to submit billing for a house call.

## WEBSITES

- American Academy of Home Care Physicians www.aahcp.org
- National Association of Home Care and Hospice www.nahc.org

## REFERENCES

1. Aging in the United States-Past, Present, and Future. Department of Commerce Report. 1997. Available at: http://www.census.gov/ipc/prod/97agewc.pdf. Accessed November 15, 2008
2. Roberts D, McKay MP, Shaffer A. Increasing Rates of Emergency Department Visits for Elderly Patients in the United States, 1993–2003. Annals of Emergency Medicine, Vol. 51, No. 6, pp. 769–774, 2008
3. Baker DW, Einstadter D, Husak SS, et al. Trends in Postdischarge Mortality and Readmissions, Has Length of Stay Declined Too Far? Archives of Internal Medicine, Vol. 164, pp. 538–544, 2004
4. Holtz-Eakin D. High-Cost Medicare Beneficiaries. Congressional Budget Office. May, 2005, pp. 1–12. Available at: http://www.cbo.gov/ftpdocs/63xx/doc6332/05-03-MediSpending.pdf. Accessed October 26, 2008
5. Murkofsky RL, Alston K. The Past, Present, and Future of Skilled Home Health Agency Care. Clinics in Geriatric Medicine, Vol. 25, pp. 1–17, 2009
6. Levine SA, Boal J, Boling P. Home Care. Journal of the American Medical Association, Vol. 290, pp. 1203–1207, 2003
7. Verbrugge LM, Jette AM. The Disablement Process. Social Science Medicine, Vol. 38, No. 1, pp. 1–14, 1994
8. Billings JA, Ferris FD, Macdonald N, et al. The Role of Palliative Care in Medical Education: Report from a National Consensus Conference. Journal of Palliative Medicine, Vol. 4, No. 3, pp. 361–371, 2001
9. Coleman EA, Berenson RA. Lost in Transition: Challenges and Opportunities for Improving the Quality of Transition Care. Annals of Internal Medicine, Vol. 140, pp. 533–536, 2004
10. Kripalani S, LeFevre F, Phillips CO, et al. Deficits in Communication and Information Transfer Between Hospital-Based and Primary Care Physicians, Implications for Patient Safety and Continuity of Care. Journal of the American Medical Association, Vol. 297, No. 8, pp. 831–841, 2007
11. Kuo Y-F, Sharma G, Freeman JL, Goodwin JS. Growth in the Care of Older Patients by Hospitalist in the United States. The New England Journal of Medicine, Vol. 360, No. 11, pp. 1102–1112, 2009
12. Toto P. Success Through Teamwork in the Home Health Setting: The Role of Occupational Therapy. Home Health Care Management and Practice, Vol. 19, No. 1, pp. 31–37, 2006

13. Mager DR. Medication Errors and the Home Care Patient. Home Healthcare Nurse, Vol. 25, No. 3, pp. 151–155, 2007
14. Forster A, Muriff H, Peterson J, et al. The Incidence and Severity of Adverse Events Affecting Patients After Discharge from the Hospital. Annals of Internal Medicine, Vol. 138, pp. 161–167, 2003
15. Feldman MS, Frey P, Giammarco I, et al. Improving Medication Use in Newly Admitted Home Healthcare Patients: A Randomized Controlled Trial. Journal of the American Geriatric Society, Vol. 50, No. 9, pp. 1597–1598, 2002
16. Coleman EA, Smith JD, Raha D, Min SJ. Posthospital Medication Discrepancies. Archives of Internal Medicine, Vol. 165, pp. 1842–1847, 2005
17. Bruce ML, McAvay GJ, Raue PJ, et al. Major Depression in Elderly Home Health Care Patients. The American Journal of Psychiatry, Vol. 159, pp. 1367–1374, 2002
18. Boult C, Reider L, Frey K, et al. Early Effects of "Guided Care" on the Quality of Health Care for Multimorbid Older Persons: A Cluster Randomized Control Trial. Journal of Gerontology, Vol. 63A, No. 3, pp. 321–327, 2008
19. Stevens JA, Thomas K, Teh L, et al. Unintentional Fall Injuries Associated with Walkers and Canes in Older Adults Treated in U.S Emergency Departments. Journal of the American Geriatric Society, Vol. 57, pp. 1464–1469, 2009
20. Fortinsky RH, Baker D, Gottschalk M, et al. Extent of Implementation of Evidence-Based Fall Prevention Practices for Older Patients in Home Health Care. Journal of the American Geriatric Society, Vol. 56, pp. 737–743, 2008
21. Kashem A, Droogan MT, Santamore WP, et al. Managing Heart Failure Care Using an Internet-Based Telemedicine System. Journal of Cardiac Failure, Vol. 14, No. 2, pp. 121–126, 2008
22. Frey KA, Bratton R. Role of Telemedicine in the Health Care Delivery System. Journal of the American Board of Family Practice, Vol. 15, No. 2, pp. 170–171, 2002
23. Myers S, Grant R, Lugn NE, et al. Impact of Home-Based Monitoring on the Care of Patients with Congestive Heart Failure. Home Health Care Management and Practice, Vol. 18, No. 6, pp. 444–451, 2006
24. Leff B, Burton JR. The Future History of Home Care and Physician House Calls in the United States. Journal of Gerontology, Vol. 56A, No. 10, pp. M603–M608, 2001
25. Leff B, Burton L, Mader S, et al. Hospital at Home: Feasibility and Outcomes of a Program To Provide Hospital-Level Care at Home for Acutely Ill Older Patients. Annals of Internal Medicine, Vol. 143, pp. 798–808, 2005
26. Sheppard S, Doll H, Angus R, et al. Avoiding Hospital Admission Through Provision of Hospital Care at Home: A Systematic Review and Meta-Analysis of Individual Patient Data. Canadian Medical Journal, Vol. 180, No. 2, pp. 175–182, 2009

# Chapter 2
# Assisted Living and Residential Care

Daniel Haimowitz

**Keywords:** Assisted living • Assisted living residents • Assisted living costs • Assisted living facilities • Assisted living physicians

## INTRODUCTION

Assisted living (AL) is becoming an increasingly important component of the long-term care continuum. The continued trend is for a greater number of people to choose to reside in assisted living communities (ALC). There are over 36,000 licensed facilities and over 950,000 residents (Robert Mollica, personal communication, 2007).

AL is usually significantly less expensive than nursing home care and can offer more autonomy and privacy. Due to a variety of factors, including patients' desires to age in place and remain independent as long as possible and avoid nursing home placement, AL residents have experienced an overall increase in the prevalence of frailty and ADL dependence. Many practitioners have commented that residents in AL today have characteristics similar to nursing home residents of several decades ago. The increased number of AL beds along with some publicity of poor care has caused increased scrutiny of the AL industry from state legislators and regulatory agencies, as well as federal lawmakers. Along with changing state regulations, there has been improvements in staff education and facility oversight, and new concepts to improve affordability and facility designs. AL may serve as a bridge for some between independent living and the nursing home, but there are important differences between the nursing home and the AL setting.

## ASSISTED LIVING HISTORY

AL has experienced rapid growth over the past two decades. ALCs were opened initially to respond to consumer need when patients could not be cared for at home, yet did not require nursing home services. Core values include autonomy and choice, privacy and dignity, and the ability to age in place, within a home-like environment that differs from more formal institutional settings. This dramatic increased use of AL is in contrast to a much smaller rise in nursing home bed utilization over the past 15 years. A wide variety of ALCs have developed over this time, ranging from small "mom and pop" four to eight resident homes to large ALCs housing several hundred residents. Most of these facilities are for profit. This has contributed to the multitude of names for AL nationally (Table 2.1), which will be hereafter referred to as ALCs. The needs of consumers and variety of options drive the AL market.

TABLE 2.1. Various names for assisted living communities (ALC)

Adult Congregate Living Care
Adult Foster Care
Adult Homes
Adult Living Facilities
Basic Care Facilities
Board and Care
Catered Living Services
Community-Based Retirement Facilities
Community Residence Facilities
Community Residential Care Facilities
Congregate Care
Domiciliary Care
Elder Care Homes
Enhanced Care
Enhanced Living
Home for the Aged
Old Age Homes
Personal Care
Residential Care Facilities for the Elderly
Residential Facilities for Groups
Retirement Residences
Service-enriched Housing
Shared Housing Establishments
Sheltered Housing
Supportive Care
Supported Living

There has been conflict in the past between facility owners/providers and consumers groups. Providers have vigorously defended a "social" model for ALCs due to a wish to keep facilities as home-like as possible and not have requirements that would entail costly and time-consuming paperwork. Unfortunately, there have been multiple instances of elder abuse, poor care, and malpractice, which have led consumer advocates to favor more of a "medical" model. This underscores the increasing medical problems of AL residents. The trend has been towards more conciliatory attitudes between these two positions. Recent interest has been on person-centered care, and research geared specifically towards AL.

National organizations have worked together to improve care in AL. The national Assisted Living Workgroup (ALW), an initiative formed at the request of the U.S. Senate Special Committee on Aging, presented 110 recommendations in order to assure quality in AL. An outgrowth of the ALW is the Center for Excellence in Assisted Living (CEAL). CEAL is an ongoing effort at the national level to promote high-quality AL. CEAL also serves as an ongoing informational clearinghouse, bringing together research, best practices, and policy. There are multiple provider, consumer, profit, and nonprofit groups currently focusing on AL.

## DEFINITION OF ASSISTED LIVING

The variation among the different facilities makes it difficult to establish a uniform definition of AL. The ALW developed the following definition:

Assisted living is a state regulated and monitored residential long-term care option. Assisted living provides or coordinates oversight and services to meet the residents' individualized scheduled needs, based on the residents' assessments and service plans and their unscheduled needs as they arise [1].

Services required by state law and regulation must include but are not limited to:

- 24-h awake staff to provide oversight and meet scheduled and unscheduled needs
- Provision and oversight of personal and supportive services (assistance with activities of daily living and instrumental activities of daily living)
- Health-related services (e.g., medication management services)
- Social services
- Recreational activities
- Meals
- Housekeeping and laundry
- Transportation

A resident has the right to make choices and receive services in a way that will promote the resident's dignity, autonomy, independence, and quality of life. These services must be disclosed and agreed to in the contract between the ALC and resident. AL does not generally provide ongoing, 24-h skilled nursing. However, residents are eligible to receive home health services on an intermittent basis according to skilled nurse needs when these are unable to be provided by the AL staff.

## FACILITY CHARACTERISTICS

One of the key differences between nursing facilities and AL is that there are no federal regulations for AL. Each state has developed their own specific regulations, thereby avoiding onerous federal regulations that would likely lead to increased cost to both facilities and residents. Some advocate that there are potential benefits to federal oversight that would establish more clear and uniform enforceable standards in order to maintain quality patient care.

ALCs differ widely in size, capabilities of care, and philosophy. The adage "if you've seen one assisted living facility, you've seen one assisted living facility" applies. Many are freestanding facilities, while others may be part of a continuing care retirement community (CCRC). Rooms are typically a private or semiprivate studio and one- or two-bedroom apartments. As part of resident rights, recent proposals call for emphasis on private rooms for all residents. There are many AL chains, with a total occupancy capacity up to 50,000 beds. In 2009, the largest chains were Sunrise Senior Living, Emeritus Corporation, Brookdale Senior Living, Atria Senior Living Group, Five Star Quality Care, and Assisted Living Concepts. One third of all ALCs and beds are located in California, Florida, and Pennsylvania.

Staffing in ALCs may widely vary. There is no usually requirement for a nurse on site. There is also typically no social worker or dietician. Depending on size, there may be no activities staff. Documentation and charting also vary, with state-specific regulations and scope of practice issues dictating which staff, if any, are able to take verbal physician orders. State regulations and facility-specific policies also vary on which medical conditions may prohibit admission to or give cause for discharge from an ALC, such as ventilator dependency, stage IV decubiti, continuous intravenous fluids, and communicable airborne infections requiring isolation. Most ALCs will admit residents with moderate need for assistance, such as needing help with or using wheelchairs (62–71%). However, only 44% would admit those needing assistance with transfers, and 53% would not admit residents with moderate-to-severe dementia [2].

There is an increasing prevalence of dementia seen in AL residents that is to be expected with advancing age, with estimates ranging from 30 to 67%. Many ALCs have dementia-specific units, while other facilities care only for residents with dementia. State regulations have begun focusing on dementia care in areas such as resident safety, staff training, and provision of dementia-specific activities. The Alzheimer's Association has developed AL-specific criteria and guidelines for dementia care [3]. Practitioners may notice a phenomenon in dementia-specific units that if a significant number of residents with dementia are admitted in a similar stage over the same period, after a time of "aging in place" and disease progression, many of these residents will need to be discharged from the AL facility to a nursing facility for more complex care or end of life care. If anticipatory marketing has not been done, the facility may experience a significant drop in occupancy rates and subsequent financial crisis. However, AL residents may receive hospice care and continue to reside in the ALC depending on state regulation and the individual facility's capabilities.

## RESIDENT CHARACTERISTICS

Similar to nursing facilities, AL residents are typically female, white, and average 87 years of age [4]. They have increasing ADL needs (Table 2.2), which generally correlate with worsening overall health. This ADL dependency is not as severe as that of nursing facility residents, but does exceed that of community-dwelling elderly. Data indicate that AL residents generally need assistance with two ADLs and have an average length of stay of 28 months.

Three quarters of residents are either entirely (22%) or partially (49%) responsible for making the decision to move into an ALC, while for other residents their adult child, child's spouse, or other family member commonly makes this decision. More than 70% of residents move into an ALC from their own private home or apartment and relocate within 10 miles of their previous permanent residence more than 60% of the time [4].

TABLE 2.2. ADL dependence

| Assistance with | ALC (%) | NH (%) |
|---|---|---|
| Bathing | 64 | 95 |
| Eating | 12 | 51 |
| Dressing | 39 | 89 |
| Toileting | 26 | 82 |
| Transferring | 19 | 77 |

AL residents often suffer from multiple medical problems. Almost half have chronic conditions in three or more different general disease categories [5]. As noted, there is an increasing incidence and prevalence of dementia. Some studies suggest that up to half of AL residents are demented. Other common conditions include impaired mobility, incontinence, hypertension, arthritis, and osteoporosis.

Medication usage is an important issue in AL. Residents take an average of seven to eight prescriptions and two OTC medications daily, and 80% require assistance with taking these medications [4]. Unlike skilled nursing facilities, there is no federal mandate for a consultant pharmacist medication review, though many ALCs may provide this service. Use of over-the-counter medicines and alternative and herbal therapy are other potential concerns for the practitioner [6].

Overall, 60–90% of residents are satisfied with their care. The main reason(s) for residents moving from the ALC are a change in health status or death. About 60% move to a nursing facility, 13% move back home or to a child's or relative's home, 10% transfer to another ALC, and 7% go to a nonshort stay hospital [4]. Understanding resident admission and discharge patterns is often helpful for physicians when they are discussing with residents and families where the AL option falls in the resident's care/illness trajectory.

## PHYSICIANS AND OTHER PROVIDERS

There is no federal mandate for having a medical director in AL, although some organizations have established this position. The ALW did not reach a majority consensus to recommend having a medical director – but has recommended use of an "external professional consultant." However, one quarter to one third of ALCs have acquired a medical director [4]. In general, most attending physicians see residents in their private office. In ALC there is usually not a well-established "medical staff." Unlike nursing facilities, where there are mandatory visits no less than every 60 days, an AL resident is required to be seen at a minimum of only once yearly. Facilities can contract with different services, including home health care and hospice agencies. Despite the lack of regulation in most states, a consultant pharmacist provides medication review and monitoring at 64% of ALCs. [4]

## FINANCING

Payment for AL is generally private pay, with residents and families financing the majority of costs. AL costs are significantly lower than nursing facility costs. Unlike the skilled nursing facility, there

TABLE 2.3. Variations in base rate costs for ALC

| City | Low | High | Average |
|---|---|---|---|
| Southern Maine | $3,300 | $5,682 | $4,708 |
| Boston, MA | $2,724 | $6,275 | $4,143 |
| New York | $1,125 | $6,250 | $4,146 |
| Philadelphia area, PA | $1,600 | $4,200 | $3,098 |
| Miami, FL | $2,000 | $4,263 | $2,936 |
| Dallas/Fort Worth | $1,700 | $4,475 | $2,849 |
| Chicago, IL | $2,200 | $4,000 | $2,939 |
| Indianapolis, ID | $1,650 | $3,885 | $2,448 |
| Des Moines, IA | $1,400 | $3,300 | $2,550 |
| South Dakota | $1,680 | $2,867 | $2,194 |
| Portland, OR | $2,350 | $4,500 | $3,044 |
| Seattle, WA | $1,900 | $3,900 | $2,965 |
| Los Angeles, CA | $1,300 | $3,000 | $2,235 |
| San Francisco, CA | $2,000 | $5,670 | $3,669 |

are no Medicare payments to ALCs. Costs vary widely, depending on size of the home, care requirements, and geographic region (Table 2.3). The average (mean) cost for a single occupancy unit is $3,000/month [4]. The basic AL rate cost was $2,873/month in 2008, compared to $4,267/month for residents who require Alzheimer's disease and dementia-specific care [7]. Fees usually include rent, meals, and some level of basic services.

Many states have developed Medicaid waiver programs under CMS to cover personal and skilled care services for qualified, low-income patients. Medicaid funds can only be used for those rendered services, *not* room and board charges. These waivers are only available when a resident meets both the state's criteria for being "nursing home eligible" and the Medicaid financial eligibility requirement. Residents may experience a long delay before receiving such a waiver and some ALC providers state they receive inadequate reimbursement under the waiver. Long-term care insurance is an infrequent primary payment source. The lack of funding for AL makes affordability a major concern for the future viability of the AL industry.

Another affordability concern is "a la carte" pricing policies at ALCs where facilities may charge extra when residents need additional help (i.e., a higher level of care/assistance) due to progressive or advanced illness. Since many residents have limited funds, their families may be reluctant or even refuse to pay the increased fees and often subconsciously deny the existence of increasing frailty and medical risk.

Despite all these concerns about affordability, residents' move-out of an ALC due to financial reasons occurs only 6% of the time [4]. This may be a difficult time for families and, not infrequently, residents may be transferred to the hospital, which in turn then assumes the responsibility of placing the resident at another health care facility.

## PHYSICIAN BILLING

Readers are referred to Part IV, Chapter 14, Table 14.9 on coding. Of note, the custodial care codes should be used (99324-99326 and 99334-99337), *not* the home visit codes when practitioners see the resident in the ALC.

## ASSISTED LIVING CARE

### Direct Care Services

AL residents generally require initial assessment by a physician prior to move-in, with specifics varying by state. Unlike a formal mandatory plan of care in a nursing facility, the ALC may develop a "service plan," which is similar in nature and customized to the needs and preferences of the resident. Some service plans, however, may not incorporate a health care plan. Residents cannot be forced to move out of a facility against their wishes, but instead need to meet discharge criteria exemplified by not being able to be cared for appropriately and safely. As previously mentioned, home care and even hospice care may be available in the facility if the resident qualifies for these services.

### Medication Management

Medication management is a significant issue in AL. As in other settings, this should involve evidence-based prescribing, delivery of medications, and e-prescribing. Health care providers taking care of AL residents should be knowledgeable about the basic tenets of geriatric prescribing (see Chap. 15 for a more detailed review). This includes the five "R's" – the *r*ight medication at the *r*ight time, the *r*ight dose, and the *r*ight route of administration for the *r*ight patient. The Beers Criteria of "potentially inappropriate" medications for the elderly is a useful guide [8]. Many facilities have a contract with a consultant pharmacist that can assist the facility with medication management. Medication over- and undertreatment [9] is a problem in AL that consultant pharmacists often address. The pharmacist may be especially helpful if they have advanced qualifications in geriatric pharmacy patient care.

Another medication management concern in AL is that in many instances, nonlicensed staff members give or assist with the dispensing of medications without adequate nurse supervision. Requirements for level of staff training and oversight of medication administration vary among states. Staff may lack assessment skills, so medication side effects may be unrecognized. Unlike the nursing facility, physicians may not be notified when a resident has refused to take medications at the ALC.

AL residents often self-administer medications, which over time can become unsafe, exemplified by the resident with dementia and increasing problems with memory loss and executive function. Even the definition of "self-administer" may be unclear – in some facilities, this could simply mean that staff takes a medication out and places it into the resident's hand.

Record keeping varies in ALCs, though some have more traditional patient charts. There is also no standardization in the way medications are delivered and stored in AL facilities. Order changes, monitoring, and multiple prescribers present a challenge to safe medication management. Practitioners may have no influence on a particular facility's structure, staff competency, ongoing quality improvement processes, and accountability in regard to medication administration and management, but could (and should) offer their expertise as a resource.

When applying the basic principles of medication management in the elderly, careful consideration must be given to the fact that the resident resides in AL. Any medication can cause almost any side effect in an elderly patient. Since the AL staff may not have formal training, common geriatric syndromes that may be caused by medications (such as falls, urinary incontinence, change in appetite, and new or worsened confusion) may not be recognized. Without a formal chart or well-established notification channels, the attending physician may be unaware that new medications were prescribed or doses changed by another practitioner.

As in nursing facilities, medications may be prescribed without a face-to-face examination by the practitioner. AL residents may receive unnecessary medications if the AL staff lacks good assessment skills, or if underlying disease states go undiagnosed or untreated. The resident's quality of life needs to be carefully and continuously evaluated. As in all settings where the frail elderly receive care, a condition may not need treatment if its potential side effects or risks outweigh the potential benefits.

Since the government categorizes an AL resident as the same as a community-dwelling resident in regard to Medicare Part D, residents and their families may be presented with the problem of dramatically higher pharmacy costs when reaching the "donut hole" where residents are expected to pay for medications that are usually covered by pharmacy benefits. This essentially means that residents end up paying more out of pocket for medication costs, which when combined with facility fees may entail significant financial hardship for the resident and perhaps their family as well.

### Resident Rights
A common concern of residents and their family is that they are often unaware of facility practices and costs. Marketing information should be consistent, and ideally, residents should receive open disclosure of all ALC fees and services when signing the admission contract. They should also be aware of facility policy on transfer or discharge out of the ALC, and there should be a fair appeals policy at every facility. The ALW recommendations regarding resident rights and provider responsibilities are noted in Tables 2.4 and 2.5, where the ALC is also called an ALR.

### Staff Training
Some stress that sufficient and experienced 24-h staffing be available in the ALC. Not only should the staff be aware of principles of normal aging but they should also be familiar with drug pharmacology and common problems seen in the elderly resident. Staff also needs to be able to determine when qualified professionals should be contacted when a significant change of condition occurs in a resident [10]. In general, state regulations are requiring more rigorous staff and administrative training in AL.

### Facility Operations
State regulations generally address various areas affecting ALCs and their residents. These include resident activities, food preparation, transportation, environmental management, fire safety, disaster and emergency planning, life safety, and building codes [1].

## BARRIERS TO CARE
Previous studies have noted that the most common resident/family complaints and survey deficiencies reported in AL are related to medication administration (48%), staff quality and qualifications (41%), and insufficient staff (36%) [11].

Lack of education in basic geriatrics principles can be a problem in some AL facilities. For example, some AL residents with dementia may lack that diagnosis, and untrained staff may be unable to identify and report observations that would lead to

TABLE 2.4. Resident rights

Within the boundaries set by law
- Be shown consideration and respect
- Be treated with dignity
- Exercise autonomy
- Exercise civil and religious rights and liberties
- Be free from chemical and physical restraints
- Be free from physical, mental, fiduciary, sexual and verbal abuse, and neglect
- Have free reciprocal communication with and access to the long-term care ombudsmen program
- Voice concerns and complaints to the ALR orally and in writing without reprisal
- Review and obtain copies of their own records that the ALR maintains
- Receive and send mail promptly and unopened
- Private unrestricted communication with others
- Privacy for phone calls and right to access a phone
- Privacy for couples and for visitors
- Privacy in treatment and caring for personal needs
- Manage their own financial affairs
- Confidentiality concerning financial, medical, and personal affairs
- Guide the development and implementation of their service plans
- Participate in and appeal the discharge (move-out) planning process
- Involve family members in making decisions about services
- Arrange for third party services at their own expense*
- Accept or refuse services
- Choose their own physicians, dentists, pharmacists, and other health professionals
- Choose to execute advance directives
- Exercise choice about end of life care
- Participate or refuse to participate in social, spiritual, or community activities
- Arise and retire at times of their own choosing
- Form and participate in resident councils
- Furnish their own rooms and use and retain personal clothing and possessions
- Right to exercise choice and lifestyle as long as it does not interfere with other residents' rights
- Unrestricted contact with visitors and others as long as that does not infringe on other residents' rights
- Come and go rights that one would enjoy in their own home

In addition, residents' family members have the right to form and participate in family councils

---

*An ALR may require that providers of third party services ensure that they and their employees have passed criminal background checks, are free from communicable diseases and are qualified to perform the duties they are hired to perform.

TABLE 2.5. Provider responsibilities

In the context of resident rights
- Promote an environment of civility, good manners, and mutual consideration by requiring staff, and encouraging residents, to speak to one another in a respectful manner
- Provide all services for the resident or the resident's family that have been contracted for by the resident and the provider as well as those services that are required by law
- Obtain accurate information from residents that is sufficient to make an informed decision regarding admission and the services to be provided
- Maintain an environment free of illegal weapons and illegal drugs
- Obtain notification from residents of any third party services they are receiving and to establish reasonable policies and procedures related to third party services
- Report information regarding resident welfare to state agencies or other authorities as required by law
- Establish reasonable house rules in coordination with the resident council
- Involve staff and other providers in the development of resident service plans
- Maintain an environment that is free from physical, mental, fiduciary, sexual and verbal abuse, and neglect

earlier recognition and treatment. As noted, most physicians see AL residents as outpatients, probably due to time constraints. These physicians may not be geriatricians, nor have specialized training in geriatrics. Some may bring an age bias to their practice and may not recognize the special challenges or needs of the aging patient. In addition, they may not be cognizant of the dangers inherent to hospitalization of these residents, such as delirium, inappropriate prescribing, and nosocomial infections. There are a myriad of benefits for physicians who travel to see residents at the ALC, including:

- Physician learns about AL capabilities
- Sees resident in their own environment
- Improved communication with AL staff
- Increased reimbursement from CMS for domiciliary codes
- No need for facility transportation/escort costs
- No need for family transport time/costs
- More efficient use of physician and staff time
- Increased resident/family/facility satisfaction
- Potential for more patients for the physician
- Potential for improved resident care
- Potential for reduced medical errors
- Better marketing/public relations for facility

Effective communication is a goal in all medical environments, not just AL. Communication problems in the AL setting are seen on multiple levels – staff may not have a formalized "sign out" between shifts, physicians may not get accurate information (especially after hours), staff may not have sufficient assessment skills or know when to contact physicians, and multiple physicians involved in care may not be aware of what the other physicians are ordering. In addition, many hospital emergency room physicians, like those in the community, are unaware of the differences between ALCs and nursing facilities and lump them all into one category.

Accordingly, with the impending large increase in the elderly population, and a corresponding increase in the number of persons in AL, some warn that the federal and state governments need to address concerns regarding the AL industry [12].

## OPTIMAL MEDICAL CARE

### Physician Practice

The physician's role in AL has been largely undefined, due in part to the industry's history of distinguishing between the "medical" vs. "social" models of care [13]. At this time, there is scant data in the literature, but Schumacher [14] advocates for proactive development of relationships between ALCs and residents' medical providers. He notes that "some ALCs appear to mistakenly interpret a 'social model' of care as one that discourages the ALC's involvement with any medical providers due to concerns about medicalization, staff time constraints, and cost issues." He recommends clear and timely communication with medical providers regarding medication management, availability of accurate information and documentation regarding residents' health status longitudinally, and development of a focused medical provider education packet describing the relevant services of each ALC.

The American Medical Directors Association (AMDA) convened a consensus conference to address the needs and issues related to frail AL residents with multiple chronic conditions. The main areas of concern were medication management, communication to practitioners, AL clinical practice guidelines, clinical direction, and the physician's role. Recommendations were made to develop standard assessment tools and clinical protocols in order to improve the clinical care residents receive in the AL setting [15].

Several of the issues and concerns mentioned in this chapter, including recommendations for both physicians and facilities, are elaborated upon in the AMDA Policy Statement "Physicians Role in Assisted Living" (March 2009).

**Transitions of Care**
Errors in care commonly occur when patients are either newly admitted to an ALC or readmitted from a hospital or a SNF to an ALC. Renewed attention has become focused on this event. The National Transitions of Care Coalition website includes information and tools for both consumers and health care professionals. ALCs should facilitate resident transitions to other settings. When a resident is hospitalized, the physician can educate hospital staff about the capabilities of the ALC. Physicians through communication can also help assure that residents are being transferred back to an ALC only when it is safe to do so based on a particular ALC being capable to meeting the resident's needs. Similar to a discharge from hospital to home, additional services from home care agencies and geriatric care or companion services may be necessary to help the resident stay in the ALC. On occasion, staff from the ALC may be able to evaluate the resident prior to their return from hospital or a skilled nursing facility in order to ensure a safe and appropriate transition of care. AMDA has published a clinical practice guideline on care transitions that is available through their website (www.amda.com) at no cost.

**Technology**
While most ALCs lag behind hospitals and nursing facilities in the use of technology, advances are expected in the future. The impact of electronic health record usage in AL, an example of operational technology, could assist in seamless transitions of care. A few ALCs already use high-tech sensor devices to better monitor residents, as well as other smart home technology. One type of smart home technology is the e-pill Monitored Automatic Pill Dispenser (MD.2) that can organize, remind, and track dispenses, as well as allowing reports to be viewed by medical professionals. Smart shirts, smart toilets, and bladder scanners are all available for monitoring residents in the ALC. Robot "companions" can enable some AL corporations to virtually visit facilities; telemedicine can enable clinicians to promptly assess residents in remote areas, while saving extensive travel time and expense in both instances. Future residents can be expected to be increasingly familiar with use of the Internet and the use of communication technology can let residents speak with distant family members. Game systems are also currently being used to supplement resident activities and therapy.

## SUGGESTIONS ON IMPROVING CARE

The following lists suggestions for physicians and other health care providers that are aimed at optimizing their practice in AL. Some of the suggestions may be easier to address if a medical director position has been established.

1. Adapt already established and evidence-based procedures to the AL setting.

   Many health care practitioners familiar with the workings of nursing facilities also take care of AL residents. Residents of nursing facilities are required to be seen at a minimum of every 60 days – with the increasing acuity and frailty of ALC residents approaching that in nursing facilities, it behooves physicians to establish a routine of seeing AL residents on at least a quarterly basis or more often if medically necessary. Pertinent guidelines areas can be adopted for use in ALCs, such as fall prevention, notification protocols, and reduction of antipsychotic medication. Use of a consultant pharmacist for monthly or quarterly medication reviews is encouraged. Suggestions for efficient time management in LTC are still applicable to physician care in AL (Table 2.5) [16].

2. Meet regularly with the facility administrator.

   Getting buy-in from the administrator is an important strategy that helps improve resident care. The physician may bring up topics for discussion or ask the administrator how physician involvement can help with state survey compliance and marketing of the facility's image in the community. Improvement in physician communication and documentation is generally an area of mutual interest. Scheduled meetings can vary, from monthly to less often. Minutes from previous meetings should be kept, and the focus on an identified area of concern is continued until the problem is resolved, prior to addressing another area of concern. If the administrator is unable to make meetings, physicians should at least keep in regular contact with the head of the nursing staff. A physician could also participate as a member of an "advisory committee" for the rehabilitation, hospice, and/or home care agency that is working with a large percentage of the ALC's residents.

3. Provide in-services to staff/residents.

   It is widely accepted that a well-educated staff is a critical component of providing good care. Accordingly, the physician or the physician's PA/NP can present educational sessions for front-line staff about such topics as geriatric principles, medication administration and drug side effects, best practices in communication, and common illnesses in the elderly (dementia, hypertension, diabetes, stroke, mental health disorders, etc.). Residents and families are often eager to learn more about common geriatric conditions and medication issues. Some ALCs have "family nights" where physician-led "Q & A" or "Ask the Doc" sessions can be valuable. Many facilities have resident and/or family councils. Physician attendance at these can be of great value, whether to improve education and communication, or to help to identify other issues within the community.

4. Ensure communication is effective.
Physicians can help facilities establish a process so that the attending physician is notified in a timely manner about a change in patient status, medication errors, and any treatments ordered by consultants. Implementation of a standardized process (such as the SBAR method, or use of guidelines available through AMDA and the CEAL) can improve communication between AL staff and the attending physician. The facility should include standard information whenever a resident leaves the facility to see a different physician (Table 2.6) and even more importantly that this and perhaps other critical resident information is conveyed accurately during urgent or emergency transfers. The current medication regimen is vitally important, as is advance directive status. Physicians can help facilities develop a packet of information that includes copies of items such as insurance information, family contact numbers, past medical history, pertinent consultant reports and lab work, activity and diet, and current treatments that would be readily available in an emergency. Developing relationships and communicating with local emergency department providers and emergency medical services can be helpful. Inappropriate use of these resources can lead to unnecessary transfers, hospitalizations, patient/family stress, and excess costs [14]. Transferred residents should have clear identification that they reside in an

TABLE 2.6. Standard information recommended for AL transfer/communication forms

Patient name
Patient date of birth
Attending physician
Facility name
Facility phone number
Medication list
Reason for transfer/consultation
Relevant H&P/progress notes/labs/X-rays

ALC. As mentioned, a facility may not have a resident medical chart. If so, a physician can bring an office chart with them to the ALC. A communication book in the facility can be a useful place to leave messages from the facility nurse/staff. If there is a facility chart, a physician may ask for a separate physicians section for progress notes. It may be useful to make a copy of the physician note, or fax it to the office, in order to make certain the physician visit record is preserved. Physicians must also assume responsibility for returning calls promptly and professionally. One of the major problems identified by facilities is the poor response time from physicians. Physicians should establish a protocol where the facility knows how to contact the physician for non-urgent and emergent calls. Identification of a point person to contact at the ALC is useful. The physician returning a call during the same shift can decrease miscommunication between shifts. Some facilities prefer that the physician calls back regularly at a certain time of day.

Good communication with families can prevent many problems and increase resident, family, and staff satisfaction. Calls received from the family should be returned, as promptly as possible and with respect. Family should be contacted when there is a change in status, and when a resident is transferred out of the facility. Discussing family expectations upon resident admission can help identify unrealistic expectations. Medication issues and costs are a frequent concern and should be discussed with the family at appropriate intervals.

5. Focus on high-risk medications and medical problems.
Certain common geriatric disease states lend themselves well to risk reduction strategies. As in nursing facilities, special attention should be given to fall prevention, decubitus ulcers, diabetic management (especially hypoglycemia), and resident elopement. Some medication errors may have more potential for significant harm than others, such as warfarin, diabetic (both oral and injectable), and antipsychotic medications.

6. Initiate discussion on advanced directives.
While a recent report notes that advance care planning is 5–10% higher in residential care/AL than in nursing facilities [17], many ALC residents either have no advance health care directives or have them be unrecognized in an emergency situation. A physician's focus on facility process and resident and staff education can be instrumental in championing use of orders for life-sustaining treatments such as the POLST (Physician Orders for Life Sustaining Treatment) forms.

7. Encourage preventive medicine.
   The importance of health promotion, disease prevention, and wellness services for AL residents has been well recognized. ALCs represent exceptional opportunities for treatment and management of chronic conditions, with the potential for enormous benefit to their residents. [18] Examples include screening for Alzheimer's disease, hypercholesterolemia and osteoporosis, implementation of immunization protocols, and promotion of exercise programs.

8. Urge hiring of a medical director.
   The ALC administration or corporation may be unaware of the advantages of a medical director versus their concern about the financial burden of paying the physician. Appropriate medical direction includes improved patient care, communication and marketing, and lowered liability risk.

   A significant number of ALCs neither have written policies and procedures for a quality improvement regarding medication management, nor policies regarding drug regimen review and monitoring for adverse drug events [19]. Improving medication management is an ideal opportunity for medical director leadership. AMDA's *Position Statement on Assisted Living* lists some potential roles and responsibilities of an AL medical director (the ALC is referred to as an ALR – Table 2.7). The challenge to the physician is convincing the facility of the significant benefits this may provide. There is evidence that having a full-time physician at the facility by itself improves care. One study showed statistically significant decreases in hospitalizations and hospital days, and a suggestion of decrease in falls [22]. Many ALCs often have a physician who sees a majority of the residents, becoming a sort of "de facto" medical director. This position will not have any coverage for administrative liability; however, the physicians may find themselves empowered to suggest or enact changes beneficial for resident care.

9. Guide families/colleagues towards available resources.
   Physicians may play a role when patients are no longer able to be cared for at home. Several organizations offer information about the ALCs in the community and guide to choosing a facility (CCAL, National Center for Assisted Living (NCAL), AARP, Assisted Living Federation of American). Hospital social workers may not be aware of some of these resources or of the existence of the CEAL or AL-specific consumer groups. Some areas of the country have literature available to families that list housing options including AL (such as the SourceBook: Guide to Retirement Living for several eastern states).

TABLE 2.7. Potential roles and responsibilities of AL Medical Director

Practitioner services
  Assist the ALR in ensuring that residents have appropriate physician coverage and ensure the provision of physician and health care practitioner services
  Assist the ALR in developing a process for reviewing physician and health care practitioners' credentials
  Provide specific guidance for physician and health care practitioner performance expectations
  Assist the ALR in ensuring that a system is in place for monitoring the performance of health care practitioners
  Facilitate feedback to physicians and other health care practitioners on performance and practices
  Assist ALR with resident assessment and development of the clinical component of the service plan, when necessary
Clinical care
  Participate in administrative decision-making and the development of policies and procedures related to resident care and medication management
  Participate in administrative decision-making on staffing levels, coverage, licensing, and training requirements for resident-care staff
  Assist in developing, approving, and implementing specific clinical practices for the ALR to incorporate into its care-related policies and procedures, including areas required by laws and regulations
  Review, respond to, and participate in federal, state, local, and other external inspections
  Assist in reviewing policies and procedures regarding the adequate protection of residents' rights, advance care planning, and other ethical issues
Quality of care
  Assist the ALR in establishing systems and methods for reviewing the quality and appropriateness of clinical care, medication management, and other health-related services and provide appropriate feedback
  Participate in the ALR's quality improvement process
  Advise on infection control issues and approve specific infection control policies to be incorporated into ALR policies and procedures
  Assist the facility in providing a safe and caring environment with optimal levels of family and community involvement
  Assist in the promotion of employee health and safety
  Assist in the development and implementation of employee health policies and programs
Education, information, and communication
  Promote a learning culture within the facility by educating, informing, and communicating
  Assist the ALR in developing medical information and communication systems with staff, residents, families, and others
  Assist in establishing appropriate relationships with other health care professionals

TABLE 2.8. Factors influencing AL growth and structure

Shifting population demographics
Evolving patient mix and acuity levels
Health status and lifespan of target populations
Cost structure (e.g., liability insurance and higher costs to serve patients with more demanding service needs)
Regulatory landscape
Medical and technological advances
Adequacy of public financing
Availability of small ALCs

10. Champion state "mini-ALWs."
    One of the recommendations from the national ALW was to have state-level public meetings to review their recommendations. Virginia has already convened such a meeting. A physician interested and involved in AL may be able to spearhead a "mini-ALW" in their state. This can be a moving target, as many different factors influence the growth and structure of the AL industry (Table 2.8) [20].

## SUMMARY

Physicians play an essential role in the treatment of patients in the AL setting. Understanding the capabilities of the ALC where residents live is critical. The potential for clinician collaboration in AL facilities in establishing seamless community-based care, promotion of preventive care and wellness, early identification of patient sentinel events, and contribution to quality of life outcomes shows great promise [21]. Ideally, the physician can be a "middle man," advocating for resident care and helping to establish a safety net for patient care [15] while understanding facility concerns and trying to keep the facility affordable for residents.

## PEARLS FOR THE PRACTITIONER

- ALCs are regulated by the states and there are no mandatory federal regulations. This leads to significant state-to-state variability in rules, requirements, and terminology.
- Facilities themselves vary significantly in size, patient characteristics, philosophy, staff, and patient care capabilities.
- Staff number, availability, training, and capabilities also vary greatly by state and location, leading to potential problems with communication, medication management, and overall patient care.

- Seeing patients in the ALC has many benefits for all concerned.
- Many of the barriers to care in AL can be addressed and overcome by increased physician attention and involvement.

## WEBSITES

- AARP www.aarp.org
- Alzheimer's Association www.alz.org
- American Medical Directors Association (AMDA) www.amda.com
- Assisted Living Consult www.assistedlivingconsult.com
- Assisted Living Federation of America (ALFA) www.alfa.org
- Center for Excellence in Assisted Living (CEAL) www.theceal.org
- CCAL www.ccal.org
- National Center for Assisted Living (NCAL) www.ncal.org
- National Transitions of Care Coalition www.ntocc.org
- POLST website www.ohsu.edu/polst
- Snap for Seniors www.snapforseniors.com
- U.S. Department of Health and Human Services Office of Disability, Aging, and Long-Term Care Policy http://aspe.hhs.gov/daltcp/home.shtml

## REFERENCES

1. The Assisted Living Workgroup. Assuring Quality in Assisted Living: Guidelines for Federal and State Policy, State Regulation and Operations. A Report to the US Senate Special Committee on Aging, April 2003.
2. Hawes C, Phillips CD, Rose M, et al. A national survey of assisted living facilities. Gerontologist, 2003;436(6):875–882.
3. Alzheimer's Association Campaign for Quality Residential Care. Dementia Care Practice Recommendations for Assisted Living Residences and Nursing Homes.
4. 2009 Overview of Assisted Living, a Collaborative Research Project of AAHSA, ASHA, ALFA, NCAL & NIC.
5. McNabney M, et al. The spectrum of medical illness and medication use among residents of assisted living facilities in central Maryland. J Am Med Dir Assoc, 2008;9(8):558–564.
6. Carder P. Beyond the Radar Screen: Access to and Use of OTC and As-Needed Medication by AL Residents. AMDA Annual Symposium presentation, 2009.
7. The MetLife Market Survey of Nursing Home and Assisted Living Costs, October 2008.
8. Fick DM, et al. Updating the Beers criteria for potentially inappropriate medication use in older adults: results of a US consensus panel of experts. Arch Intern Med, 2003;163:2716–2724.

9. Sloane PD, et al. Medication undertreatment in assisted living settings. Arch Intern Med, 2004;164:2031–2037.
10. Stefanacci R, Podrazik, P. Assisted living facilities: optimizing outcomes. J Am Geriatr Soc, 2005;53:538–540.
11. State Residential Care and Assisted Living Policy: 2004 U.S. Department of Health and Human Services, April 2005.
12. Levenson S. Assisted living: shall we learn from history or repeat it? J Am Med Dir Assoc, 2008;9:539–541.
13. Utz R. Assisted living: the philosophical challenges of everyday practice. J Appl Gerontol, 2003;22:379–404.
14. Schumacher J. Assisted living communities and medical care providers: establishing proactive relationships. Sr Hous Care J, 2005;13(1):35–48.
15. Vance J. Proceedings of the AMDA Assisted Living Consensus Conference, Washington, DC, October 24, 2006. J Am Med Dir Assoc, 2008;9(6):378–382.
16. Anderson EG. Nursing home practice: 10 tips to simplify patient care. Geriatrics, 1993;48:61–63.
17. Daaleman T, et al. Advance care planning in nursing homes and assisted living communities. J Am Med Dir Assoc, 2009;10(4):243–251.
18. Schumacher J. Examining the physician's role with assisted living residents. J Am Med Dir Assoc, 2006;7(6):377–382.
19. Mitty E. Medication management in assisted living: a national survey of policies and practices. J Am Med Dir Assoc, 2009;10(2):107–114.
20. The Senior Care Source Facts Figures & Forecasts. Novartis, 2008;5: 34–44.
21. Schumacher J. Physicians and Their Assisted Living Residents: Adventures in Falls (Mis)Communication. AMDA Annual Symposium presentation, March 2009.
22. Pruchnicki A. Full Time Primary Care in an Assisted Living Facility. AMDA Poster Submission, Annual Symposium, 2005.

# Chapter 3
# Nursing Facilities

Richard G. Stefanacci

**Keywords:** Nursing facility • Short-term skilled care • Nursing facility regulations • State Operations Manual • Nursing facility payment • Omnibus Reconciliation Act

The provision of care for the elderly in nursing facilities is an integral part of long-term care. There are over 16,000 Medicare and Medicaid-certified nursing facilities in the US with almost 1.5 million residents. State Medicaid programs pay for the majority of the frail elderly care. Residents of nursing facilities have a need for management of multiple chronic conditions taking an average 8–10 medications per day. Care in nursing facilities is highly regulated through both state and federal regulations in order to assure appropriate resident care. This care is provided through an interdisciplinary team that strives to have each resident attain the highest practicable level of well-being.

A transition of care often occurs when an older person, living at home, has an acute change in condition that requires that the person be admitted to a hospital and then discharged to a nursing facility. During their stay at the nursing facility, it is not uncommon that another acute event occurs that then requires transfer back to the hospital and subsequently back to the nursing facility. Such transitions in care require careful coordination to protect against adverse outcomes. Medicare is requiring improvements in transitions of care and has funded several pilot projects related to this.

## THE INTERDISCIPLINARY TEAM

An interdisciplinary team of health care professionals who provide a comprehensive and coordinated assessment and management of each resident's medical, psychological, social, and functional needs can best care for residents in LTC. This is mandated in nursing facilities, but is also a helpful way to care for the elderly in the assisted living facility and home as well (Table 3.1).

## REGULATIONS: OBRA '87

Prior to 1987, nursing facility care was characterized by the prevalent use of physical restraints, inappropriate use of psychotropic medication, overuse of urinary catheters, and a high occurrence of urinary incontinence, pressure ulcers, weight loss, and behavioral problems. Because of this widespread poor quality of care in nursing facilities, Congress requested that the Institute of Medicine (IOM) study how to improve the quality of care in the nation's Medicaid and Medicare-certified nursing facilities. In its 1986 report, *Improving the Quality of Care in Nursing Homes*, the IOM expert panel recommended:

- A stronger federal role in improving quality
- Revisions in performance standards, and the inspection, i.e., survey process
- Better training of staff
- Improved assessment of resident needs
- And a dynamic and improved regulatory process [1]

The Omnibus Reconciliation Act of 1987 (OBRA '87) contained the Nursing Home Reform Act, which was created by federal legislators in response to these recommendations by the IOM. The "Campaign for Quality Care" was organized by the National Citizens' Coalition for Nursing Home Reform in order to implement the IOM recommendations and to support Federal reforms. National organizations representing consumers, nursing facilities, and health care professionals have worked and continue to work together to create consensus positions on major nursing facility issues.

Under OBRA '87, surveyors of nursing facilities shifted focus from the nursing facility to resident outcomes. The quality of life and the quality of care of each resident then became the two basic areas of review. Under quality of life, the concept of the living environment maintaining or improving the residents' "well-being" became the major focus. In addition to physical and mental health, well-being includes the resident's functional status, self-esteem, relationships, appearance as well as their social and spiritual needs.

The changes that OBRA brought to the care of residents in nursing facilities are noteworthy. Some of the most important provisions include:

TABLE 3.1. The interdisciplinary care team in nursing facilities

| Title | Scope of practice | Education | Salary |
|---|---|---|---|
| Certified nurses aids | Work under the supervision of a nurse and provide assistance to patients with daily living tasks | In addition to a high school diploma or GED, completion of a 6–12 week CNA certificate program at a community college or medical facility | $23,663–$29,801 |
| Licensed practical nurse | Provide the patient care on a personal level. They usually report directly to physicians and RN's and are responsible for collecting data such as taking vital signs and monitoring Input and output. Additionally, they are responsible for performing procedures such as wound care, ostomy care and Foley catheter insertion. In some, but not all states, LPNs and LVNs may administer medications or start IV fluids. | Required to pass a licensing examination, known as the NCLEX-PN, after completing a State-approved practical nursing program. A high school diploma or its equivalent usually is required for entry | $31,080–$43,640 |
| Registered nurse | Work directly with patients and their families. They are the primary point of contact between the patient and the world of health care, both at the bedside and in outpatient settings. RNs perform frequent patient evaluations, including monitoring and tracking vital signs, performing procedures such as IV placement, phlebotomy, and administering medications. Because the RN has much more regular contact with patients than physicians, the RN is usually first to notice problems or raise concerns about patient progress | The three major educational paths to registered nursing are a bachelor's degree, an associate degree, and a diploma from an approved nursing program. Nurses most commonly enter the occupation by completing an associate degree or bachelor's degree program. Individuals then must complete a national licensing examination in order to obtain a nursing license | $47,710–$69,850 |

(continued)

TABLE 3.1. (continued)

| Title | Scope of practice | Education | Salary |
|---|---|---|---|
| Registered nurse assessment coordinator (RNAC) | RNAC will assist the Director of Nursing (DON) with ensuring that documentation in the center meets Federal State and Certification guidelines. The RNAC will coordinate RAI process assuring the accuracy timeliness and completeness of the MDS RAPS and Interdisciplinary Care Plan. The RNAC conducts the nursing process – Assessment Planning Implementation and Evaluation – under the state's Nurse Practice Act for Registered Nurse Licensure | | $77,000 |
| DON | The Director of Nursing has the responsibility of overseeing the standards of nursing practices for the organization's nursing services. The DON participates with other members of Nursing Services and Administration in the development of patient care programs, policies, and procedures to meet all requirements including ethical and legal concerns | | $97,000 |

| | | |
|---|---|---|
| Social worker | Assist people by helping them cope with issues in their everyday lives, deal with their relationships, and solve personal and family problems | All States and the District of Columbia have licensing, certification, or registration requirements regarding social work practice and the use of professional titles. Although standards for licensing vary by State, a growing number of States are placing greater emphasis on communications skills, professional ethics, and sensitivity to cultural diversity issues. Most States require 2 years (3,000 h) of supervised clinical experience for licensure of clinical social workers | $29,590–$62,530 |
| Dietitian | Plan food and nutrition programs, supervise meal preparation, and oversee the serving of meals. They prevent and treat illnesses by promoting healthy eating habits and recommending dietary modifications. They perform nutrition screenings for their clients and offer advice on diet-related concerns such as weight loss and cholesterol reduction | At least a bachelor's degree. Licensure, certification, or registration requirements vary by State | $38,430–$57,090 |

(continued)

TABLE 3.1. (continued)

| Title | Scope of practice | Education | Salary |
|---|---|---|---|
| Physical therapist | Physical therapists provide a variety of medical services to help individuals who have been injured or physically affected by illness to recover or improve function. A physical therapist must be able to evaluate a patient's condition and devise a customized physical rehabilitation and treatment plan to enhance strength, flexibility, range of motion, motor control, and reduce any pain, discomfort, and swelling the patient is experiencing | Graduate from a physical therapist educational program with a master's or doctoral degree | $65,005–$75,670 |
| Occupational therapist | Occupational therapists help patients improve their ability to perform tasks in living and working environments. They work with individuals who suffer from a mentally, physically, developmentally, or emotionally disabling condition. Occupational therapists use treatments to develop, recover, or maintain the daily living and work skills of their patients. The therapist helps clients not only to improve their basic motor functions and reasoning abilities, but also to compensate for permanent loss of function. The goal is to help clients have independent, productive, and satisfying lives | A master's degree or higher in occupational therapy is the minimum requirement for entry into the field | $61,713–$75,230 |

| | | |
|---|---|---|
| Recreational therapist | Recreational therapists devise programs in art, music, dance, sports, games, and crafts for individuals with disabilities or illnesses. These activities help to prevent or to alleviate physical, mental, and social problems | Bachelor's degree with some additional training is usually required for this field | $38,775–$49,342 |
| Attending primary care physician | Responsibility for initial patient care and support discharges and transfers. Also make periodic, pertinent on-site visits to patients and insure adequate ongoing coverage | In addition to 4 years of medical school, most nursing home attending physicians complete a primary residency, which is typically 1–3 years. Some go on to complete a geriatric fellowship as well | $147,516–$205,096 |
| Medical director | Roles and responsibilities of the medical director in the nursing home can be divided into four areas: physician leadership, patient care-clinical leadership, quality of care, and education. Nursing facilities are required to have a medical director as outlined in OBRA '87 | Currently Maryland is the only State that requires Medical Directors to be a Certified Medical Director (CMD) in Long-Term Care or have similar training. CMD was established by the American Medical Directors Association to professionalize the field of medical direction | $18,000–$30,000[a]. Part-time position |
| Nurse practitioner | Advanced practice nurses who provide high-quality health care services similar to those of a doctor. NPs diagnose and treat a wide range of health problems. They have a unique approach and stress both care and cure. Besides clinical care, NPs focus on health promotion, disease prevention, health education, and counseling | The entry-level training for NPs is a graduate degree. At this time, NPs complete a master's or doctoral degree program. This means that NPs earn a bachelor's degree in nursing (4 years of education), then their graduate NP degree (2–4 years of education) | $75,838–$89,392 |

(continued)

TABLE 3.1. (continued)

| Title | Scope of practice | Education | Salary |
|---|---|---|---|
| Consultant pharmacists | Focuses on reviewing and managing the medication regimens of patients, particularly those in institutional settings such as nursing homes. Consultant pharmacists ensure their patients' medications are appropriate, effective, as safe as possible, and used correctly and identify, resolve, and prevent medication-related problems that may interfere with the goals of therapy | The Doctorate of Pharmacy (Pharm.D.) is the only professional Pharmacy degree, and the 5-year Bachelors of Science in Pharmacy is being phased out as a professional degree. Since this program traditionally follows 2 years of Prepharmacy education, students typically take 6 years of postsecondary education to obtain their Pharm.D. | $97,505–$107,100 |
| Nursing home administers | Responsibility as the managing officer of the facility to plan, organize, direct, and control the day-to-day functions of a facility and to maintain the facility's compliance with applicable laws, rules, and regulations.<br><br>The administrator shall be vested with adequate authority to comply with the laws, rules, and regulations relating to the management of the facility | Typically a certificate program of about 120 h is required before sitting for a licensing examination. Most are required to have completed a bachelor degree program as well as preceptor training as a NHA | $82,327–$101,025 |

- Emphasis on residents' quality of life as well as the quality of care
- A resident assessment process leading to development of an individualized care plan
- New expectations that each resident's ability to walk, bathe, and perform other activities of daily living will be maintained or improved unless an underlying medical condition precludes it
- The right to be free of unnecessary and inappropriate physical and chemical restraints
- The right to choose a personal physician and to access their medical records
- The right to organize and participate in a resident or family council
- The right to return to the nursing facility after a hospital stay or have an overnight visit with family and friends
- The right to safely maintain personal funds with the nursing facility
- The right to remain in the nursing facility unless nonpayment, dangerous resident behavior, or a significant change in the resident's medical condition occurs
- Prohibitions on asking family members to pay for Medicare and Medicaid services
- Uniform certification standards for Medicare and Medicaid homes
- Seventy-five hours of training for paraprofessional staff
- New opportunities for residents with mental retardation or mental illness to access services inside and outside the nursing facility
- New penalties for certified nursing facilities that fail to meet minimum federal standards

Under OBRA, state surveyors no longer spend their time exclusively with staff or with review of facility records. Conversations with residents and families are now an important survey event. Observations of dining and medication administration are other focal points of the survey. Since OBRA has been implemented, it has changed the care and lives of residents of nursing facilities across the United States. Significant improvements in the comprehensiveness of care planning have occurred, antipsychotic drug use has declined by 28–36%, and physical restraints have been reduced by 40%.

## NURSING FACILITY REGULATIONS

The Resident Assessment Instrument (RAI) provides a comprehensive assessment of each resident's functional capabilities and helps the nursing facility staff identify each resident's health problems. Resident Assessment Protocols (RAPs) are a major part of this process and provide the foundation upon which a resident's individual care plan is developed by the interdisciplinary team. Use of the Minimum Data Set (MDS) is part of the federally mandated process for clinical assessment of each resident and usually "triggers" several RAPs. With implementation of MDS 3.0 on October 1, 2010 the RAPs have been replaced by the Care Area Assessment (CAA) process.

MDS assessments are required to be completed on admission to the nursing facility and updated quarterly and annually, as well as when there is a significant change in condition (worsened or improved). These assessments focus on many areas including: tasks of daily living (ADLs), mobility, cognition, continence, mood, behaviors, nutritional status, vision and communication, recreational activities, psychosocial well-being, pain, falls, and injuries.

Once the MDS information is entered into a computer database by the MDS or RAI coordinator, it is then transmitted from the nursing facility to the state database. From the state database, it is then sent to the national database at the Centers for Medicare and Medicaid Services (CMS). The information in the MDS determines the resident's Resource Utilization Group (RUG) that then determines the per diem rate paid to the facility for the resident's stay under Medicare Part A, i.e., skilled care. The MDS data also determine each facility's quality indicator (QI) and quality measure (QM) report, some of which are publicly reported and are routinely used by surveyors during the presurvey and survey process:

## CURRENT USES OF THE MDS INCLUDE
- Payment
  - RUGs
  - Facility Prospective Payment System (PPS)
- Care Planning
  - RAI (CAA)
- Quality Indicators and Quality Measures
  - Quality improvement activities
  - Available to State surveyors
  - Available for posting at the Medicare "Nursing Home Compare" website

MDS 3.0 and the Quality Indicator Survey (QIS) process has become mandatory in all states. Specifics of the MDS 3.0 can be obtained at the CMS website at http://www.cms.hhs.gov/NursingHomeQualityInits/25_NHQIMDS30.asp (Table 3.2).

## REGULATIONS: STATE OPERATIONS MANUAL
The State Operations Manual (SOM) sets out survey investigative protocols and interpretive guidelines to provide guidance to state

TABLE 3.2. MDS 3.0: goals, changes, and anticipated results[a]

| Goal of MDS 3.0 | MDS 3.0 changes | Anticipated results |
| --- | --- | --- |
| Improving the:<br>Reliability<br>Accuracy<br>Usefulness<br>Length<br>Staff satisfaction and perception of clinical utility | Introduce advances in assessment measures:<br>Increase the clinical relevance of items<br>Improve the accuracy and validity<br>Increase the resident's voice by introducing more resident interview items<br>Briefer assessment periods for clinical items | Improve identification of resident needs<br>Enhance resident-focused care planning<br>Enhance communication among providers |

[a] http://www.cms.hhs.gov/NursingHomeQualityInits/25_NHQIMDS30.asp

surveyors. These serve to clarify and explain the intent of the federal regulations. Furthermore, these protocols and guidelines direct the surveyor's attention when preparing for the survey, conducting the survey, and evaluating the survey findings. The survey is conducted to determine whether a citation of noncompliance is appropriate. Deficiencies are based on a violation of the state and/or federal regulations, as supported by surveyor observations of the nursing facilities' staff performance and care practices.

The SOM Interpretive Guidelines include three parts:

1. Survey tag number
2. Wording of the regulation
3. Guidance to surveyors, including additional survey procedures and probes

The regulations emphasize the need for continued, rather than annual, cyclical compliance. The enforcement process mandates that policies and procedures are established to remedy deficient practices and to ensure that correction is lasting. Facilities must take the initiative and responsibility for continuously monitoring their own performance to sustain compliance. Measures to meet the requirements for an acceptable plan of correction in response to survey deficiencies emphasize the need to achieve and maintain compliance. A second requirement is that all survey deficiencies will be addressed promptly. A third requirement is that all residents will receive the care and services they need to meet their highest practicable level of functioning.

## QUALITY INITIATIVE: MEDICARE FIVE STAR PROGRAM

With three million older Americans admitted to nursing facilities each year of which 1.5 million stay long enough to consider the nursing facility their main residence, it should come as no surprise that nursing facilities are strictly surveyed in order to assure appropriate care. Despite this, one in five nursing facilities nationwide was cited for deficiencies that caused actual harm or immediate jeopardy to their residents [2].

Some major areas of quality focus that were identified by nursing facility medical directors include the following [3]: telephone conversations, transitional care, falls and hip fractures, warfarin usage, pressure ulcers, inappropriate medications, pain control, urinary incontinence, weight loss, and exercise of residents. The CMS "Nursing Home Compare" website reviews the survey deficiencies received by nursing facilities, but does not reflect the entire inspection report (form HCFA-2567). The complete survey inspection report and the nursing facility's subsequent *plan of correction* to address the deficiencies are available either from the State survey agency or from the nursing facility itself.

The Department of Health and Human Services (DHHS) has a national Nursing Home Quality Initiative for improving nursing facility care. A critical part of this initiative is CMS's public posting of the quality indicators for every nursing facility, also known as "report cards" [4]. These report cards are supposed to be used by consumers to make better-informed decisions and motivate providers to improve care; but, there is concern that these nursing home report cards fail to adjust for risk differences in resident populations of various long-term care facilities [5]. The CMS quality initiative continues to redirect focus on the care needs of frail elders who reside in nursing facilities. Under CMS, the Nursing Home Quality Initiative has also expanded and refined its measures to improve resident outcomes and care effectiveness, like reducing the occurrence of pressure ulcers and avoiding potentially preventable hospital admissions.

CMS, under its 2007 Action Plan [6], is now focusing on nursing facility quality improvement through:

- Refining the web-based report card at "Nursing Home Compare"
- Expanding the certification and survey process
- Establishing a pilot demonstration project on pay-for-performance under the term "value-based purchasing"

Hypothetically, the Nursing Home Value-Based Purchasing Demonstration would result in cost savings for Medicare through reductions in hospitalizations and subsequent skilled nursing facility (SNF) stays. The problem is that cost savings may not occur even if a nursing facility performs well; therefore, no performance incentive payments will be made to that facility [7].

## FINANCING

The complexity of nursing facility care is further complicated by a fragmented payment system (Table 3.3).

Within most nursing facilities, residents are typically receiving either skilled or nonskilled nursing care. Skilled care occurs when a resident requires more intensive nursing and rehabilitation services. Skilled care is available to Medicare beneficiaries following a hospitalization under Medicare part A. Nonskilled general nursing facility care is typically paid for by state Medicaid programs or privately (Table 3.4).

TABLE 3.3. Medicare benefit coverage

| Medicare part | Title | Coverage |
|---|---|---|
| A | Hospital insurance | Hospital, subacute care, hospice |
| B | Medical insurance | Physician and nurse practitioner services Certain vaccines |
| C | Medicare advantage | Managed care |
| D | Prescription drug coverage | Prescription drugs |

TABLE 3.4. Skilled versus nonskilled nursing facility care

|  | Eligibility | Room and board | Physician services | Medication |
|---|---|---|---|---|
| Skilled | For Medicare beneficiaries requiring skilled nursing care following a 3-day acute hospitalization | Part A | Part B | Part A |
| General nursing care (nonskilled) | ADL/IADL needs | Medicaid LTC insurance private payment | Part B Part C | Part D |

TABLE 3.5. Medicare daily base rates for fiscal year 2009 (MedPAC)

| Rate component | Nursing | Therapy | Room and board | Total |
|---|---|---|---|---|
| Urban | $151.74 | $114.30 | $77.44 | $343.48 |
| Rural | $144.97 | $131.80 | $78.87 | $355.64 |

**Medicare Part A**

Medicare beneficiaries who need short-term skilled care (nursing or rehabilitation services) following a hospital stay require at least 3 days of hospitalization. Hospital observation days do not count towards this requirement. The Medicare SNF benefit pays facilities a predetermined daily rate for each day of care up to 100 days (Table 3.5). The PPS rates are determined through RUGs. Residents are assigned to one of 66 RUGs based on resident characteristics and expected service use (skilled nursing, rehabilitation). After the first 2 weeks of a skilled facility stay, Medicare Part A no longer covers 80% of the cost, which is financially difficult for some elderly.

**Medicare Part B**

Also known as Medical Insurance, Medicare Part B covers practitioner (physician, physicians' assistant, and nurse practitioner) and rehabilitation services (OT, PT, or ST) for nonskilled residents. Medicare Part B also covers vaccines like the influenza and pneumococcal.

**Medicare Part C**

Medicare is expanding programs that care for beneficiaries in and outside of the traditional nursing facility. Under Medicare Part C (also called Medicare Advantage), managed care organizations are responsible for providing all the benefits available under Medicare Part A, B, and D. United Healthcare launched the Evercare program in 1987. Evercare utilizes NPs within nursing facilities to provide timely care and has been shown to reduce emergency room evaluations, hospital admissions, and increase preventive care. The Evercare program is also able to provide a skilled level of services at nursing facilities without Medicare's 3 days of hospitalization requirement.

More recently, the Medicare Modernization Act allowed for the continuing development of these types of programs as well as a broader range of options under Medicare Advantage (MA) and Special Needs Plans (SNPs). SNPs are authorized to focus on one of three distinct patients groups: residents of nursing homes, dually eligible seniors (those who are entitled to Medicare Part A and/or Part B *and* are eligible for some form of Medicaid benefit), or those suffering from multiple chronic illnesses. The SNFs receive financial incentives to provide care that improves health outcomes and prevents hospitalizations.

### Medicare Part D
Medicare Part D is the prescription drug benefit that started January 1, 2006. Medicare Part D moved drug coverage from Medicaid to Medicare. Residents enrolled in Medicaid receive their Medicare Part D medications without any copayments or premiums.

### Medicaid
All state Medicaid programs have two eligibility requirements that regulate which persons may obtain Medicaid financial support for their nursing facility stay(s). The first is financial eligibility, and the second, medical eligibility. With respect to medical eligibility, states adopt their own procedures and set of criteria because CMS grants determination of medical necessity to the States. While Medicaid no longer pays for Part D-covered medications for the dually eligible, Medicaid does cover non-Part D medications such as benzodiazepines that were excluded from Part D coverage. Medicaid also covers the daily cost of nursing facility room and board for nonskilled stays.

## TRANSITIONS OF CARE
Quality of care can be affected (for better or worse) during the transition of care from one setting to another. When residents transition from the long-term care facility to other settings or vice versa, they are at high risk for the adverse effects of prescribing or transcription errors. Overlooked appointments, diagnoses, or laboratory tests as well as a missed or duplicated medication are just a few of the potential errors that can lead to poor outcomes. Seamless transitions from the hospital to home, skilled nursing care, or home health care will reduce these errors. Selected QIOs under contract with CMS are trying to improve care coordination, promote seamless transitions, and reduce rehospitalizations. Medicare is striving to improve these transitions by encouraging provider investments in health information technology as well as anticipating a "bundled" payment system that would financially tie hospitals and nursing facilities together for an episode of resident care. Medicare is also encouraging the development of systems that will hold hospitals financially accountable for poor outcomes during transitions of care in a system that will have interdisciplinary teams that will work on assuring improved transitions.

## FUTURE CHANGES

Proposed changes to Medicare also present challenges for LTC pharmacy providers. These challenges involve every aspect of the Medicare program from Part A through Part D and include promotion of quality outcomes with an incentivized payment system based on outcomes and integration of care systems. CMS announced plans to launch a 3-year Medicare pilot demonstration project in 2009 that is testing a bundled-payment system where physicians and hospitals are paid a single amount for all services associated with surgical procedures. Currently, CMS pays hospitals a predetermined amount (related to DRGs) for nonphysician services. Under the pilot program, providers would receive a single payment for Medicare Part A (which covers hospital services) and Medicare Part B (which covers physician services). CMS's explained reason for the pilot project: "physicians who care for a patient during a hospital stay are paid separately under the Medicare Physician Fee Schedule for each service they provide and the separate payment systems can lead to conflicting financial incentives that may affect decisions about what care will be provided." A similar program could easily be applied to nursing facilities where the nursing facility would receive payment for physician's services, thus providing a path for greater integration of physician services with the nursing facility providing care.

Medicare has also been expanding care options beyond that provided by a solo nursing facility practitioner working in a fee-for-service system. Medicare LTC increases the scope of practice of physician extenders, such as nurse practitioners and physician assistants, by expanding their practice to alternative sites of care such as assisted living facilities and the beneficiaries' home. Not only is Medicare working on SNPs and improvements in transitions of care, but also working to better integrate the long-term care system through home and community-based waivers. These waivers pay for care of nursing facility eligible people in nonnursing facility settings. The changes that Medicare LTC has proposed will pose both challenges and opportunities for providers dedicated to serve this growing frail elderly population.

## SUMMARY

As a result of concern over quality of care in the nation's nursing facilities, the focus of regulation and payment has shifted to the attainment of better quality outcome at less cost. Changes in payment are occurring in every aspect of the Medicare system: Medicare which covers the initial skilled stay within a nursing facility called Part A, the Medicare physician services Part B, the

Medicare managed care program of Part C, and the Medicare prescription drug program of Part D are all undergoing changes. Not only is payment reform occurring, but the reporting of data both to Medicare and to the public is undergoing improvement. Through the establishment of the Medicare Five Star Program hospital discharge planners, patients and their families can better identify nursing facilities that deliver higher quality services.

## PEARLS FOR THE PRACTITIONER

- The OBRA '87 changed the focus of care in nursing facilities to quality outcomes.
- Beyond the regulatory focus of OBRA, health care reform envisions financial incentives to encourage ever-improving quality outcomes.
- Reporting changes are occurring to quality data: to Medicare through the MDS and to the public through Medicare's Five Star Program.
- Care in nursing facilities is best delivered through an Interdisciplinary Care Team.
- Knowledge of the benefits under Medicare's Parts A, B, C, and D is crucial to improve the development of relationships and processes between health care providers.
- Practitioners and nursing facilities need a positive attitude and work ethic toward future change in order to insure their future success.

## WEBSITES

- Annals of Long-Term Care www.annalsoflongtermcare.com/
- Medicare www.medicare.gov
- Clinical Geriatrics www.clinicalgeriatrics.com/
- American Geriatrics Society www.americangeriatrics.org
- Kaiser Family Foundation www.kff.org
- American Society of Consultant Pharmacist www.ascp.com

## REFERENCES

1. Federal Nursing Home Reform Act (OBAR 87 Summary). Available at http://www.docstoc.com/docs/25984550/Federal-Nursing-Home-Reform-Act.
2. Nursing home reform: Continued attention is needed to improve quality of care in small but significant share of facilities. Testimony before the Special Committee on Aging, US Senate. Washington, DC: General Accounting Office, 2007.
3. Morley JD. Rapid Cycles, an Essential Part of the Medical Director's Role. J Am Med Dir Assoc 2008. 8(1):535–538.

4. Nursing Home Compare. Medicare: The official U.S. government site for people who have Medicare website July 2002: Available at http://www.medicare.gov/NHCompare/home.asp.
5. Mukamel DB, Glance LG, Li Y, et al. Does risk adjustment of the CMS quality measures for nursing homes matter? Med Care 2008; 46: 532–541.
6. Center for Medicare and Medicaid Services. Action Plan for (Further Improvement of) Nursing Facility Quality 2006. Available at http://www.cms.hhs.gov/surveycertificationgeninfo/downloads/2007actionplan.pdf.
7. White, A., Hurd, D. Moore, T., Warner, D., Wu, N., and Sweetland, R. (2006). Quality monitoring for Medicare global payment demonstrations: nursing home quality-based purchasing demonstration, final design report. Centers for Medicare & Medicaid Services Contract #500-00-0032, T.O. #1. Cambridge, MA: Abt Associates.

# Chapter 4
# The Role of Practitioners and the Medical Director

Steven A. Levenson

**Keywords:** Practitioners • Medical director • Medical director role • Medical director responsibilities • Nursing facility quality

## INTRODUCTION

The role of nursing facilities in the United States has changed along with the health care system. Traditionally, nursing facilities provided a significant amount of personal and health care in a residence primarily for cognitively and functionally impaired elderly. Today, nursing facilities still provide this residential care, but in recent years they have admitted more people from acute or specialty hospitals. The long-term care residents and postacute care patients are often unstable, having many active medical comorbidities as well as risk factors for syndromes such as anorexia and falling. Nursing facilities therefore require more physician involvement in assessing and managing symptoms and condition changes in the people under their care [1].

Long-term residents often need acute and chronic medical care and short-stay patients may have an extended stay or even become residents after completing their postacute care. Individuals who live in nursing facilities are commonly referred to as residents; those who come to nursing facilities primarily to receive short-term medical care after an acute care stay at a hospital are often referred to as patients. Both medical directors and treating physicians need to be flexible, as they are often involved in caring for individuals with both chronic and acute problems. Physicians play a vital role in providing nursing facility care, serving either as a medical director and/or the primary physician for residents, or as a consultant. The attending physician is a crucial part of the LTC team because of their primary responsibility for their patient's medical care [2].

While many medical directors also serve as attending physicians, the roles and functions of a medical director are separate from those of an attending physician. The attending physician provides direct resident care; the medical director oversees and coordinates the facility's medical care and helps the facility oversee and improve that care. As of 2009, at least one state had implemented substantial regulations regarding their medical director and physician expectations [3]. Other states have developed, or are considering developing, more limited oversight. Although concern related to physician performance and practice is enduring and widespread, perspectives about the desirability and impact of these requirements vary considerably [4].

## THE ROLE OF THE PRACTITIONER

Physicians have a decidedly mixed history of involvement in long-term care. Many physicians have shown lack of interest in the care of the chronically ill and unwillingness to take care of nursing facility residents [5]. Physicians may be unaware of pertinent approaches to the care of the complex frail elderly patient or the current standards required for postacute and long-term medical care.

According to the Omnibus Reconciliation Act of 1987 regulatory requirements, every nursing facility resident must have an attending physician to supervise his or her medical care [6]. "Supervising the care" means participating in the assessment and management of patients, monitoring changes in their medical status, and providing consultation or treatment when needed. It also includes such things as prescribing new treatment as indicated, conducting required routine visits, or delegating and supervising nurse practitioners or physician assistant visits. In addition, it means reviewing the pertinence and effectiveness of care provided by other physicians and licensed health care professionals and practitioners involved in the care of their resident. Table 4.1 describes the basic physician's functions and tasks based on federal OBRA'87 requirements.

Table 4.2 identifies key practitioner responsibilities in long-term care that are integral to quality resident care in the LTC setting [7]. The practitioners should work with the facility's leadership, including the medical director, director of nursing, and administrator in order to perform and act appropriately and address any conflicts or problems that may arise.

TABLE 4.1. Attending physician's functions and tasks in the nursing facility based on federal OBRA'87 regulations

| Roles | Related functions and tasks |
| --- | --- |
| Supervise individual resident care | Approve a resident's admission to the facility; e.g., this may be done by giving and approving orders upon admission |
| | Be aware of, and contribute to, a patient's assessment and care planning; e.g., by helping staff identify and manage underlying causes of impaired function and significant condition changes |
| | Ensure that there is backup medical coverage if the attending physician is unavailable; e.g., by providing the facility with information about on-call coverage and addressing any issues with that coverage |
| Make resident visits | Take an active role in supervising their residents' care |
| | At the time of each visit: |
| | Review the total program of care, including medications and treatments rendered by other disciplines |
| | Write, sign, and date a progress note |
| | Sign and date all orders except immunization orders that may be periodic without a new order |
| | Evaluate the resident's condition and continued appropriateness of the current medical regimen |
| Make timely visits | See a patient at least once every 30 days for the first 90 days after admission, and at least once every 60 thereafter (the next scheduled visit date should be determined by this interval, not by the actual date that the last visit occurred; a visit is timely if it occurs not later than 10 days after the date it was required) |
| | Make all required physician visits personally (required visits after the initial visit may alternate between visits by the attending physician and visits by a physician assistant, nurse practitioner, or clinical nurse specialist under the physician's supervision) |
| Arrange for provision of emergency services | Designate backup coverage, e.g., individual physician, physician group, or advance practice nurse |
| | Ensure that backup coverage is available as needed |
| | Address issues related to backup coverage, as needed by the facility |
| Delegate tasks appropriately | Delegate tasks to physician assistants, nurse practitioners, or clinical nurse specialists consistent with OBRA'87 requirements and state requirements related to licensure and scope of practice |

TABLE 4.2. Practitioner's roles and related functions and tasks

| Practitioner's role | Related functions and tasks |
| --- | --- |
| Accept responsibility for resident care | Assess new admissions in a timely fashion<br>Seek, provide, and analyze information regarding a patient's current status, recent history, medications, and treatments<br>Provide information and documentation that helps staff determine appropriate level of care for a new admission<br>Authorize admission orders in a manner that enables the facility to provide safe, appropriate, and timely care<br>If pending transfer to another physician's service, continue to provide all necessary medical care and services, until another physician takes over the care |
| Support discharges and transfers | Follow up, as needed, when an acutely ill or unstable patient is transferred<br>Provide necessary documentation and/or other information needed at the time of transfer to enable care continuity<br>Provide a pertinent discharge summary within 30 days of patient discharge or transfer from the nursing facility |
| Make periodic, pertinent resident visits | Visit patients in a timely fashion, based on their needs and on regulatory requirements, including an alternate visit schedule as appropriate<br>Maintain progress notes that cover pertinent aspects of a patient's condition, current status, and goals<br>Review and approve a patient's treatment and care program<br>Determine a patient's medical condition and address active issues at visits<br>Respond to issues requiring a physician's expertise, such as assessment of recent condition changes and review of current medications and treatments for continued relevance and safety<br>Provide legible progress notes in a timely manner |
| Provide adequate ongoing coverage | Designate alternate coverage<br>Update the facility about communicating with his/her practice and designated alternate coverage<br>Help ensure that alternate coverage provides adequate and timely support<br>Notify the facility of any extended absence and related coverage arrangements |

(continued)

TABLE 4.2. (continued)

| Practitioner's role | Related functions and tasks |
| --- | --- |
| Provide appropriate resident care | Perform accurate, timely, and relevant medical assessments |
| | Define and describe resident symptoms and problems, clarify and verify diagnoses, and help establish realistic prognosis and care goals |
| | Help determine appropriate services and programs for the patient |
| | Verify the medical necessity and appropriateness of treatments and services, including rehabilitation services, in accordance with relevant practice standards and regulatory requirements |
| | Respond in an appropriate time frame to emergency and routine notification by staff |
| | Analyze and respond to laboratory and other diagnostic test results |
| | Assess and promptly manage significant acute changes in a patient's condition when notified |
| | Guide ethics-related decisions (for example, options for life-sustaining treatments) |
| | Order appropriate comfort and supportive measures as needed |
| | Periodically review continued relevance of all prescribed medications for patients and monitor for possible medication-related adverse consequences |
| Provide appropriate and timely medical orders | Provide timely and legible medical orders |
| | Sign and verify the accuracy of verbal orders |
| Provide appropriate, timely, and pertinent documentation | Document required explanations of medical decisions, helping the facility comply with its legal and regulatory requirements |
| | Complete all physician information required on death certificates in a timely manner |
| Perform and act appropriately | Abide by pertinent facility and medical policies and procedures, and collaborate with the medical director/facility leadership to help the facility provide high-quality care |
| | Contact the medical director/facility leadership about issues and concerns |
| | Keep the well-being of patients in mind in all situations |
| | Be alert to any observed or suspected violations of resident rights, including abuse or neglect |
| | Interact in a courteous, professional manner with facility staff, patients/residents, family/significant others, facility employees, and management |
| | Inform the medical director/facility leadership of disputes or problems that cannot be readily resolved by the involved parties |

## THE ROLE OF THE MEDICAL DIRECTOR

Medical directors serve in various settings, including hospitals, insurance companies, specialty programs or services (e.g., dialysis, hospice, wound care), and assisted living facilities (only some of which have medical directors). However, they are predominantly in nursing facilities as a result of federal requirements. In federal nursing facility regulations and related surveyor guidance, the medical director is defined as "a physician who oversees the medical care and other designated care and services in a health care organization or facility" [6].

### Medical Director Characteristics

The background, characteristics, and performance of medical directors have been researched over the years [8, 9] and also investigated by the American Medical Director's Association (AMDA). However, only some of these characteristics have been identified to date. Most medical directors have an internal medicine or family medicine background, and approximately 23% of medical directors are also geriatricians [10]. A medical director may cover one or several facilities. Although most medical directors also serve as attending physicians in their facilities, a significant number act solely as a medical director.

### Origins of the Medical Director Role

The nursing facility medical director concept evolved out of government investigations stemming from a 1970 *Salmonella* outbreak in a Maryland nursing facility [11, 12]. In the 1970s, the American Medical Association's Committee on Aging attempted to define the roles and functions of a medical director and promote educating physicians about these basic roles and responsibilities [13]. By 1974, every skilled nursing facility (those certified to provide skilled nursing services to Medicare beneficiaries) was required to retain a full- or part-time medical director [14].

The 1987 Omnibus Budget Reconciliation Act (OBRA) and related regulations expanded the medical director requirements to include residential as well as skilled portions of nursing facilities. For regulatory purposes, both skilled and residential facilities were referred to as "nursing facilities." Subsequently, surveyor guidance (including that found at 42 CFR 483.75(i) Medical Director [F501]) has clarified expectations. In the late 1980s and 1990s, both physicians serving as medical directors [15, 16] and their representative organizations (AMDA) [17] increasingly pulled together the scattered information and perspectives on medical direction, In 2001, the Institute of Medicine recommended that nursing facilities give medical directors greater authority and develop structures and processes not only to enable, but also to require a more focused and dedicated physician participation [18].

**Key Medical Director Responsibilities**
Based on these diverse initiatives, there are regulatory and professional sources of a medical director's job responsibilities. Collaboration among physician organizations and regulatory agencies has helped to make those requirements more consistent throughout the United States. In contrast, requirements for medical direction in assisted living facilities vary among states. As of 2009, most states did not require a medical director in assisted living facilities.

*Regulatory Foundation*
As of 2009, federal regulations require every nursing facility in the United States to retain a physician to serve as its medical director. The primary source of medical director regulations is the federal OBRA'87 regulations and related surveyor guidance, but there are also some state regulations regarding medical director's responsibilities [19]. Under federal nursing facility regulations, requirements are broken into discrete segments called "F-Tags." These federal tags relate to one or more specific regulatory requirements and are used for survey purposes.

A specific section of federal regulations (F-Tag 501) covers the medical director. The actual regulations regarding medical direction are brief, requiring that the medical director implements resident care policies and coordinate medical care in the facility. The Centers For Medicare and Medicaid Services (CMS) gives surveyors-related guidance. This surveyor guidance provides additional information and instructions on how to survey a facility for compliance with federal regulations, including the medical director (F-Tag 501) (Table 4.3) [20]. A nursing facility can be cited for a deficiency if it does not have a medical director who is fulfilling these requirements. The surveyor guidance for F-Tag 501 requires nursing facilities to have medical directors who:

- Are licensed physicians
- Coordinate medical care in the facility and oversee the implementation of resident care policies
- Help the facility develop, implement, and evaluate resident care policies and procedures that reflect current standards of practice

TABLE 4.3. Medical director's responsibilities based on F-Tag 501

| Roles | Related functions and tasks |
| --- | --- |
| Coordination of medical care | Help the facility obtain and maintain timely and appropriate medical care that: |
| |   Supports the health care needs of the residents |
| |   Is consistent with current standards of practice |
| |   Helps the facility meet its regulatory requirements |
| | Help the facility identify, evaluate, and address/resolve medical and clinical concerns and issues that: |
| |   Affect resident care, medical care, or quality of life |
| |   Are related to the provision of services by physicians and other licensed health care practitioners |
| | Help the facility develop a process to review basic physician and health care practitioner credentials (e.g., licensure and pertinent background) |
| | Help the facility develop systems to ensure that other licensed practitioners (e.g., nurse practitioners) who may perform physician-delegated tasks act within the regulatory requirements and within the scope of practice as defined by State law |
| | Help the facility ensure that residents have primary attending and backup physician coverage |
| Implementation of resident care policies | Collaborate with facility leadership, staff, and other practitioners and consultants to help develop, implement, and evaluate resident care policies and procedures that reflect current standards of practice |
| | Review and help revise existing policies |
| | Provide clinical leadership regarding application of current standards of practice for resident care and new or proposed treatments, practices, and approaches to care |
| | Advise on availability, qualifications, and clinical functions of staff necessary to meet resident care needs |
| Support for improving quality of care | Help coordinate and evaluate the medical care within the facility |
| | Review and evaluate aspects of practitioner care and services |
| | Help the facility identify, evaluate, and address health care issues related to the quality of care and quality of life of residents |
| | Promote attainment of optimal resident outcomes |
| | Guide facility staff regarding when to contact a practitioner, including information that should be gathered prior to contacting the practitioner regarding a clinical issue/question or change in condition |

(continued)

TABLE 4.3. (continued)

| Roles | Related functions and tasks |
|---|---|
| Survey-related support | Provide input to surveyors on physician issues, individual residents' clinical issues, and the facility's clinical practices<br>Clarify clinical questions or information about the care of specific residents for surveyors<br>Attend exit conference or otherwise demonstrate interest and help the facility analyze the nature and scope of its deficiencies<br>Help the facility identify corrective actions for survey citations |

And

Help the facility address:

- Medical and clinical concerns
- Issues that affect resident care, medical care, or quality of life
- Issues related to the provision of services by physicians and other licensed health care practitioners

The F-Tag 501 medical director guidance emphasizes the medical director's role in helping facilities identify whether their care is consistent with current standards of practice. The guidance defines "current standards of practice" as "approaches to care, procedures, techniques, treatments, etc., that are based on research and/or expert consensus and that are contained in current manuals, textbooks, or publications, or that are accepted, adopted or promulgated by recognized professional organizations or national accrediting bodies" [20]. The facility is expected to obtain the medical director's input into all clinical policies, including those from other disciplines.

### *Professional Foundations of the Medical Director Role*

The medical director's responsibilities also originate from the recommendations of professional associations or the specific needs of the medical director's organization or facility; e.g., serving as a liaison to a specific referral source. AMDA is a national organization that represents long-term care medical directors and has produced consensus statements on many topics including medical director roles and related functions and tasks (Table 4.4) [21]. AMDA recommendations go beyond those delineated in the federal regulations to include aspects of medical direction that the organization has identified as vital for high-quality medical direction in LTC.

Table 4.4. Medical director's responsibilities as identified by American Medical Director's Association (AMDA)

| Role | Related functions and tasks |
| --- | --- |
| Physician leadership | Help ensure appropriate physician coverage and provision of physician and health care practitioner services |
| | Help develop a process for reviewing practitioner credentials |
| | Give practitioners performance expectations |
| | Help develop and implement a system to monitor practitioner performance |
| | Help give performance-related feedback to practitioners |
| Patient care/ clinical leadership | Help develop policies and procedures related to resident care |
| | Help identify specific clinical practices for the facility to incorporate into its care-related policies |
| | Help guide staff about contacting practitioners and the medical director |
| | Review and consider consultant recommendations that affect the facility's care-related policies and procedures or individual resident care |
| | Help protect resident rights, including advance care planning and other ethical issues |
| Quality of care | Review and be available for external surveys and inspections |
| | Help develop effective ways to review the quality and appropriateness of clinical care and services |
| | Participate in quality improvement processes |
| | Advise on infection control issues and approve specific infection control policies |
| | Help the facility provide a safe and caring environment |
| | Help promote employee health and safety |
| | Help develop and implement employee health policies and programs |
| Education, information, and communication | Promote a learning culture within the facility |
| | Provide information to help the facility provide care consistent with current standards of practice |
| | Help develop medical information and communication systems |
| | Represent the facility to the professional and lay community on medical and resident care issues |
| | Maintain knowledge of social, regulatory, political, and economic factors that affect medical and health services of long-term care residents |
| | Help establish appropriate relationships with other health care organizations |

## MEDICAL DIRECTOR RELATIONSHIPS WITH PRACTITIONERS

The medical director is responsible for the coordination of medical care in the facility. As identified in the federal surveyor guidance for F-Tag 501, the medical director "helps the facility obtain and maintain timely and appropriate medical care that supports the healthcare needs of the residents, is consistent with current standards of practice, and helps the facility meet its regulatory requirements" [20]. The medical director is expected to help the facility:

- Ensure that residents have primary attending and backup physician coverage.
- Obtain physician and other health care practitioner services to help residents attain and maintain their highest practicable level of functioning, consistent with regulatory requirements
- Develop a process to review basic physician and health care practitioner credentials (e.g., licensure and pertinent background)
- Address and resolve concerns and issues between the physicians, health care practitioners, and facility staff
- Help the facility address issues related to continuity of care and transfer of medical information between the facility and other care settings.

The medical director needs to define the lines of accountability between the administration, governing body or owner, and the physicians. According to the OBRA'87 surveyor guidance, the practitioners are responsible to the medical director for their performance and practice. As with the medical director, physicians may also be accountable to others for their performance as attending physicians; for example, a program director in academia or a supervisor of a group practice.

In order to oversee physician practice and care, the medical director must identify the practitioner's responsibilities and performance expectations. Therefore, the medical director must understand and convey federal and state requirements (e.g., requirements for frequency of patient visits) and other standards of practice to the physicians and practitioners in the facility.

### Defining Practitioner Responsibilities

The medical director addresses practitioner's responsibilities by:

- Identifying expectations
- Explaining how to fulfill those expectations
- Identifying criteria for satisfactory performance
- Determining whether those expectations are being met
- Giving practitioners feedback about their performance and practice

The practitioner's responsibilities in nursing facilities relate to the needs of the population and to the specific requirements of the practice setting. Medical practice in long-term care is a hybrid of ambulatory, office-based, and hospital-based practice. Nursing facility residents and subacute care patients are often medically complex. Their care often involves those of other disciplines in assessment and monitoring, identifying problems, and conveying symptoms to the physician. Assisted living residents may be less functionally impaired and medically complex, but assisted living facilities typically have fewer direct care staff than nursing homes do.

The medical director provides clinical leadership by educating practitioners about providing care in the proper context. Medical care must take into account that facilities are expected to identify and address various risk factors (e.g., impaired nutrition, fall risk) and explain the basis for clinical decisions that impact outcomes (e.g., decisions not to hospitalize, choice of medications and treatments). Clinicians who are flexible enough to recognize these factors can be more supportive and provide more effective medical care compared to those who are not.

The medical director helps the facility educate and inform the staff and practitioners about medical conditions and current geriatrics practices. Appropriate clinical practices for the long-term care population have been identified and discussed in the literature for several decades [22]. Practitioners should try to minimize complications (secondary and tertiary prevention), including those related to iatrogenic illness. In conjunction with the staff, the medical director identifies clinical conditions and risks pertinent to the facility's population such as adverse drug reactions (ADRs), common causes of acute changes in condition, fall risks, exacerbation of heart failure, altered mental status, and decline in function. The medical director's clinical knowledge and understanding of a facility's population can help the facility develop relevant policies and procedures.

## THE MEDICAL DIRECTOR'S RELATIONSHIP WITH THE FACILITY

The administrator, director of nursing, and medical director are the key management leadership in the nursing facility. The management leadership is ultimately responsible for the facility's care processes and practices. Unlike a medical staff president or chief of staff, who are primarily representing the physicians to a facility or organization, a medical director in LTC plays a meaningful role for the facility as well as for the practitioners.

Through its administrator, a facility should give their physician leader guidance on how to perform the job of medical director. The facility leadership must know what is needed from their medical director by understanding regulatory requirements and professional recommendations that affect the medical director's responsibilities.

Across the country, medical directors' performance varies considerably. Many facilities are challenged to find qualified and competent physicians who can become attending physicians and medical directors.

The OBRA'87 surveyor guidance does not specify how a nursing facility must arrange for medical director services. It simply requires that each nursing facility designates a medical director who must be currently licensed as a physician in the state where a facility is located. The facility may employ or contract directly with the medical director or may contract with a company or academic program that employs the physician. In multifacility organizations, arrangements for such services may be made by corporate or regional offices, and policies may be developed at a corporate level. In these instances, it is still expected that the medical director will be involved in the facility to ensure that clinical policies are applied appropriately.

It is desirable for the medical director to develop a job description in conjunction with the administrator. This job description should describe specific functions and tasks of the medical director and should be developed after reviewing the facility's needs, as well as required and desired medical director's responsibilities. A medical director should review the job description and consider whether it is realistic, pertinent, and clearly delineates expectations. The facility should give the medical director adequate support and compensation.

The medical director may be accountable to others in addition to the facility administrator. In academia, the medical director is accountable to a program director; other medical directors may be accountable to the supervisor or owner of a practice or company that contracts out the medical director services, or to a corporate medical director in a chain.

Facilities may have diverse criteria for choosing a medical director and may vary in their expectations of the medical director. For example, some facilities are primarily interested in physicians who will fulfill medical director roles regardless of whether they also provide primary patient care, while many facilities want the medical director to be the attending physician for a number of residents and a referral source for their facility.

Medical directors need facility support to fulfill their job responsibilities. As pointed out in the OBRA'87 surveyor guidance on medical direction, the medical director may not have control over some things that influence outcomes; e.g., performance of nursing and other disciplines. A facility can also assist the medical director by creating an environment conducive to practicing competent medicine. For example, before contacting a practitioner, the staff should be expected to:

- Perform proper assessments and coordinate phone calls
- Provide accurate information to describe a situation in detail
- Be prepared to answer the physician's questions
- Know what questions to ask the physician
- Know when to notify the medical director about physician issues and clinical concerns

## THE MEDICAL DIRECTOR'S ROLE IN FACILITY QUALITY

Medical directors are a key part of a facility's management, in that they oversee and coordinate medical care. They should also be considered part of a facility's leadership, in that they help clarify and support the goals and objectives of care, help the organization articulate and strive to meet its goals, show the staff and practitioners how to achieve desired performance, help solve and prevent problems, and help improve employee and patient health, safety, and welfare.

There is some tangible evidence of the medical director's potential impact on facility quality. Facilities with a certified medical director (a medical director who has met the AMDA's certification requirements) have been shown to have greater improvements in their quality results as compared to nursing facilities that do not have a certified medical director [23].

Surveyor guidance related to F-Tag 501 acknowledges various factors that may influence optimal outcomes, such as resident characteristics and preferences, individual attending physician actions, and facility support. While some uncorrectable factors influence outcomes, the medical director should help the facility identify and address potentially remediable issues, such as the impact of physician performance and practices. The medical director should guide the facility in determining whether clinical policies and protocols are consistent with applicable standards of medical and geriatric practice. The medical director should help the facility evaluate the care of individual patients and act on quality of care concerns and should advise the facility about clinical risk management concerns such as ADRs, medication errors, and falls. The medical director should also help review accidents and incidents and advise on infection control issues as well as give input into specific infection control policies and practices.

In order to improve care and assess problems in a facility, the medical director can help the facility identify quality measures and indicators, e.g., rates of unplanned hospital transfers and the incidence of adverse consequences related to specific medications. The medical director should help staff review and discuss quality data and clinical topics such as pressure ulcers and unplanned weight loss as part of the quality assurance process and at quality assurance meetings. The medical director can also help a facility develop and implement a program to evaluate the care and performance of physicians and other licensed health care practitioners whom the medical director oversees.

In appropriate circumstances, the medical director may intervene directly in the care of other physicians' patients by examining a patient or giving orders; for example, if another practitioner's actions or inactions are considered to be jeopardizing the individual's life, health, or safety, or if the physician is preventing the facility from meeting its legal and regulatory requirements.

## PEARLS FOR THE PRACTITIONER

- Physicians play an important role in long-term care, both in providing direct care and providing oversight as medical directors.
- Expectations for performance and practice by both practitioners and medical directors come from both regulatory and professional sources and have increasingly become more uniform and widely known.
- A facility's approach to its practitioners greatly influences the success of practitioner participation and, in turn, many aspects of the facility's results. This includes – but is not limited to – support for the medical director and holding practitioners accountable for resident care.
- Practitioners should view their roles in the proper context, related to both the system in which they operate and to medical decision making about individual residents.
- Clinician performance and participation have varied substantially over the years, ranging from excellent to highly problematic.
- The medical director can have a major impact on a facility's care, by influencing both the facility's practices and the practitioners' performance.

- The medical director is accountable to the facility administrator and the licensed health care practitioners – including physicians – should be accountable to the medical director.
- The medical director informs and educates the practitioners about expectations and then reviews and gives them feedback about their performance.
- Effective medical direction and attending physician care can go far towards improving and sustaining high quality care. Less effective participation can be problematic.

## WEBSITE
- Medical Directors Association Management Tools http://www.amda.com/managementtools/index.cfm

## REFERENCES
1. Levenson SA. Subacute care. In Capezuti E, Siegler G, Mezey MD (eds.). The Encyclopedia of Elder Care (2nd ed.). New York: Springer, 2007.
2. Dimant J. Roles and responsibilities of attending physicians in skilled nursing facilities. J Am Med Dir Assoc 2003;4:231.
3. Boyce BF, Bob H, Levenson SA. The preliminary impact of Maryland's medical director and attending physician regulations. J Am Med Dir Assoc 2003;4:157.
4. Levenson SA. The impact of laws and regulations in improving physician performance and care processes in long-term care. J Am Med Dir Assoc 2004;5:268.
5. Mitchell JB, Hewes HT. Why won't physicians make nursing facility visits? Gerontologist 1986;26:650.
6. Centers for Medicare and Medicaid Services (CMS). State Operations Manual: Appendix PP – Guidance to Surveyors for Long Term Care Facilities, Revision 52. Physician Services (F483.40). http://www.cms.hhs.gov/manuals/downloads/som107ap_pp_guidelines_ltcf.pdf. Accessed on 10/6/2010.
7. Levenson SA. Medical Director and Attending Physicians Policy and Procedure Manual for Long-Term Care. Dayton, OH: Med-Pass, 2005.
8. Zimmer JG, Watson NM, Levenson SA. Nursing facility medical directors: ideals and realities. J Am Geriatr Soc 1993;41:127.
9. Department of Health and Human Services, Office of Inspector General. Nursing Facility Medical Directors Survey. http://oig.hhs.gov/oei/reports/oei-06-99-00300.pdf. Accessed on 10/6/2010.
10. Resnick HE, Manard B, Stone RI, Castle NG. Tenure, certification, and education of nursing facility administrators, medical directors, and directors of nursing in for-profit and not-for-profit nursing facilities: United States 2004. J Am Med Dir Assoc 2009;10:423.
11. Gladue JR. Evolution of the Medical Director concept. J Am Geriatr Soc 1974;22:43.

12. Reichel W. Role of the medical director in the skilled nursing facility: historical perspectives. In Reichel W (ed.). Clinical Aspects of Aging (2nd ed., p. 570). Baltimore, MD: Williams and Wilkins, 1983.
13. Gruber HW. The medical director in the nursing facility – a catalyst for quality care. J Am Geriatr Soc 1977;25:497.
14. HEW guidelines and survey procedures – medical director. J Am Health Care Assoc 1975;1:29.
15. Levenson SA. Medical Direction in Long-Term Care. A Guidebook for the Future (2nd ed.). Durham, NC: Carolina Academic Press, 1993.
16. Pattee JJ, Otteson O. Medical Direction in the Nursing Facility. Minneapolis, MN: Northridge, 1991.
17. Pattee JJ, Altemeier TM. Results of a consensus conference on the role of the nursing facility medical director. Annu Med Direct 1991;1(1):5.
18. Institute of Medicine. Improving the Quality of Long-Term Care. Washington, DC: National Academy Press, 2001.
19. Levenson SA. The Maryland regulations: rethinking physician and medical director accountability in nursing facilities. J Am Med Dir Assoc 2002;3:79.
20. Centers for Medicare and Medicaid Services (CMS). State Operations Manual: Appendix PP – Guidance to Surveyors for Long Term Care Facilities, Revision 52. F501-Medical Director (F483.75(I)). http://www.cms.hhs.gov/manuals/downloads/som107ap_pp_guidelines_ltcf.pdf. Accessed on 10/6/2010.
21. American Medical Directors Association. Roles and responsibilities of the medical director in the nursing facility: position statement A03. J Am Med Dir Assoc 2005;6:411.
22. Ouslander JG. Medical care in the nursing facility. JAMA 1989;262:2582.
23. Rowland FN, Cowles M, Dickstein C, Katz PR. Impact of medical director certification on nursing facility quality of care. J Am Med Dir Assoc 2009;10:431.

# Part 2
Common Clinical Conditions in Long-Term Care

# Chapter 5
# Common Clinical Conditions in Long-Term Care

Naushira Pandya

**Keywords:** Hypertension • Anemia • Heart failure • COPD • Type 2 diabetes • Hypothyroidism • Vitamin $B_{12}$ deficiency • Scabies • Herpes zoster

## INTRODUCTION

The management of medical conditions in the frail elderly population that resides in long-term care (LTC) can be quite challenging. This chapter touches on some of the common clinical conditions that are frequently encountered in residents of the LTC continuum. This discussion focuses on the frail elderly LTC resident. The treatment and especially the treatment goals of these conditions in the frail elderly resident often differ from those of other patient settings and populations. The conditions that will be discussed are:

- Hypertension
- Anemia
- Heart failure (HF)
- COPD
- Type 2 diabetes
- Hypothyroidism
- $B_{12}$ deficiency
- Skin disorders
  - Scabies
  - Herpes zoster (HZ)

## HYPERTENSION

Although hypertension (HTN) is not a normal part of aging, its prevalence increases steadily with age. Many physiologic changes that occur with aging are thought to contribute to elevated blood pressure; arterial stiffness, decreased baroreceptor sensitivity, increased activity of the sympathetic nervous system, decreased alpha and beta-adrenergic receptor responsiveness, decreased ability to excrete a sodium load, low plasma rennin activity, obesity, and insulin resistance. Systolic HTN is a highly prevalent condition which is more common than diastolic HTN in older adults and more closely related to cardiovascular risks in LTC. The National Health and Nutritional Examination Survey reported a 50–75% prevalence of HTN among those aged 65 years or older, and 75% prevalence of HTN among women aged 75 years and older. In a nursing facility study of 3,600 individuals, HTN was present in 57% of older men (mean age 80 years) and in 60% of older women (mean age 81 years) [1].

### Benefits of Treatment

In addition to the well-ascribed risk factors of stroke and cardiovascular disease, people with HTN are also at risk for atrial fibrillation, congestive heart failure (CHF), peripheral arterial disease (PAD), chronic kidney disease (CKD), and cognitive impairment (each with a relative risk between two to four). Cardiovascular morbidity and mortality have been shown to increase as the systolic and diastolic blood pressures become higher, and the benefits of treating this HTN in the elderly have been firmly established. The Cochrane Review of essential HTN treatment in elderly patients (15 trials with 24,055 subjects ≥60 years) reported a reduction in total mortality, RR 0.90 (0.84, 0.97), and a reduction in total cardiovascular morbidity and mortality, RR 0.72 (0.68, 0.77), with HTN treatment. In very elderly patients ≥80 years, the reduction in total cardiovascular mortality and morbidity was similar, RR 0.75 [0.65, 0.87]; however, there was no reduction in total mortality, RR 1.01 [0.90, 1.13] [2]. Residents with more cardiovascular risk factors (e.g., diabetes, family history of heart disease, left ventricular hypertrophy [LVH]) will have more cardiovascular events prevented in the near future by antihypertensive therapy than those at lower risk. The benefit of antihypertensive treatment in patients of age 80 years and older has been clarified by results of the HYVET study in which 3,845 healthy community individuals over age 80 years with a sustained SBP of ≥160 mmHg were randomized to indapamide or placebo with the addition of perindopril or placebo to achieve a target BP of 150/80. The benefits of treatment were apparent at 1 year and increased at 2 years with a 30% reduction in the incidence of fatal or nonfatal stroke, a 39% reduction in fatal stroke, and a 21% reduction in all-cause mortality [3]. The PROGRESS, Syst-Eur, and the Rotterdam studies showed that antihypertensive therapy also reduced vascular dementia and cognitive impairment.

### Evaluation

The diagnosis of HTN should be made carefully. In addition to using an appropriate cuff size and measuring blood pressure in the seated and rested position, it is important that HTN should be diagnosed on the basis of the average of two readings that are obtained on at least three occasions. This is especially important in older adults because there is an increase in blood pressure variability with aging. Stage I HTN is defined by the Joint National Committee on the Prevention, Detection, Evaluation and Treatment of High Blood Pressure (JNC7) as a SBP of 140–159 mmHg or DBP of 90–99 mmHg [4]. Over 90% of elderly with elevated BP will have essential HTN, and the majority will have a systolic elevation of their BP. Because many drugs are known to increase blood pressure, a careful medication review should be performed when a resident's BP is found to be newly elevated. Nonsteroidal anti-inflammatory drugs including COX-2 inhibitors, erythropoietin, alcohol, and corticosteroids are commonly implicated in elevating BP.

A resident with HTN should also be evaluated for comorbid medical problems that are common in the elderly and are also known to cause HTN, such as renovascular HTN and sleep apnea. Those who present with diastolic HTN should be evaluated for renovascular HTN if it is clinically appropriate. Sleep apnea is common in this population and may provide the pathophysiological explanation of elevated blood pressure in some. But elderly with unexplained hypokalemia accompanied by metabolic alkalosis may have primary hyperaldosteronism as a cause of their HTN. Although the incidence of pheochromocytoma is small, it may warrant consideration as well if a resident's BP is unusually labile [5].

### Treatment Goals

The goals of therapy may differ for each person and need to be defined within the context of their overall clinical situation and comorbidities, as well as the effect on the quality of life. Overall cardiac risk factors should be modified to the extent possible. The elderly should be encouraged to increase activity if possible and to stop smoking. The treatment plan should include screening for diabetes and hyperlipidemia, and salt restriction if this is appropriate. But the clinician should realize that even a relatively simple intervention such as dietary sodium restriction could affect nutritional status and contribute to weight loss. The following treatment plan can be used to guide pharmacological treatment:

- Thiazide diuretics should be used as the initial drugs if they are not contraindicated, since these agents have been shown to be effective in reducing cardiovascular events and mortality.
- An alternative drug may be selected as the initial agent based on comorbid clinical conditions (type 2 diabetes mellitus (DM), CHF, or CKD).
- If blood pressure goals are not met, add low doses of a second drug chosen from another class depending on the resident's other medical problems. Begin therapy with half of the usual recommended dose and increase gradually.
- In Stage 2 HTN, when a person's SBP is 160–179 mmHg or DBP 100–109 mmHg, usually two drugs are required, such as a thiazide diuretic combined with an angiotensin converting enzyme (ACE) inhibitor.

Most of the elderly with HTN will require two or more antihypertensive agents to control their blood pressure. Although beta-blocker therapy is not recommended as first-line therapy in older adults with HTN alone, it benefits people with HTN and many comorbid conditions including CAD, CHF, hyperthyroidism, essential tremor, and arrhythmias. Supraventricular tachyarrhythmias, such as atrial fibrillation with a rapid ventricular rate benefit from beta-blockers therapy. Alpha-blockers or calcium channel blockers should not be used for elderly with prior myocardial infarction (MI) and left ventricular dysfunction. Elderly people with DM, CKD, or proteinuria should be given ACE inhibitors or angiotensin II receptor blockers (ARB). When adverse effects of cough, altered taste, rash, or angioneurotic edema occur from an ACE inhibitor, an ARB may be substituted. One study showed that combining an ACE inhibitor and an ARB, ramipril and telmisartan, increased hypotension, syncope, and renal dysfunction while not improving cardiovascular outcomes [6]. Aliskiren is the first approved drug in a new class of direct renin inhibitors. In a study of 900 people aged 65 and older, it lowered blood pressure by an additional 2.3 mmHg compared to the ACE inhibitor ramipril. Although it appears to be well tolerated, its use in the frail elderly has not been studied. The advantages, disadvantages, indications, and cautions of antihypertensive medication classes are listed in Table 5.1.

TABLE 5.1. Advantages and disadvantages of antihypertensive medication classes [5]

| Antihypertensive class | Advantages | Disadvantages | Recommended indications | Cautions |
|---|---|---|---|---|
| Thiazide diuretics | Greater reduction of systolic BP<br>Daily use<br>Improve bone mineral density | Hypokalemia<br>Urinary frequency | Systolic hypertension | Hyponatremia<br>Gout |
| ACE inhibitors and angiotensin receptor blockers | No CNS side effects<br>Preserve renal function<br>Reduce proteinuria | Cough<br>Hyperkalemia | CHF<br>Type 2 diabetes | Chronic kidney disease (CKD)<br>Renal artery stenosis |
| Calcium channel blockers | No CNS side effects<br>No metabolic effects | Constipation<br>Peripheral edema<br>Heart block | Systolic hypertension<br>CAD | Left ventricular dysfunction |
| Beta-adrenergic receptor blockers | None (not recommended as monotherapy) | CNS (central nervous system) side effects<br>Increased glucose and lipids with cardioselective | Post MI | COPD (chronic obstructive pulmonary disease)<br>PAD<br>Heart block<br>Depression<br>Hyperlipidemia<br>Type 2 DM |
| Alpha adrenergic receptor blockers | Improved urinary symptoms in benign prostatic hypertrophy (BPH) | Increased CHF hospitalization | Prostatism | Left ventricular dysfunction |

Adapted from Geriatric Medicine and Gerontology, Sixth Edition McGraw Hill [41]

When HTN is poorly controlled, the following factors should be considered:

- Inadequate dosing of antihypertensive drugs
- Inappropriate drug combinations
- Polypharmacy and increased incidence of adverse drug effects
- Unrecognized contributing medical conditions or drugs
- Practitioner inertia and failure to modify treatment

### Implications for LTC

The advantage of lowering blood pressure in the LTC population that is very old (>85 years), frail, and has multiple competing comorbidities is not clearly established. At this time there are no data to support lowering of blood pressure to levels recommended by JNC7 (less than 140/90 mmHg, and less than 130/80 mmHg in those with diabetes) in persons over 80 years of age. Because our population in LTC often has a limited life expectancy and is prone to developing orthostatic and postprandial hypotension, syncope, and falls, the risk of lowering blood pressure with medication is increased and its potential benefit is reduced. More data are required to help us determine how best to treat elevated BP in residents with high-risk conditions such as DM, recent stroke, functional impairment, and aortic aneurysm.

## ANEMIA

Anemia is caused by decreased hematopoetic reserve, reduced absorption of essential nutrients, decline in GFR and erythropoietin secretion (EPO), increased concentrations of cytokines, and a relative EPO deficiency; however, anemia is *not* considered a normal part of aging. Anemia may have an insidious onset with nonspecific symptoms until it is advanced. Mild anemia in a LTC resident is often perceived as being benign or attributed to the presence of chronic comorbidities. However, studies in community dwelling elders show that anemia may be an independent risk factor for adverse outcomes that may increase synergistically if DM, CKD, or cardiovascular disease is present.

Several complications have been associated with anemia and they may be grouped as impairments or outcomes:

### Impairments
- Decline in exercise tolerance
- LVH

# 5 COMMON CLINICAL CONDITIONS IN LONG-TERM CARE

- Decline in renal function
- Autonomic dysfunction
- Sarcopenia

**Outcomes**
- Frailty
- Falls
- Cognitive impairment
- Impaired physical performance
- Increased care needs
- Increased mortality

**Definition**

The World Health Organization defines anemia as a hemoglobin (Hb) level of less than 12 g/dL in older women and less than 13 g/dL in older men. These cutoffs are based on statistical distributions and a self report of clinical diseases and do not take into account the direct relationship of hemoglobin and clinical outcomes. In the Women's Health and Aging Study, a risk gradient for adverse outcomes (mortality, frailty, disability) was present with Hb in the "normal range" as was a rise in the erythropoietin level [7]. In a recent multifacility study, 56% of residents reviewed were anemic; prior estimates have ranged from 34.4 to 60% [8].

**Signs and Symptoms**

Signs and symptoms in LTC residents may be nonspecific. Residents may not offer specific complaints and it can be useful for members of the interdisciplinary care team to report some of the following findings to the practitioner if they are observed during care. Signs and symptoms of anemia affect multiple systems and are listed below:

- Anorexia, nausea
- Bleeding gums
- Chest pain, palpitations, tachycardia
- Cold intolerance
- Dizziness
- Decreased activity level or endurance
- Dyspnea
- Fatigue
- Increase in falls
- Increased confusion, headache
- Jaundice

- Melena
- Hematuria
- Pallor (skin, conjunctivae)

**Causes of Anemia**

Anemia is generally due to an underlying clinical disorder and warrants an evaluation in LTC residents unless the resident has a reduced life expectancy, is receiving palliative care, or declines further evaluation. A systematic evaluation in the appropriate resident can help the practitioner make rational treatment decisions. Using empiric iron replacement, for example, can potentially overlook a significant underlying treatable disorder. The causes of anemia may be classified by etiology, bearing in mind that more than one cause may be present in a given person:

- Nutrient deficiency anemia (iron, folate, $B_{12}$). (Iron deficiency due to chronic blood loss is included)
- Anemia of CKD
- Anemia of chronic inflammation
- Unclassified (may require a repeat, more comprehensive evaluation)

However, an alternative approach based on clinical decision-making is more useful in most clinical settings. It includes assessing the resident's medical history and comorbidities, current and recent medication use, physical findings, and reviewing their laboratory tests. Anemia can then be classified by considering kinetics (decreased production, increased destruction, or loss of RBCs) or by considering red cell morphology. The following algorithm (Figure 5.1) suggests a diagnostic approach using the mean corpuscular volume (MCV), first classifying the anemia as macrocytic, normocytic, or microcytic before performing further targeted tests.

Noninvasive diagnostic tests that may be used in a selective manner depending on the clinical evaluation and red cell morphology are listed below:

- Complete blood count with reticulocyte count
- Examination of peripheral blood smear
- Ferritin, serum iron, total iron-binding capacity, serum soluble transferrin receptor
- Serum folate (RBC folate)
- Vitamin $B_{12}$ (methylmalonic acid, homocysteine)
- Renal function (eGFR)

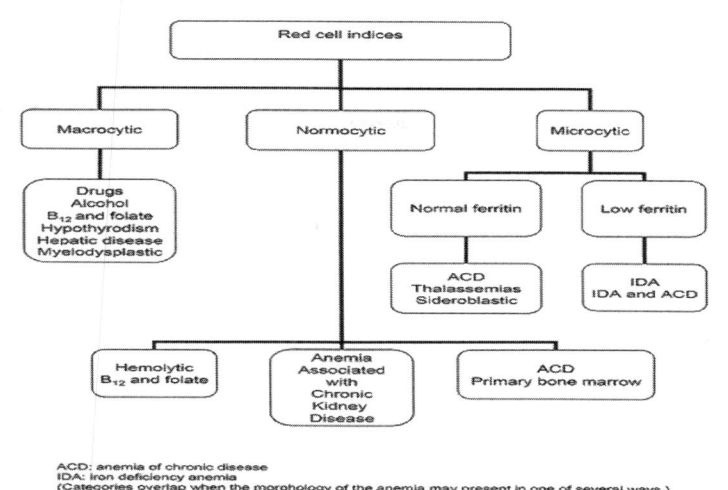

**Algorithm for Diagnosis of Anemia Using Red Cell Morphology**

```
                          Red cell indices
         ┌───────────────────────┼───────────────────────┐
    Macrocytic              Normocytic               Microcytic
         │                       │              ┌────────┴────────┐
      Drugs                      │         Normal ferritin    Low ferritin
     Alcohol                     │              │                 │
  B₁₂ and folate                 │             ACD               IDA
  Hypothyrodism                  │         Thalassemias      IDA and ACD
  Hepatic disease                │         Sideroblastic
  Myelodysplastic                │
         │                       │                            
  ┌──────┴──────┐         ┌──────┴──────┐           ┌──────┴──────┐
   Hemolytic              Anemia                        ACD
  B₁₂ and folate       Associated with            Primary bone marrow
                      Chronic Kidney
                         Disease
```

ACD: anemia of chronic disease
IDA: iron deficiency anemia
(Categories overlap when the morphology of the anemia may present in one of several ways.)

FIGURE 5.1. Algorithm for the diagnosis of anemia using red cell morphology. Adapted from: Thomas, 2006. Copyright John Wiley & Sons Limited. Reproduced with permission.

- Liver function
- Sedimentation rate
- Tests for hemolysis (serum LDH, bilirubin, and haptoglobin)
- Serum protein electrophoresis
- Stool for occult blood (endoscopy if appropriate)
- Thyroid-stimulating hormone (free T4)

(Adapted from American Medical Directors Association (AMDA). Anemia in the Long-term Care Setting clinical practice guideline 2007) [9].

It is sometimes difficult to differentiate iron deficiency anemia from anemia of chronic inflammation since the typical abnormalities of advanced iron deficiency occur at a later stage and both types of anemia can coexist. Table 5.2 will assist in analyzing equivocal studies. Measurement of the soluble transferrin receptor in conjunction with iron studies and ferritin is gaining some acceptance in differentiating iron deficiency anemia and anemia of chronic inflammation in difficult cases.

TABLE 5.2. Differentiating iron-deficiency anemia from anemia of chronic disease on the basis of lab values [42]

| Blood test | ACI | IDA | ACI + IDA |
|---|---|---|---|
| Iron | ↓ | ↓ | ↓ |
| TIBC | ↓ | ↑ | LN or ↓↑ |
| % Transferrin saturation | ↓ or N | ↓ | ↓ |
| Ferritin | ↑ or N | ↓ | ↓ or N |
| Soluble transferrin receptor | N | ↑ | ↑ or N |

## Anemia of CKD

As renal function declines in people with CKD, their Hb declines progressively. This drop in Hb is especially noticeable as the GFR trends below 60 mL/min per 1.73 m$^2$. The anemia of CKD is typically normochromic and normocytic due primarily to a deficiency of erythropoietin production. About 40–44% of nursing home residents have a GFR below 60 mL/min per 1.73 m$^2$, and in one recent study, 60% of residents with Stage III CKD were considered anemic.

## Acute or Chronic Immune Activation (ACI)

ACI causes disturbances of iron homeostasis that limits the availability of iron for erythropoiesis. There is increased uptake of iron by macrophages with impaired release of this nutrient. This disturbance in iron homeostasis is mediated by the proinflammatory cytokine interleukin-6, which increases the production of the polypeptide hepcidin in the liver. Hepcidin then decreases duodenal absorption of iron. Hematopoeisis is impaired as is the response to EPO.

## Treatment

Treatment for nutritional deficiencies and hypothyroidism should begin when possible, once the noninvasive tests have been completed. If anemia is related to medication use, chronic bleeding, CKD, chronic inflammation, malignancy, or hemolysis, then the underlying condition should be stabilized to the extent possible and any offending drugs discontinued. Treatment options for specific types of anemia and cautions to consider when treating the various anemia types are presented in Table 5.3.

Blood transfusions are generally given for acute significant blood loss associated with hypotension and cardiovascular compromise. For chronic anemia, blood transfusion is recommended if the Hb drops to 7 g/dL or the hematocrit reaches 21%, or in the presence of angina, HF, dyspnea, tachycardia, or hypotension.

TABLE 5.3. Treatment options for anemia based on cause

| Cause of anemia | Treatment options | Cautions |
|---|---|---|
| Iron deficiency | Ferrous sulfate 325 mg 1–2× daily (200 mg elemental iron) Parenteral iron (in cancer, CKD) | Constipation GI distress Consider blood loss |
| Vitamin B$_{12}$ deficiency | Vitamin B$_{12}$ 1,000 µg IM weekly ×1 month, then monthly Oral B$_{12}$ 500–1,000 µg daily | Check for concurrent folate deficiency |
| Folate deficiency | Folate 1mg orally, daily for 2–3 weeks, then reevaluate the need for continued therapy | Check for concurrent B$_{12}$ deficiency |
| Anemia of chronic inflammation | Treat or stabilize the underlying disease | Anemia may persist Erythropoeitin use is not approved |
| Anemia of CKD | Epoetin alfa or darbepoetin alfa SC Control diabetes and HTN | Maintain Hb 10–12 g/dL Weekly Hb till stable then monthly Monitor BP |
| Hemolytic anemia | Identify underlying cause Discontinue any contributing medications | |

## HEART FAILURE

Cardiovascular disease was the primary diagnosis for 24.7% of admissions to nursing facilities in 2004. It is responsible for significant morbidity, readmissions to the hospital, and impacts function as well as quality of life. In one large nursing facility study, 29% of men (mean age 80 years) and 26% of women (mean age 81 years) developed HF. The lifetime risk of HF doubles for people with BP >160/90 mmHg. HTN is therefore a major risk factor for the development of HF, especially diastolic HF in LTC residents. Diastolic dysfunction with preserved ejection fraction (EF) was present in 50% of nursing facility residents with HF in one study. Moreover, HF incidence increases significantly in older adults with diabetes and obesity, especially if female. Elderly with HF and an either markedly high or low BP have a worse prognosis [10]. An abnormal left ventricular ejection fraction (LVEF) is a strong independent predictor of mortality in elderly nursing facility residents (74%, 5-year mortality in those with normal LVEF and 92%, 5-year mortality in those with abnormal LVEF) [11].

**Evaluation**

The American College of Cardiology (ACC)/American Heart Association (AHA) guidelines for the evaluation and management of HF have classified this condition in four stages (A-D) as shown in Table 5.4 [12]. The first two stages are not HF, but are designed to help practitioners identify those at risk for developing HF.

The clinical differentiation between diastolic and systolic dysfunction, although challenging, may be helpful in decision-making. A complete history and physical examination should be performed in residents with shortness of breath, reduced exercise tolerance, edema, or other symptoms suggestive of HF. Current medications, use of alcohol, illicit drugs, and alternative therapies as well as chemotherapy agents should also be considered.

The manifestations of HF may be atypical in LTC residents. Frail elderly may be noted to have malaise, lethargy, declining function, or neurological symptoms such as confusion or sleep disturbance when they develop an exacerbation of HF. Gastrointestinal manifestations of HF may include anorexia, nausea, and abdominal discomfort.

TABLE 5.4. Staging of HF

|  | Stage A | Stage B | Stage C | Stage D |
|---|---|---|---|---|
| Definition | High risk for HF. No structural disease or symptoms | Structural heart disease without signs or symptoms of HF | Structural heart disease with prior or current symptoms of HF | Refractory HF requiring specialized interventions |
| Examples | HTN ASCVD DM Obesity Metabolic syndrome *Or* Cardiotoxin use FHx of CM | Previous MI LVH, dilation Low EF Asymptomatic valvular disease | Known structural heart disease *And* Shortness of breath Fatigue Reduced exercise tolerance | Marked symptoms at rest despite maximal therapy (cannot be discharged without special interventions) |

Diastolic dysfunction patients are more often female, have a fourth heart sound, sustained PMI, absence of jugular venous distension, absence of peripheral edema, normal heart size on chest X-ray, and LVH on the electrocardiogram (EKG). By contrast, patients with systolic dysfunction are more often male, have a third heart sound on examination, displaced PMI, jugular venous distension, pitting edema, and Q waves on the EKG.

**Laboratory Testing**
The most useful test in the evaluation of elderly with HF is the comprehensive 2-dimensional echocardiogram with Doppler flow studies to assess whether the LVEF is preserved or reduced and check for the presence of valvular, pericardial, or right ventricular abnormalities. Mobile diagnostic teams can perform echocardiograms in nursing facilities, assisted living communities, or in the home, but they may also have been performed during a hospitalization. A chest X-ray is useful to estimate cardiac size, assess pulmonary congestion, and detect other pulmonary disease. The presence of Q waves, LVH, arrhythmias, or conduction disorders may be revealed by an EKG. Both chest X-ray and EKG should be performed initially in residents presenting with HF, but should not be used as the primary basis of the identification of the cause of HF.

Screening for thyroid disease is also recommended (see Sect. "Hypothyroidism"), but screening for other disorders such as hemochromatosis, HIV, connective tissue diseases, and infectious causes should only be performed when the clinical suspicion is high. Serum assays for natriuretic peptides (BNP and NT-proBNP) are readily available and are associated with abnormal ventricular hemodynamics causing symptomatic HF. In addition to the clinical examination, they may lend weight to the suspicion of HF in residents in whom the cause of dyspnea is not clear. While BNP tests have a strong negative predictive value, they are less elevated in HF with a normal EF. They are normal in stable treated HF, but levels are often elevated in renal failure, chronic hypoxia, and pulmonary HTN as well. BNP levels cannot be used to adjust therapy [12].

Electrolytes and renal function should be measured regularly since hypokalemia is an adverse effect of diuretics and may cause fatal arrhythmias or digoxin toxicity. Many residents with hypokalemia also have hypomagnesemia and may not respond adequately to potassium supplementation. Hyperkalemia can become a complication of ACE inhibitors, ARB, or worsening renal function that requires HF therapies and other medications to be adjusted. The development of hyponatremia may be an indication of disease progression and is associated with reduced survival in elderly with HF.

Serial chest X-rays are not recommended, but monitoring weights 2–3 times a week during an exacerbation of HF is a useful practice when treating a LTC resident. The residents' functional status can also be followed at scheduled visits in addition to the physical examination, including sitting and standing BP. Edema found on physical exam may also be due to noncardiac causes.

## Common Precipitants of Heart Failure in LTC Patients

In addition to attempting to identify the cause of HF, it is also important to be aware of the common conditions that may precipitate an exacerbation of HF so that the medication regimen and coexisting medical conditions can be optimized, and specialist input obtained if indicated. Precipitators of HF in LTC residents are listed below:

- MI or ischemia
- Excess of dietary sodium
- Arrhythmias (atrial fibrillation or flutter with rapid rate, sick sinus syndrome, ventricular arrhythmias)
- Pulmonary embolism
- Hypoxia due to chronic lung disease
- Infections (pneumonia, viral illness, sepsis)
- Fever
- Anemia
- Hyperthyroidism or hypothyroidism
- Chronic kidney disease
- Poorly controlled HTN
- Thiamine deficiency
- Medications (alcohol, beta-blockers, calcium channel blockers, NSAIDS, corticosteroids, antiarrhythmic drugs, clonidine, and minoxidil)

## Process of Care Considerations

Close observation and early detection by the care team are important for elderly who develop new or recurrent HF. Timely intervention with evaluation of weights, chest X-ray, electrolytes and renal function, adjustment of therapy, and regular monitoring by nursing staff may prevent hospitalization. Practitioners should evaluate the resident and reassess the medication regimen to detect any cause of the HF exacerbation. Prior records of cardiac investigations and echocardiograms will assist in better defining the type of HF in terms of LVEF, LVH, or valvular dysfunction. A study of 156 episodes of HF in 4,693 Medicare nursing facility admissions within the first 90 days of stay reported that symptom presentation and evaluation by nursing staff at night increased the odds of rehospitalization fourfold. The presence of hypotension and delirium was predictive of death. After adjusting for these, residents who received ACE inhibitors and orders for skilled nursing observations more than once a shift decreased the odds of dying by 70% [13]. Residents with anemia (Hb < 9.8 g/dL) were twofold more likely and those with CKD (stage III or greater) were fivefold more likely to be rehospitalized from a nursing facility HF rehabilitation unit.

**Management**

Table 5.5 represents consensus recommendations for the treatment of HF which should be applied to each resident in an individualized manner [12].

TABLE 5.5. Treatment of heart failure

| Stage A | Stage B | Stage C | Stage D |
| --- | --- | --- | --- |
| Treat HTN | All measures for stage A | All measures for stage A and B | Appropriate measures for stages A, B, and define goals of care |
| Treat lipid disorders | ACEI or ARB if history of MI and low EF | Dietary salt restriction | Options |
| Smoking cessation | Beta-blockers if history of MI | Drugs for routine use | Palliative care/hospice |
| Control DM and metabolic syndrome | Valve replacement or repair | Diuretics for fluid retention | Extraordinary measures |
| Avoid alcohol | | ACEI | Heart transplant |
| ACEI or ARB for ASHD or DM | | Beta-blockers | Chronic inotropes |
| | | Drugs for selected patients | |
| | | Aldosterone antagonist | |
| | | ARB | |
| | | Digoxin | |
| | | Nitrates/hydralazine | |
| | | Devices in selected patients | |
| | | Biventricular pacing | |
| | | Implantable defibrillator | |

*Cautions*
- Encourage moderate activity and physical therapy if possible.
- Thiazides are ineffective if GFR is <30 mL/min/1.73 m$^2$; use loop diuretic.

- If symptoms persist and ACEI or ARB cannot be given due to fall in GFR or hypotension, give isosorbide plus hydralazine, especially in African Americans.
- Use an aldosterone antagonist in patients with preserved renal function and normal serum potassium.
- Avoid calcium channel blockers.

### *Digoxin*

Many residents may receive digoxin (sometimes for years) as a standard part of the treatment regimen for HF, despite the presence of sinus rhythm, and normal LVEF. The evidence indicates that digoxin has no significant effect on mortality or all-cause hospitalization of patients with EF greater than 45%, but is a reasonable addition in those elderly who do not have an adequate response to ACE inhibitors, beta-blockers, and diuretics for fluid retention.

The elderly are at increased risk of digoxin toxicity due to renal insufficiency, hypoalbuminemia, and hypokalemia with hypomagnesemia as well as drug interactions. Drug interactions between digoxin and antiarrythmics. And erythromycin and tetracycline, can be especially problematic. Close monitoring is recommended and serum concentrations should be maintained between 0.5 and 0.8 ng/mL [14].

### Refractory HF

HF in LTC residents has an unpredictable course that may be altered by intensive medical management, but has a high incidence of sudden death. Palliative care should be considered for those with refractory HF and persistence of distressing symptoms such as dyspnea, fatigue, pain, sleep disturbance, and severe functional decline.

## CHRONIC OBSTRUCTIVE PULMONARY DISEASE

Chronic obstructive pulmonary disease (COPD) is an insidious, progressive lung disease characterized by airflow obstruction that is not fully reversible. COPD may be difficult to diagnose because people often will modify their lifestyle gradually to compensate for symptoms and the dyspnea of COPD may be difficult to differentiate from that of asthma, HF, or other comorbidities that may limit activities. COPD is the fourth leading cause of death in the United States. One in six patients admitted to a nursing facility may have COPD or emphysema, which is thought to be responsible for 1% of deaths in LTC [15].

### Identification of COPD

Smoking (90% of cases), advanced age, repeated pulmonary infections, prior tuberculosis, occupational or environmental causes, and alpha-1 antitrypsin deficiency are all thought to be risk factors for COPD. Early identification of COPD is important since 50% of lung function is lost by the time dyspnea occurs with mild exertion and only 30% of lung function remains when there is dyspnea at rest. All new admissions to LTC and long-term residents with recurrent pulmonary problems should be screened for COPD by utilizing the following clinical indicators [16]:

- Dyspnea (progressive, worse with exertion)
- Cough (may be intermittent and unproductive)
- Chronic sputum production (any pattern)
- Avoidance of activities that lead to dyspnea
- History of smoking
- Recurrent pulmonary infections
- Occupational or environmental exposure to particles
- Weight loss, anxiety, or sleep disorders

On examination, residents may be barrel-chested, have prolonged expiration or pursed lip breathing, make use of accessory muscle of respiration, and have wheezing, rhonchi, or distant heart sounds. The signs of *cor pulmonale* include jugular venous distension, hepatic congestion, pedal edema, and a loud P2 component of the second heart sound.

**Diagnosis of COPD**

The clinical evaluation and review of past records may be very helpful in diagnosing COPD, but the definitive method of diagnosis is by spirometry which usually measures $FEV_1$ (volume of air exhaled in 1 s) to FVC (total volume of air exhaled).

Normal: $FEV_1/FVC \geq 70\%$ or $FEV_1 \geq 80\%$ of predicted
COPD: $FEV_1/FVC \leq 70\%$
Restrictive lung disease: $FEV_1/FVC \geq 90\%$ (pulmonary fibrosis, severe kyphosis)

However, not all LTC facilities will have bedside spirometers and their use in very frail or demented residents is usually not feasible. Measurement of alpha-1 antitrypsin deficiency, arterial blood gases, and response to bronchodilators or methacholine challenge are not usually required. Instead, other diagnostic tests are commonly used and provide useful clues regarding the presence of COPD or other conditions with similar signs. A complete blood count may reveal an abnormally high Hb level due to hypoxia, and a chemistry profile may have high bicarbonate indicating a metabolic compensation for hypercapnea. Even though chest X-rays are not diagnostic, they may reveal HF, bullae, pneumonia, pulmonary scarring, or low flat diaphragms, retrosternal airspace, and a teardrop-shaped heart suggestive of COPD. An EKG may show atrial arrhythmias, or right heart strain, and occasionally a BNP may be helpful in differentiating dyspnea due to COPD from HF. Pulmonary consultation may be helpful if the cause of dyspnea is not clear or the resident exhibits a poor response to treatment. The following are the GOLD Spirometric Criteria for COPD Severity [17]:

I: Mild COPD
- FEV1/FVC < 70%
- FEV1 ≥ 80% predicted

II: Moderate COPD
- FEV1/FVC < 70%
- 50% ≤ FEV1 < 80% predicted

III: Severe COPD
- FEV1/FVC < 70%
- 30% ≤ FEV1 < 50% predicted

IV: Very severe COPD
- FEV1/FVC < 70%
- FEV1 < 30% predicted *or* FEV1 < 50% predicted *plus*
Chronic respiratory failure

### Management of COPD

Since staging of COPD by spirometry criteria is not usually possible in LTC, clinical presentation will be utilized to guide the approach to management. The general approach to the management of COPD is shown in Figure 5.2.

Encouraging smoking cessation by counseling or with pharmacotherapy is important at any stage of the disease, as are measures to improve nutrition and encourage physical activity and immunization with influenza and pneumococcal vaccinations. Complications such as polycythemia, hypoxia, and HF should be treated concurrently, and goals of care should be discussed with the resident and their family.

Pharmacological treatment should be stepwise and cumulative. The medications for COPD currently available can reduce symptoms, increase exercise capacity, and reduce the number and severity of exacerbations; but no treatment has been shown to modify the progressive decline in lung function. Three types of

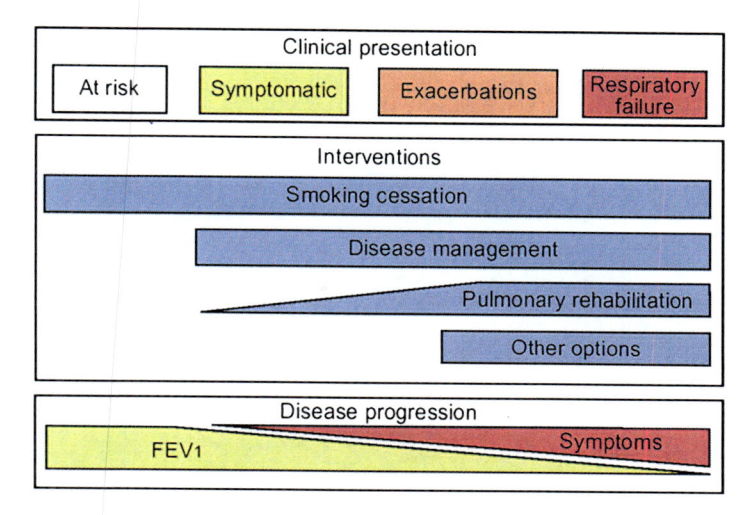

FIGURE 5.2. General approach to the management of COPD [18].

bronchodilators are in common clinical use: β-agonists, anticholinergic drugs, and methylxanthines.

- Long-acting bronchodilators are more effective than short-acting bronchodilators or anticholinergics.
- Anticholinergics given 4 times a day can improve health status.
- A combination of short-acting agents (salbutamol/ipratropium) produces a greater change in lung function than either agent alone.
- Bronchodilators from different classes may improve efficacy, understanding that treatment needs to be long-term.
- An inhaled corticosteroid combined with a long-acting beta-2 agonist is more effective than either agent alone and may reduce the frequency of exacerbations, as well as improve health status.
- The inhaled route of treatment is preferred.

The following algorithm (Figure 5.3) proposed by the American Thoracic Society and the European Respiratory Society in 2004 is a feasible one for use in LTC patients [18].

If forced expiratory volume <50% predicted and exacerbations of COPD requiring a course of oral corticosteroid or antibiotic occurred at least once within the last year, consider adding regular ICS. If an ICS and a long-acting beta agonist are used, prescribe a combination inhaler.

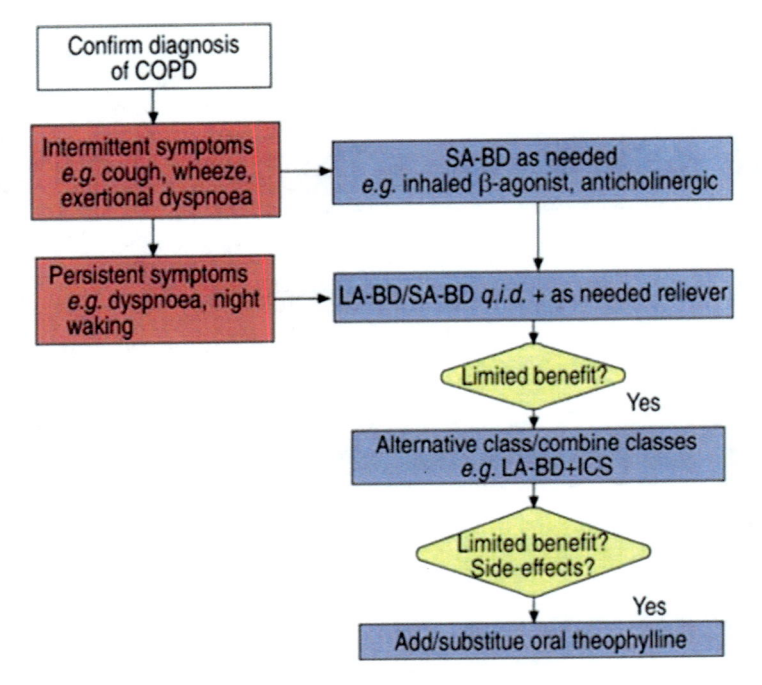

FIGURE 5.3. Algorithm for the use of bronchodilators for COPD [3]. SA-BD: short-acting bronchodilator; LA-BD: long-acting bronchodilator; ICS: inhaled corticosteroid. [18].

Commonly used pharmacological treatments, both inhaled and oral are identified in Table 5.6, with dosage recommendations and cautions.

The routine use of antibiotics is not recommended other than for acute exacerbations. Mucolytics are not recommended either, but may be considered for patients with viscous mucous. Although cough is troublesome, the regular use of antitussives is only recommended if it impairs daily activities and the prolonged use of oral glucocorticoids should be avoided.

## Acute Exacerbations

Acute exacerbations are often characterized by an increase in dyspnea and cough, chest tightness, fever, and delirium, with a change in sputum color and consistency. The cause may be an acute respiratory infection, but the situation may be difficult to distinguish from pneumonia, HF, or thromboembolic disease. The dose and frequency of inhaled bronchodilators should be increased

TABLE 5.6. Commonly used pharmacological agents; benefits and cautions

| Drug class | Drug example | Dosage | Cautions |
|---|---|---|---|
| Short-acting β agonists | Albuterol MDI<br>Albuterol 2.5 mg for nebulization<br>Levalbuterol 0.6 mg | 1–2 inhalations every Q 4–6 h, <br>3 mL TID-QID<br>3 mL TID | All three drugs may be used for acute bronchospasm |
| Long-acting β agonists | Formoterol DPI<br><br>Salmeterol DPI | 1 inhalation (12 µg) every Q 12 h<br>1 inhalation (50 µg) every Q 12 h | Not for acute bronchospasm. Palpitations, tremor, bronchospasm |
| Anticholinergics | Ipratropium bromide MDI<br>Ipratropium bromide 500 µg for nebulization<br>Tiotropium DPI | 2–3 inhalations QID<br><br>2.5 mL TID-QID<br><br>1 inhalation daily | May be used for acute exacerbation<br>For maintenance treatment. Not for acute bronchospasm<br>Caution with BPH and glaucoma |
| Glucocorticoids<br>Inhaled corticosteroids (MDI or DPI) | Beclomethasone diproprionate 40 µg/inhalation<br>Fluticasone DPI | 1–2 inhalations BID<br><br>2 inhalations BID | For severe COPD with repeated exacerbations; added to routine bronchodilator therapy |
| Oral corticosteroids | Prednisone 5 mg<br>Prednisolone 4 mg | 30–40 mg/day for 10 day<br>24–32 mg/day for 10 day | Monitor glucose in patients with DM Osteoporosis, myopathy, and cataracts |
| Methylxanthines | Theophylline ER | 400 mg/day | Toxicity and multiple drug interactions. Caution with liver and cardiac disease. Check levels |

and it is advisable to have PRN orders for nursing staff to initiate treatment with rescue medications while the practitioner is being contacted. If a resident has difficulty using a metered dose inhaler (MDI), hand-held nebulizers should be used for bronchodilator therapy. Oral prednisone (30–40 mg for 10 days) may improve lung function and shorten the course of the acute illness. A short course of oral antibiotics (amoxicillin, cephalosporins, doxycycline, or macrolides) is helpful, although amoxicillin/clavulanate or respiratory fluoroquinolones should be used if prior treatments have failed. Some residents may benefit from suctioning of excess sputum and chest percussion. Ideally, oxygen saturation should be checked and supplemental oxygen is given to maintain $SaO_2$ above 90%. A chest X-ray, CBC, electrolytes, sputum culture, or EKG may provide additional information regarding precipitating causes, but a sputum culture is often difficult to obtain in this population.

The decision to hospitalize residents should be individualized and based on the LTC setting and its ability to handle the resident. In general, hospitalization should be considered for any patient who fails to respond to treatment, develops tachypnea (respirations >28 breaths /min), remains hypoxic, develops delirium or high fever, has significant difficulty sleeping or eating, or has serious comorbidities (HF, DM, CKD, liver disease) [19].

Nonpulmonary complications of COPD increase the morbidity and reduce functional status of the affected person. Cardiovascular and skeletal muscle changes contribute to reduced exercise capacity. Residents frequently have a reduced BMI, lean body mass, and hypogonadism. These factors, in addition to vitamin D deficiency, glucocorticoid use, and sedentary lifestyle, lead to the development of osteoporosis which may only be recognized after the occurrence of a fracture. In addition, residents may experience anxiety, depression, weight loss, sleep disturbance, and cognitive dysfunction. All these problems should be addressed individually as well as by appropriate stepwise and timely treatment of COPD. Because of the progressive and insidious nature of COPD, especially in residents with advanced disease, it is important to have an ongoing discussion with the resident and/or their family about realistic expectations and treatment goals [15].

## DIABETES

Diabetes affects over 26% of LTC residents [20]. Diabetes care accounts for an estimated 32% of Medicare expenses and is an independent predictor of LTC facility placement in the elderly. Diabetic residents are a heterogeneous group characterized by a higher degree of cardiovascular comorbidities, infections, lower extremity complications, pain, pressure ulcers, urinary incontinence, injurious falls, oral problems, cognitive dysfunction, and functional dependency. The majority of residents in LTC have Type 2 diabetes, but there is little consistency in the management of this condition and paucity of data to guide the practitioner in terms of goals of glycemic control and its impact on clinical outcomes. Many elderly have diabetes-related complications secondary to accelerated microvascular and macrovascular disease as well as other comorbidities requiring multiple medications. Complications of diabetes in older adults include [21]:

- Increased susceptibility to infections
- Dehydration
- Delayed wound healing
- Worsening cardiac ischemia/ silent ischemia
- Recurrent CHF
- Oral dryness, infections, burning, caries, periodontal disease
- Urinary retention, incontinence, UTI's
- Weight loss

Hence, effective diabetes management is multifaceted and requires a protocol-driven, team-based, individualized approach to care in the nursing facility. Diabetes care that is able to approximate this approach may be more effective. Goals of treatment are affected by life expectancy, risk of disease, and complications vs. risk of treatment, particularly hypoglycemia. National organizations have formulated clinical guidelines to streamline care of people with diabetes. The clinical guidelines were formulated in an attempt to improve metabolic control and reduce detrimental effects of both hyper and hypoglycemia, and to potentially reduce debilitating complications of DM [21–23].

The challenges of managing diabetes in LTC may be attributed to resident and disease, institution, staff and practitioner, and medication management factors as noted in Table 5.7.

Although laboratory tests may be obtained frequently, abnormal glucose values indicating impaired fasting glucose (fasting plasma glucose [FPG] 100–125 mg/dL, 5.6–6.9 mmol/L) or impaired glucose tolerance (2-h postload glucose 140–199 mg/dL, 7.8–11.1 mmol/L) may not be recognized or followed appropriately. Elderly with undiagnosed diabetes are at risk of coronary heart disease, stroke, and complications of DM. Low physical activity, medications, and concurrent medical conditions such as obesity, pancreatic disorders, and hyperthyroidism can all increase the risk of diabetes. Some commonly used medications, which cause

TABLE 5.7. Challenges of managing diabetes in LTC

| Resident and disease | Institution | Staff and practitioner | Medication management |
| --- | --- | --- | --- |
| Altered pharmacokinetics and pharmacodynamics | Staff turnover and lack of familiarity with residents | Knowledge deficits (disease, complications, selection and modification of therapies) | Multiple and changing treatment approaches |
| Increased risk of hypoglycemia | Restricted dietary practices | Lack of team communication (hyperglycemia, glucose excursions) | Reliance on sliding-scale insulin protocols |
| Irregular meal consumption | Inadequate review of glucose logs | Therapeutic nihilism | Inappropriate dosing or timing of insulin |
| Cognitive dysfunction and depression | Lack of facility – specific diabetes treatment algorithms | Failure to individualize care (A1C, BP, lipids) | Hypoglycemia management (delayed recognition or overcorrection) |
| Psychological insulin resistance | Lack of established blood glucose parameters for physician notification | Failure of timely and stepwise rational advances in therapy | Lack of comfort with newer insulins and injectable agents, and delivery systems |
| Impaired vision and manual dexterity | | | |
| Greater potential for adverse effects and drug interactions | | | |

hyperglycemia, are glucocorticoids, anti-psychotics, β adrenergic agonists, thiazides, and dilantin [21].

In July 2009, the International Expert Committee on Diabetes recommended that the A1C be used for the diagnosis of diabetes. This assay is now standardized and is a clinically convenient and biologically stable index of chronic glycemic exposure over time and risk for diabetic complications. Diabetes is diagnosed when the A1C is ≥6.5% and should be repeated to confirm the diagnosis. Those with an A1C below the threshold for diabetes, but ≥6.0%, should receive attention to existing cardiovascular risk factors to the extent feasible if clinically appropriate [23].

**Treatment Selection**

The general principles of treating diabetes in LTC residents are similar to those used for treating diabetes in the community. While lifestyle changes are effective, dietary restriction is not recommended in LTC since food enjoyment, quality of life, and prevention of weight loss take precedence. Ambulation, seated exercise, and any physical activity possible should be encouraged. Type 2 diabetes is a progressive disease and combination treatment with oral agents is often required as is the use of insulin because the insulin secretion rate in older adults is reduced and delayed. Important considerations in the selection of therapies are the resident's age, renal impairment, hepatic impairment, and weight loss. The following algorithm suggested by the ADA and the European Association for the Study of Diabetes represents a feasible approach (Figure 5.4).

Medications with the least risk of hypoglycemia are metformin, acarbose, miglitol, DPP-4 inhibitors (sitagliptan), GLP-1 analogs (exetanide), short-acting beta-cell enhancers (repaglinide, nateglanide), and long-acting insulin analogs. Management of blood pressure, lipids, nutritional status, pain control, neuropathic symptoms, and lower extremity infections, ulcers and limb loss should also be considered in the overall care of the resident.

**Insulin**

Prolonged severe hyperglycemia leads to glucotoxicity that increases insulin resistance and impairs insulin secretion. The usual course of DM is for the efficacy of oral hypoglycemics to decline with time and the A1C to rise by 0.2–0.3% per year. Timely use of insulin beginning with basal insulin analogs (10 U daily with weekly increases of 2–3 U) is simple and effective, especially in the elderly over age 80 with liver disease or CKD. Insulin should be used acutely if there is marked hyperglycemia, significant weight loss, severe

**Tier 1: Well-validated core therapies**

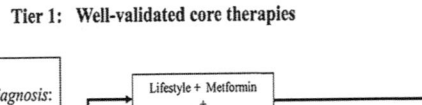

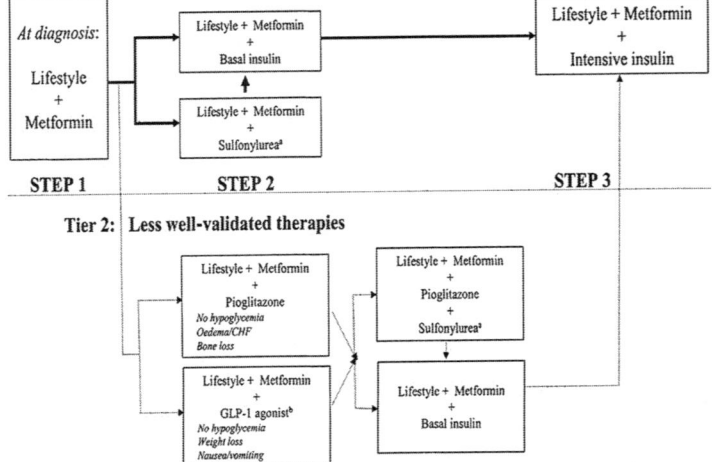

```
At diagnosis:              Lifestyle + Metformin
                                  +                              Lifestyle + Metformin
Lifestyle              →       Basal insulin           →                 +
    +                              ↑                            Intensive insulin
Metformin                   Lifestyle + Metformin                        ↑
                                  +
                              Sulfonylurea[a]

    STEP 1                      STEP 2                          STEP 3
```

**Tier 2: Less well-validated therapies**

```
                     Lifestyle + Metformin        Lifestyle + Metformin
                             +                            +
                         Pioglitazone                Pioglitazone
                       No hypoglycemia                    +
                        Oedema/CHF                  Sulfonylurea[a]
                         Bone loss

                     Lifestyle + Metformin        Lifestyle + Metformin
                             +                            +
                        GLP-1 agonist[b]              Basal insulin
                       No hypoglycemia
                         Weight loss
                       Nausea/vomiting
```

FIGURE 5.4. Algorithm for the treatment of diabetes. From [40].

symptoms, ketonuria, diabetic ketoacidosis, or hyperosmolar state. Sulfonylureas may be discontinued and the dose of thiazolidinediones reduced once the fasting glucose levels have been stabilized. If the A1C remains elevated, the glucose log should be reviewed and regular insulin or a rapid acting insulin analog added to the main meal. Basal analog insulins lower the risk of overall and possibly nocturnal hypoglycemia, whereas rapid acting analogs allow flexibility for inconsistent mealtimes and erratic intake that is not unusual in the LTC resident. It is important to be aware that these insulins should be administered 10–15 min before a meal, and insulin glulysine can be administered up to 20 min after the meal.

### Sliding-Scale Insulin

Sliding-scale insulin delivery as a method of glucose control has many disadvantages. Although it is widely used alone or as an adjunct to oral agents or insulin, it provides no basal insulin and is a reactive instead of proactive approach. This method uses hyperglycemia as a threshold (e.g., >200) and often involves "one-size-fits-all" dosing which is rarely modified. Because of a false sense of security, trends in glycemic control and glucose excursions are often not assessed; for example, the practitioner contacted if glucose is <60 or >300 mg/dL [24]. On a practical level, sliding-scale insulin delivery results in an increased number of injections, medication errors, and increased nursing time. Sliding-scale insulin may be more useful as a *supplemental scale* to schedule oral or injectable therapies in residents with newly diagnosed diabetes, when insulin requirements are unknown or when new or temporary therapies (e.g., external nutrition or glucocorticoid treatment) are initiated. When using sliding-scale insulin delivery as a supplemental scale, additional insulin requirements can be reviewed in 1–2 weeks, at which time the scheduled regimen can then be modified.

### Suggestions for Adjusting Insulin Therapy Based on Glucose Patterns

Maintaining adequate glucose control in a resident needing insulin requires frequent evaluation for targeted glucose levels and adjusting the insulin dose accordingly. The following charts (Tables 5.8 and 5.9) can be used as a guide for which insulin dose to increase or decrease based on the resident's average glucose levels at various time of the day [21].

### Goals of Treatment

TABLE 5.8. Standard human insulin therapy: regular and NPH given twice a day

| Average blood glucose | Regular AM | Regular PM | NPH AM | NPH PM |
|---|---|---|---|---|
| **Fasting** | | | | |
| Low | | | | ↓ |
| High[a] | | | | ↑ |
| **Prelunch**[c] | | | | |
| Low | ↓ | | ↓ | |
| High | ↑ | | | |
| **Pre Supper** | | | | |
| Low | | | ↓ | |
| High[b] | | | ↑ | |
| **Bedtime**[d] | | | | |
| Low | | ↓ | | ↓ |
| High | | ↑ | | |

Permission from AMDA has been requested
[a]Evaluate 3 AM BG readings to eliminate possible nocturnal hypoglycemia leading to rebound hyperglycemia
[b]Evaluate 3 PM BG readings for necessity of afternoon snack
[c]Prelunch glucose levels are influenced by both the R and NPH given in the AM
[d]Bedtime glucose levels are influenced by both the R and NPH given at supper

TABLE 5.9. Analog insulin therapy: basal insulin with rapid acting insulin at each meal

| | | Rapid | | |
| Average blood glucose | Basal | Breakfast | Lunch | Supper |
| --- | --- | --- | --- | --- |
| **Fasting** | | | | |
| Low | ↓ | | | |
| High[a] | ↑ | | | |
| **Prelunch** | | | | |
| Low | | ↓ | | |
| High | | ↑ | | |
| **Presupper** | | | | |
| Low | | | ↓ | |
| High[b] | | | ↑ | |
| **Bedtime** | | | | |
| Low | | | | ↓ |
| High | | | | ↑ |

If a correction dose (sliding-scale) is routinely being added to the patient's usual rapid insulin dose at meals due to hyperglycemia, the *average correction* dose used for any particular meal can be used as the number of units to increase the preceding rapid acting insulin dose

Note: giving rapid acting insulin up to 15 min after eating may be more appropriate if a patient's eating is unpredictable. This allows for not giving the insulin if the patient does not eat

[a] Evaluate 3 AM BG readings to eliminate possible nocturnal hypoglycemia leading to rebound hyperglycemia

[b] Evaluate 3 PM BG readings for necessity of afternoon snack

Treatment goals should be individualized and take into account the state of the disease, extent of microvascular and macrovascular complications, estimated remaining life expectancy, resident and/or family preferences, functional and cognitive status, presence of a major psychiatric disorder, and risk of hypoglycemia. In one study experienced nursing facility physicians managed diabetes less aggressively in residents who were both cognitively and functionally impaired, than those who had either cognitive or functional impairment [25]. Despite the lack of a systematic approach to diabetes care, a recent study in 13 nursing facilities ($N=372$) revealed that 88% of residents had a most recent A1C of <8%, within established guidelines. However, only 35% of residents had established glucose parameters indicating when nurses should alert practitioners for serious hypoglycemia or hyperglycemia (in 14% this was a glucose of >400 mg/dL) [26].

Recent evidence from the ACCORD, ADVANCE, and VADT trials, which investigated the effects of intensive (goal A1C ≤6.5%) vs. standard glycemic control, has not shown a significant reduction in CVD outcomes during the randomized trial periods. However, long-term follow-up of the DCCT and UKPDS cohorts suggests that treatment to A1C targets below or around 7% in the years soon after the diagnosis of diabetes is associated with long-term reduction in risk of macrovascular disease [27]. Less stringent A1C goals such as A1c between 7 and 8%, than the general goal of <7%, may be more appropriate for many of our frail elderly LTC residents that often have a history of severe hypoglycemia, limited life expectancy, advanced microvascular or macrovascular complications, or extensive comorbid conditions.

**Hypoglycemia**

Symptomatic hypoglycemia is defined by symptoms related to hypoglycemia and confirmed by PG ≤72 mg/dL (≤4.0 mmol/L). This can be problematic since symptoms may be atypical such as disorientation, poor coordination, weakness, falls, aggression, or altered behavior. These behaviors can mistakenly be attributed to dementia, or other disorders, and the hypoglycemia overlooked. Moreover, older adults have a lower glucose threshold at which they develop subjective symptoms and hence reduced reaction time.

Risk Factors for severe hypoglycemia in older adults with diabetes include:

- Age
- Unawareness of, or previous severe hypoglycemia
- High doses of insulin or sulfonylureas
- Recent hospitalization or intercurrent illness
- Polypharmacy (>5 prescribed meds)
- Poor nutrition or variable oral intake
- Chronic liver, renal, or cardiovascular disease
- Endocrine deficiency (thyroid, adrenal, or pituitary)
- Alcohol use
- Loss of normal counter-regulation

Insulin-induced hypoglycemia can result from delayed insulin clearance as in the case of renal failure, erratic absorption by injecting hypertrophic sites, and increased insulin sensitivity due to weight loss or significantly increased activity. Frequent use of sliding-scale insulin, improper timing of insulin relative to timing of food intake, inappropriately tight blood glucose control, injection of wrong type of insulin (e.g., rapid acting instead of long acting), and unawareness of hypoglycemia can also cause insulin-induced hypoglycemia [43].

Hypoglycemia may be corrected with ingestion of *15 g* of glucose or carbohydrate, which is equivalent to 1/2 cup juice, 1/2 cup apple sauce, 1 cup milk, 1 tube glucose gel, or 3 glucose tablets. Caregivers should wait *15 min*, recheck blood glucose, and, if still below the target, give another *15 g* of glucose or carbohydrate. Elderly who are obtunded may be treated with SC or IM glucagon (1 mg or 1 U) or 50% dextrose IV, usually 50 mL, although a lesser volume may be used if hypoglycemia is not severe.

## Monitoring

### Assessment of Glycemic Control

There is no consensus regarding the frequency of glucose checks in LTC. The practice of routinely checking premeal and bedtime glucose should be used only for those individuals receiving multiple insulin injections or pump therapy. For residents receiving oral agents or less frequent insulin injections, a reasonable approach to glucose monitoring would be twice daily with rotated times, 2–3 days per week. Postprandial monitoring may be helpful in situations where the fasting glucose is at goal, but the A1C remains elevated.

### Assessment of Facility Management of Diabetes

Successful implementation of facility-wide diabetes evaluation, treatment, and monitoring protocols is possible if there are buy-in from the administration and effective education and communication with practitioners, nursing staff, and medical assistants in the nursing or assisted living facility. Although in the assisted living facility buy-in from nursing and administration is equally important, it may be more difficult to accomplish this due to much more limited resources. The role of each discipline should be defined and a "diabetes nurse" or champion could ensure implementation of any protocols that are created in either setting. A quality improvement program could be devised by selecting certain process indicators (e.g., prevalence of sliding-scale insulin use or regularity of foot examinations) or outcome indicators (e.g., incidence of hypoglycemia or A1C levels) for periodic review and intervention at the facility.

## HYPOTHYROIDISM

Although thyroid disease in the elderly is common, its presentation is often subtle and varied. Because of this frequently nonspecific presentation, thyroid disease requires appropriate screening and interpretation of thyroid function tests in the context of the resident's clinical findings and medication regimen.

*Hypothyroidism* is defined as a state of reduced thyroid hormone availability to the tissues. *Overt hypothyroidism* is present when serum freeT4 levels are below the normal range in the presence of hypothyroid symptoms. Mild thyroid failure or *subclinical hypothyroidism* is a condition in which the TSH level is elevated in the presence of a normal free T4 level.

With age, there is an increase in fibrosis, lymphocyte infiltration, and nodularity of the thyroid, but in the vast majority of older adults, thyroid function remains normal. There is no change in total T4 and free T4 but a slight decrease in TSH and free T3; however, these stay within the normal range with a slight increase in reverse T3.

### Screening for Thyroid Dysfunction

The American Thyroid Association recommends screening all individuals after age 35, and every 5 years thereafter [28]. However, the American College of Physicians does not recommend routine screening, citing a lack of benefit in the treatment of subclinical thyroid disease. In the Colorado Thyroid Disease Prevalence Study, 16% of women and 21% of men over age 74 years had elevated TSH levels [29]. Older adults over age 60 have a 2.3–10% prevalence of hypothyroidism, and since symptoms may be nonspecific, it is the author' opinion that periodic screening is justified for this treatable condition. Screening for thyroid dysfunction is recommended for the following conditions or clinical situations:

- Biological agents (interferons, growth hormone treatment)
- Chronic kidney disease
- Cognitive impairment or psychiatric illness
- Down's or Turner's syndrome
- Drug therapy (amiodarone, lithium)
- Goiter
- Hyperlipidemia
- Irradiation of head and neck
- Pituitary surgery or irradiation
- Radical laryngeal/pharyngeal surgery
- Thyroid disease or surgery in the past
- Thyroid nodule
- Type 1 diabetes
- Severe head injury
- Unexplained depression
- Unexplained weight loss

## Appropriate Use of Thyroid Function Tests

In most situations, measurement of a sensitive serum TSH level will suffice since this test is sensitive enough to distinguish a normal from a low or high value. However, in the elderly with pituitary or hypothalamic disorders, the TSH may be misleading (subnormal or low normal). This is also the case in the elderly with serious acute or chronic illnesses, poor compliance, and taking drugs that alter thyroid hormone levels. There is increasing recognition of partial hypopituitarism in frail LTC residents with cardiovascular disease. Hence, measurement of a TSH and a free T4 level is a more helpful strategy. A complete "thyroid panel" is not usually necessary. Table 5.10 provides a guide for the interpretation of TSH and free T4 (FT4) levels [30].

Several medications can affect the function of the thyroid as well as thyroid function tests; hence, careful interpretation is necessary. The specific effects of medications are shown in Table 5.11.

Excess of thyroid-binding globulin (TBG) will lead to an increase in total T4 levels, whereas a deficiency of TBG levels would lead to a decrease of total T4 levels. Hence, incongruous thyroid function tests should lead to a review of possible causes of altered TBG levels and measurement of the T3 Resin Uptake. Conditions associated with altered TBG levels relevant to LTC residents are listed below.

| *TBG excess* | *TBG deficiency* |
|---|---|
| Estrogen | Androgen administration |
| Acute or chronic active hepatitis | High-dose glucocorticoids |
| Acute porphyria | Nephrosis |
| Opiates, methadone | Hypoproteinemia |
| Perphenazine | Chronic liver disease |

A T3 or free T3 level is useful to confirm the diagnosis of T3 hyperthyroidism, or in the case of nonthyroidal illness when the free T3 is low. Testing for thyroglobulin (Tg) and thyroglobulin antibodies (TgAb) is recommended in the follow-up of treatment for differentiated thyroid cancer to identify or rule out the presence of residual thyroid tissue. Thyroglobulin is undetectable in thyrotoxicosis factitia and is used in the assessment of the activity of inflammatory thyroiditis, e.g., subacute thyroiditis, or that due to amiodarone. The thyroglobulin antibody (TgAb) is an essential component of interpretation of assays for serum thyroglobulin to establish whether endogenous antibodies could be responsible for spuriously low thyroglobulin values and as secondary follow-up in differentiated thyroid cancer.

TABLE 5.10. Interpretations of the TSH and free T4

|  | Low FT4 | Normal FT4 | High FT4 |
|---|---|---|---|
| High TSH | Primary hypothyroidism | Subclinical hypothyroidism | Intermittent/poor compliance with thyroxine (common) TSH producing tumor |
| Normal TSH | Sick euthyroid Drug effect Secondary hypothyroidism | Euthyroid | Intermittent/poor compliance with thyroxine Thyroid hormone resistance |
| Low TSH | Secondary hypothyroidism (pituitary or hypothalamic) Sick euthyroid syndrome | Subclinical hyperthyroidism Thyroxine treatment T3 toxicosis | Hyperthyroidism |

TABLE 5.11. Drugs affecting thyroid function [30]

| Effect | Drugs |
|---|---|
| May cause hypothyroidism | Lithium, iodine (all forms, including kelp, contrast media, etc.), interferon-alpha |
| May cause hyperthyroidism | Iodine, interleukins, interferons |
| Reduce conversion of T4 to T3 | Glucocorticoids, iodine, propylthiouracil, beta-blockers, amiodarone |
| Suppress TSH | Dopamine, dobutamine, glucocorticoids, phenytoin, bromocriptine, octreotide |
| Increase clearance of T4 | Carbamazepine, phenytoin, rifampin, phenobarbitol |
| Reduce binding of T4 to thyroid-binding globulin | Salsalate, salicylates, nonsteroidal anti-inflammatory drugs, furosemide, heparin |
| Influence absorption of thyroxine | Cholestyramine, aluminum hydroxide, ferrous sulfate, sucralfate, cation exchange resins |

An ultrasound of the thyroid is useful for further evaluation of a palpable thyroid nodule or a goiter. Thyroid nodules greater than 1 cm in a *euthyroid and hypothyroid* resident should undergo final needle aspiration to evaluate for thyroid cancer if clinically appropriate. A radioactive iodine uptake scan is not recommended for hypothyroid elderly, but is useful in the identification of the cause of hyperthyroidism by helping differentiate between high uptake vs. low uptake types of hyperthyroidism.

## Causes of Hypothyroidism

The majority of residents with hypothyroidism have primary hypothyroidism. Central or secondary hypothyroidism is rare and accounts for less than 1% of cases. Central hypothyroidism may be due to pituitary or hypothalamic lesions, or dysfunction of other hypothalamic–pituitary axes. Causes of hypothyroidism in the elderly may be divided as disorders of the thyroid gland itself (primary), or disorders of the hypothalamus or pituitary.

### *Primary Hypothyroidism*
- Chronic autoimmune hypothyroidism (Hashimoto's thyroiditis)
- $^{131}$I treatment for hyperthyroidism
- Subtotal or total thyroidectomy
- Radiation therapy for head and neck cancer
- Drugs
- Iodine excess (radio contrast agents and amiodarone), lithium, interferon
- Ant-thyroid drugs (propylthiouracil, methimazole)
- Drugs that decrease TSH or thyroid hormone production (see Table 5.11)
- Infiltrative disorders (amyloidosis, hemochromatosis, scleroderma)

### *Central (Secondary) Hypothyroidism*
- Hypothalamic tumors or infiltrative lesions
- Pituitary tumors or infiltrative lesions
- Pituitary surgery
- Head injury or cranial surgery
- Radiation

## Clinical Evaluation

Clinical signs and symptoms may be nonspecific and be attributed to the aging process or to other comorbidities. Examples of such signs and symptoms include anorexia, cognitive decline, cold intolerance, constipation, dry skin, fatigue, paresthesias, slowed reflexes, and weakness. Hypothyroidism may present in an atypical fashion in the elderly and therefore requires a heightened clinical suspicion. A study comparing the clinical features of overt hypothyroidism in elderly vs. younger patients with a similar duration of disease showed that classical symptoms such as weight gain, cold intolerance, paresthesias, and muscle cramps were less frequent in older patients. However, fatigue was noted in 68% and weakness was noted in 53% of the elderly [31]. Neuropsychiatric symptoms may develop gradually and be particularly challenging in the LTC population in which the prevalence of dementia and the propensity for developing delirium are both high. The frail elderly may become withdrawn, disoriented, and cease to participate in usual activities, all of which may suggest a depressive disorder. Individuals with global intellectual slowing, change of personality, apathy, delusions, and psychosis should be evaluated for hypothyroidism.

The elderly may also have bradycardia, diastolic HTN, hypertriglyceridemia, hypercholesterolemia, and increased levels of creatinine phosphokinase with hypothyroidism. Pericardial effusion is found in 30–50% of cases of overt hypothyroidism. Hypothyroidism may mask typical symptoms of coronary artery disease due to bradycardia and reduced cardiac contractility. Atypical chest pain, exertional dyspnea, and reduced exercise tolerance caused by coronary artery disease can also be seen in a hypothyroid resident with CAD.

### Treatment of Clinical Hypothyroidism

The goal of treatment is to normalize thyroid function and to achieve a euthyroid state. The dose of thyroid hormone replacement depends on the age and weight of the resident, the average daily requirements for the elderly being 25% less than young adults. Synthetic thyroid hormone preparations are preferred since they have a longer half life and relatively constant serum concentrations. Older adults with cardiovascular disease should be started on 12.5–25 µg/day of levothyroxine and the dose should be adjusted by a similar amount every 6 weeks till the TSH has normalized. It can then be followed every 6–12 months to evaluate compliance or monitor dosage requirements in residents who have had a significant weight loss or change in their drug regimen. In primary hypothyroidism, the TSH alone can be used to monitor treatment, but in those with central (secondary) hypothyroidism, a free T4 level should be used. If no residual thyroid function exists, the daily replacement dose of levothyroxine is usually 1.6 µg/kg body weight (typically 100–150 µg). In hypothyroidism after the treatment of Graves' disease, there is often underlying autonomous function, necessitating lower replacement doses (typically 75–125 µg/day). There is no current data to recommend what the TSH level should be on stable treatment in LTC residents, and dosage adjustments should take into account any worsening of cardiovascular symptoms. It is important to note that linear changes in the concentration of T4 correspond to logarithmic changes in serum TSH. If a resident has had an abrupt discontinuation or omission of thyroxine therapy during a care transition, the person may have a marked rise in a subsequent TSH level. The dose of thyroxine when treatment is resumed should be the prior documented dose and not an arbitrarily high dose.

## Subclinical Hypothyroidism

This condition may also be referred as "mild thyroid failure" and is defined by an elevated TSH and normal free T4 levels. AntiTPO antibodies are positive in 67% of nursing home residents with subclinical hypothyroidism. Most elderly are usually asymptomatic and clinical detection is difficult especially in long-term residents.

Prevalence of this condition in 80-year-olds ranges from 14 to 20% and was 14.6% in one large nursing facility study. The etiology of subclinical hypothyroidism is usually chronic autoimmune thyroiditis, but poor compliance with thyroxine therapy, suboptimal treatment, recovery from severe illness, thyroiditis, and medications affecting thyroid function should also be considered.

The possible effects of subclinical hypothyroidism and treatment considerations include progression to overt hypothyroidism, elevation of lipid levels, altered mood and cognition, impaired cardiac function, coronary heart disease (CHD) events and CHD mortality. A high TSH level (>12 mU/L), presence of autoantibodies, a goiter, advanced age, and a history of radiation history are all risk factors for progression to overt hypothyroidism. Lipid levels are elevated in 50% of these individuals and may be lowered with thyroxine treatment. However, in the general population of the oldest old, elderly individuals with abnormally high levels of TSH do not experience adverse effects and may have a prolonged life span.

## Management of Subclinical Hypothyroidism

Current evidence does not support the benefit of routinely treating subclinical hypothyroidism to improve systemic hypothyroid symptoms, cardiac function, or neuropsychiatric symptoms. The current guidelines for the management of subclinical hypothyroidism are the following: [32]

- If the TDS is 4.5–10 mU/L in the *absence* of symptoms, repeat TSH in 1 month and every 6 months while asymptomatic.
- If the TDS is 4.5–10 mU/L in the *presence* of symptoms, consider trial of thyroid hormone replacement.
- If the TSH is >10 mU/L, in most circumstances administer thyroid treatment.

### *Nonthyroidal Illness*

A variety of systemic illnesses can cause changes in thyroid function tests. The commonest is a low T3 state with normal

TSH, FT4, and T4 (due to inhibition of 5'deiodinase and T4–T3 conversion). Patients who are severely ill may have a low T4 and low T3. There is also an acquired defect in binding of T4 to TBG leading to increased clearance of T4. TSH can decline also with severe illness. Transient high TSH may also be seen in some patients during the recovery phase from an acute illness.

## VITAMIN B12 DEFICIENCY

$B_{12}$ deficiency is common in older adults and leads to hematological abnormalities as well as neurological consequences that may be serious and irreversible. Population studies show a prevalence of $B_{12}$ deficiency of 10–15% in older adults, with one European study reporting a prevalence of 8.3% in nursing facility residents using serum $B_{12}$ levels alone. The signs and symptoms of $B_{12}$ deficiency are nonspecific and varied and can be attributed to other comorbid disorders or the neurological changes of aging. The classic presentation of $B_{12}$ deficiency with megaloblastic anemia and neurological dysfunction is less common and the elderly may have "subtle $B_{12}$ deficiency" with the metabolic deficiency only. On occasion, severe neurologic or hematologic signs can be seen, although $B_{12}$ deficiency can also occur with either neurologic or hematologic signs alone and without macrocytosis. However, in a population in which the prevalence of dementia as well as neurological and neuropsychiatric abnormalities is high, early recognition of $B_{12}$ deficiency is worthwhile [33]. Older age and more established symptoms of $B_{12}$ deficiency are associated with less likelihood of neurologic improvement. $B_{12}$ deficiency has also been associated with low bone mineral density and elevated $B_{12}$ metabolites have been implicated in prefrailty.

Food-cobalamin deficiency is responsible for about 40–50% of $B_{12}$ deficiency, and pernicious anemia for about 10%. Achlorhydria and atrophic gastritis is another important contributing factor for $B_{12}$ deficiency in older adults. Stomach acid is necessary to remove the vitamin from food, which then binds to haptocorin, undergoes degradation by pancreatic enzymes, and again binds to intrinsic factor in the ileum, following which the complex is absorbed in the circulation. There it binds to transcobalamin, which is the active form as holotranscobolamin or holoTC in order to reach the tissues. The causes of $B_{12}$ deficiency encountered in LTC residents are [34]:

- Atrophic gastritis and hypochlorhydria (leading to food-cobalamin malabsorption)
- Chronic proton pump inhibitor therapy
- Gastrectomy (total or partial) or gastric bypass surgery

- Ileal resection
- Small intestine and terminal ileum disorders (Crohn disease, sprue, malabsorption)
- H Pylori infection
- Bacterial overgrowth syndromes
- Strict vegetarian diet
- Pernicious anemia (positive antiintrinsic factor antibodies)
- AIDS and AIDS treatment (e.g., zidovudine)
- Metformin

## When Should B12 Deficiency be Suspected?

$B_{12}$ deficiency should be suspected in long-term residents with unexplained neurological symptoms, unexplained anemia, glossitis, anorexia, diarrhea, or other gastrointestinal manifestations. The presence of autoimmune diseases, such as thyroiditis, vitiligo, as well as any of the risk factors listed previously, should also increase the suspicion of the disorder [34]. The signs and symptoms of $B_{12}$ deficiency may be categorized as follows;

*Hematologic:* macrocytosis, anemia, neutrophil hypersegmentation
*Neurologic:* peripheral neuropathy, paresthesias, spinal column lesions (loss of vibration, position sense, ataxia), extensor plantars, orthostatic hypotension
Limb weakness
*Neuropsychiatric:* delirium with slow thinking, depression, confusion, memory loss, language difficulties

## Diagnosis

Blood levels of $B_{12}$ and folate are frequently ordered in elderly with anemia or dementia. Falsely low levels of $B_{12}$ may be seen in AIDS and multiple myeloma; falsely high levels may be seen in transcobalamin II deficiency or certain myeloproliferative disorders such as CML.

Metabolite testing for homocysteine (Hcy) and methyl malonic acid (MMA) is widely available, although the interpretation of these tests may be difficult and affected by other clinical conditions. MMA elevation is specific for $B_{12}$ and indicates tissue deficiency, whereas Hcy levels are elevated in most individuals with $B_{12}$ and folate deficiency. Holotranscobalamin (holoTC) represents $B_{12}$ bound to transcobalamin and is the fraction available for tissue uptake. This test is not widely available and may be equivalent to total $B_{12}$ in its ability to discriminate people with or without $B_{12}$ deficiency.

The elderly may have a tissue deficiency of $B_{12}$ with levels of up to 400 pg/mL, whereas some subnormal $B_{12}$ levels are associated with normal metabolite levels. Falsely elevated levels of MMA may be seen in hypovolemia and both MMA and Hcy may be falsely elevated in renal insufficiency. Hence, there is no clear gold standard for the diagnosis of $B_{12}$ deficiency, but metabolite levels may be useful if $B_{12}$ levels are borderline and symptoms are nonspecific [35].

No further evaluation is usually required after the diagnosis of $B_{12}$ deficiency is made with first-line tests. The Shilling test or other tests of gastric function are rarely performed since the treatment is cobalamin replacement. Bone marrow examination should only be done to rule out malignancy.

**Treatment**
Most patients with a borderline deficiency can also be treated and followed for biochemical reversal. A common strategy is to replace $B_{12}$ in the form of 1,000 µg cyanocobalamin by intramuscular injection weekly for 1 month and then monthly indefinitely. Residents with possible symptoms of $B_{12}$ deficiency should be replaced parenterally, whereas residents in whom $B_{12}$ was discovered incidentally may be replaced orally. Crystalline $B_{12}$ is well absorbed and at least 500–1,000 µg/day is required to reverse the biochemical signs of $B_{12}$ deficiency. Sublingual and intranasal forms of $B_{12}$ are more costly and less rigorously tested.

Monitoring recommendations vary and depend on the manifestation and severity of $B_{12}$ deficiency. Elderly with anemia due to $B_{12}$ deficiency should have a reticulocyte count in 1 week and hemoglobin levels in 1–2 months. Biochemical monitoring is not required in those receiving parenteral replacement, but $B_{12}$, MMA, or Hcy may be measured to assess absorption and compliance in anyone receiving oral supplementation. Treatment of $B_{12}$ deficiency may unmask underlying folate and iron deficiency, and as red cell production increases, they may also need to be supplemented.

## SKIN DISORDERS

### Scabies
Scabies is a contagious parasitic infestation of the skin caused by the human itch mite *Sarcoptes scabei*. It infects LTC residents and can cause large outbreaks among residents and staff unless it is treated, and systematic infection control protocols are followed. The severity of the scabies infection depends on the number of mites infesting the skin. A heavier more atypical

infection is characterized by extremely pruritic crusty skin lesions with thousands to millions of live mites and is also known as Norwegian scabies. Mental retardation, dementia, immunodeficiency states, renal failure, malnutrition, HIV, insulin-treated diabetes, and administration of topical and systemic corticosteroids increase the rate of progression of scabies.

### *Transmission and Diagnosis*

The incubation period of scabies is 3–6 weeks, and healthy individuals without prior infestation may be asymptomatic during this period. Those with previous infestation often develop pruritis within 48 h because the itching originates from an allergic reaction that develops to the mite. The itching that occurs with a scabies infestation is striking and can be particularly problematic at night. Skin areas that are typically affected are the web spaces between the fingers, breast folds, buttocks, genitalia, and flexor surfaces of the wrists, elbows, and axillae. The differential diagnosis of the rash may include eczema, folliculitis, tinea, psoriasis, insect bites, or dermatitis herpetiformis.

An outbreak may be defined as one or more confirmed cases within a finite period of time and in a defined location (e.g., a nursing unit or ward). Because a crusted or Norwegian scabies infection is teeming with mites, it has an even higher than normal rate of transmission. Transmission is from person to person by direct skin contact, or from wearing clothing of the infested resident (fomites). Chair covers, bed linens, and personal clothing play a much smaller role in a typical infestation than direct person to person spread.

Skin scrapings that show the presence of mites, eggs, or fecal pellets on microscopic exam usually make a definitive scabies diagnosis. Scrapings should be performed in areas that are typically infested by the mite. However, in recently exposed people, skin scrapings can be negative on multiple occasions and the Burrows Ink Test may provide clues to infestation. The Burrows Ink Test is performed by running a black or green felt tip pen over the waxy red raised burrows, and then wiping the skin off with alcohol to reveal a black or green zigzag line under magnification [36]. An eczematous eruption can frequently be seen covering the trunk of elderly infected with scabies, but this is usually an allergic reaction to the mite and may have little evidence of mite infestation. Skin biopsies are not recommended in scabies because of their low yield. Hence, empiric treatment based on symptoms may be necessary. A dermatology consultation may be considered for difficult cases.

## Controlling the Outbreak

Barrier precautions using gowns and gloves should be used till scabies has been eliminated as a possibility. The nursing facility medical director should be able to order diagnostic tests and treatment, and notify other practitioners. Either an infection control practitioner or designated nursing staff leader should track cases and contacts as well as implement barrier precautions in the nursing or assisted living facility. The staff may need to treat all residents in an area if multiple cases of infestation are found there. Staff education should be reinforced; and work assignments should minimize care areas in order to limit transmission. Any exposed visitors and volunteers should be treated as well. The local health department or the state regulatory agency should also be notified and isolation supplies and scabicides ordered.

Contact precautions should be used for at least 24 h after initiating treatment. Residents with crusted scabies will require several treatments and may be contagious for several weeks. In the case of crusted scabies, contact isolation in a single room should be continued till three consecutive skin scrapings are negative. Clothing, pillows, blankets, and wheelchair pads can be washed, sealed in plastic for 5–7 days, or placed in a hot dryer. Environmental surfaces, beds, assistive devices, diagnostic, and therapy equipment should be cleaned with an Environmental Protection Agency (EPA)-registered cleaning product. Furniture with fabric upholstery will need to be removed for 5–7 days, topical creams and lotions discarded, all carpets vacuumed, and the bag disposed of immediately.

## Treatment [36]

- Gamma-hexachlorocyclohexane (Lindane) is no longer recommended due to resistance of the mites and neurotoxicity concerns.
- Permethrin 5% (Elimite) cream is 90% effective after the first application, but in some patients, a second application after 7–10 days may be necessary.
- All symptomatic patients and close contact including staff should be treated with permethrin in the same 24–48 h period.
- Healthcare workers and their household contacts should be treated at the end of the work shift, leave permethrin cream on, and shower after 8–12 h.
- Permethrin should be applied into the entire area of skin from the hairline to the feet, including the palms and soles, under the fingernails and toenails; the scalp may rarely need treatment if infested.

- Topical steroid creams or antihistamines to treat pruritis should not be applied until the scabicide has been removed.
- Oral ivermectin (Stromectol) is an effective and cost-comparable alternative to topical scabicides, although it is not FDA approved for use in scabies. It may be particularly useful in demented patients, in large outbreaks, and in the treatment of severely crusted scabies lesions in immunocompromised residents or when topical therapy has failed. A single dose of 200 µg/kg is effective or a standard 6 mg dose for a 70 kg adult.

**Herpes Zoster**

The prevalence of HZ in LTC residents is unknown, but has been reported to be 1.4% in the elderly with 50% developing postherpetic neuralgia (PHN). This can be a devastating complication requiring prolonged pharmacotherapy and other pain management interventions, as well as leading to depression and decline in function. HZ is characterized by a pruritic, maculopapular vesicular rash that evolves into noninfectious dried crusts over a 5–6-day period. It is triggered by a decline in cell-mediated immunity that facilitates the reactivation of latent virus in the sensory ganglia. LTC residents are at greater risk because of age-related decline in cell-medicated immunity, malnutrition, multiple comorbidities, frailty, and functional impairment. They also have diminished reserves to respond to stressors related to an episode of HZ.

The lesion of HZ is often described as a "dew drop on a rose petal" which in HZ is found clustered in a dermatomal distribution, not crossing the midline. Most often, HZ is diagnosed clinically, but the laboratory diagnosis can be made by isolation of the varicella virus from a lesion. Rapid varicella virus identification using PCR is preferred if available, but direct fluorescent antibody (DFA) or a significant rise in varicella IgG can also be used to make the diagnosis.

*General Measures*

The nursing leadership and medical staff should educate the resident and direct caregivers regarding the nature of the infection and the risk of viral transmission to individuals who have not had chickenpox. HZ is not contagious for those who have a history of chicken pox or adequate titers of IgG to varicella. Skin lesions should be kept clean and dry to avoid bacterial superinfection. Antibiotic ointments and adhesive dressings should be avoided since healing and drying of the lesions will be delayed; and the resident's temperature should be monitored. Herpes viral replication in immunocompromised individuals and those with ophthalmic zoster should be treated with antiviral agents [37].

## Vaccination
The Advisory Committee on Immunization Practices (ACIP) recommends a single dose of zoster vaccine among persons of 60 years and older, regardless of prior history of HZ. People with a chronic medical condition may be vaccinated unless a contraindication or precaution exists for the condition; it is not recommended for pregnant or immunocompromised individuals [38]. Although zoster vaccine (Zostavax) has been associated with 51% fewer episodes of HZ, and 66% less PHN, the figures were only 18 and 26%, respectively, in those who were of 80 years and over. Also, the Shingles Prevention study did not include cognitively impaired, nonambulatory residents with less than 5 years of expected survival. Hence, response to the vaccine in LTC residents cannot reliably be predicted and currently widespread facility immunization programs for HZ cannot be recommended [39].

## Treatment
- Topical antiviral treatment is not efficacious.
- Systemic antiviral treatment recommended if ≥50 years age, moderate to severe pain or rash, or have nontruncal involvement within 72 h of rash onset. Begin after 72 h if neurologic or ocular signs, or with severe pain and/or rash.
  - Acyclovir 800 mg 5 times daily (every 4–5 h) for 7–10 days.
  - Famciclovir 500 mg 3 times daily for 7 days.
  - Valacyclovir 1,000 mg 3 times daily for 7 days.
- Supplementing antiviral therapy.
  - Analgesics (acetaminophen, opiods, tramadol).
  - Add gabapentin (up to 3,600 mg daily), pregabalin (75 mg twice daily), or a tricyclic antidepressant (nortriptyline 25 mg at bedtime, up to 150 mg daily), if no improvement in pain.
  - Oral corticosteroid (e.g., prednisone 60 mg daily for 7 day) for moderate to severe pain, polyneuropathy, cranial nerve paralysis, or CNS dysfunction.
- Referral to a pain specialist or pain center is recommended to evaluate for neural blockade if analgesics, adjunct therapies, and corticosteroids are not effective.
- Psychosocial evaluation to avoid isolation and severe depression.
- Attention to nutrition and maintenance of functional status.

## PEARLS FOR THE PRACTITIONER
- Some studies have shown that the treatment of HTN in those over age 80 has resulted in a significant reduction in fatal and nonfatal stroke and all-cause mortality within 1–2 years of starting antihypertensive treatment.

- Once diagnosed with anemia, residents should be evaluated for possible comorbid conditions such as impaired physical performance, risk for falls, and cognitive impairment.
- Residents with HF have a 74% or 92% 5-year mortality with either a normal or reduced LVEF, respectively, and are a major cause of hospital admissions and readmissions.
- COPD, the fourth leading cause of US deaths, is present in one in six people admitted to nursing facilities and yet remains either unrecognized or suboptimally treated.
- Effective management of diabetes requires an approach that is multifaceted, protocol-driven, interdisciplinary, and individualized. If used, sliding-scale insulin is best utilized as a supplement to scheduled oral hypoglycemic agents and/or basal insulin therapy and not as a primary means to control blood glucose.
- Subclinical hypothyroidism is both common and not associated with the classical signs and symptoms of hypothyroidism often seen in younger adults and is not uncommon in those already diagnosed with DM or vitamin $B_{12}$ deficiency.
- Vitamin $B_{12}$ deficiency in older age is commonly not associated with anemia or macrocytosis, so a high index of suspicion is warranted as to its possible presence.
- For scabies, permethrin 5% cream has a 90% effective cure rate after its first application. A second application may be necessary 7–10 days after initial treatment.
- In those 80 years and older, zoster vaccine (Zostavax®) is associated with only 18% fewer attacks of shingles and 26% less occurrence of PHN, while more effective in those of age 60 and over (51 and 66%, respectively).

## WEBSITES
- National Guideline Clearing House www.guideline.gov
- AHA www.americanheart.org
- American College of cardiology www.acc.org
- The Global Initiative for Chronic Obstructive Lung Disease www.goldcopd.com
- American Diabetes Association www.diabetes.org
- American Thyroid Association Professional Guidelines www.thyroidguidelines.net

## REFERENCES
1. Aronow WS, Ahn C, Gutstein H. Prevalence and incidence of cardiovascular disease in 1160 older men and 2464 older women in a long-term health care facility. J Gerontol Med Sci. 2002;57A:M45–6.

2. Musini VM, Tejani AM, et al. Pharmacotherapy for hypertension in the elderly. Cochrane Database Syst Rev. 2009;Issue 4. Art. No.: CD000028. DOI: 10.1002/14651858.CD000028.pub2.
3. Beckett NS, Peters R, Fletcher AE, et al. Treatment of hypertension in patients 80 years of age or older. N Engl J Med. 2008;358(18):1887–98.
4. Aram Chobanian V, George Bakris L, Henry Black R, William Cushman C, Lee Green A, Joseph Izzo L Jr, Daniel Jones W, Barry Materson J, Suzanne Oparil, Jackson Wright T Jr, Edward Roccella J, The National High Blood Pressure Education Program Coordinating Committee. The Seventh Report of the Joint National Committee on Prevention, Detection, Evaluation, and Treatment of High Blood Pressure (JNC 7). Hypertension. 2003;42:1206.
5. Anon. National High Blood Pressure Education Program Working Group Report on Hypertension in the Elderly. Hypertension. 1994;23:275–85.
6. Rosendorff C, et al. Treatment of hypertension in the prevention and management of ischemic heart disease: a scientific statement from the American Heart Association Council for high blood pressure research and the councils on clinical cardiology and epidemiology and prevention. Circulation. 2007;115:2761–88.
7. Chaves P, Ashar T, Guralnik JM, et al. Looking at the relationship between hemoglobin concentration and previous mobility difficulty in older women: should the criteria used to define anemia in older people be changed? J Am Geriatr Soc. 2002;50:1257–64.
8. Pandya N, Bookhart B, Mody SH, et al. Study of anemia in long-term care (SALT): prevalence of anemia and its relationship with the risk of falls in nursing home residents. Curr Med Res Opin. 2008;24(8):2139–49.
9. American Medical Directors Association (AMDA). Anemia in the long-term care setting. Columbia (MD): American Medical Directors Association (AMDA); 2007.
10. Wilbert Aronow S. Treatment of systolic and diastolic heart failure in the elderly. J Am Med Dir Assoc. 2006;7(1):29–36.
11. Wilbert Aronow S. Mortality in nursing home patients with congestive heart failure. J Am Med Dir Assoc. 2003;4(4):220–1.
12. Jessup M, Abraham WT, Casey DE, Feldman AM, Francis GS, Ganiats TG, Konstam MA, Mancini DM, Rahko PS, Silver MA, Stevenson LW, Yancy CW. 2009 Focused Update: ACCF/AHA Guidelines for the Diagnosis and Management of Heart Failure in Adults. Circulation. 2009;119:1977–2016.
13. Hutt E, Frederickson E, Ecord M, Kramer AM. Associations among processes and outcomes of care for medicare nursing home residents with acute heart failure. J Am Med Dir Assoc. 2003;4(4):195–9.
14. Chun J, Chodosh J. Controversy in heart failure management: digoxin use in the elderly. J Am Med Dir Assoc. 2006;7(9):581–6.
15. American Medical Director's Association. COPD management in the long-term care setting. Clin Pract Guidel. 2003.
16. Doherty DE. Identification and assessment of chronic obstructive pulmonary disease in the elderly. J Am Med Dir Assoc. 2003;4(5):S116–20.

17. Global Initiative for Chronic Obstructive Lung Disease. Global Strategy for the Diagnosis, Management, and Prevention of Chronic Obstructive Pulmonary Disease (updated 2008). Available at: http://www.goldcopd.org.
18. Celli1 BR, MacNee2 W, Agusti A, et al. Standards for the diagnosis and treatment of patients with COPD. Eur Respir J. 2004;23:932–46.
19. Ziment I, Yick D. Treatment of chronic obstructive pulmonary disease. J Am Med Dir Assoc. 2003;4(5):S121–6.
20. Travis SS, Buchanan RJ, Wang S, et al. Analyses of nursing home residents with diabetes at admission. JAMDA. 2004;5(5):320–7.
21. American Medical Directors Association. Diabetes management in the long-term care setting clinical practice guideline. Columbia: AMDA; 2008.
22. California Healthcare Foundation/American Geriatrics Society Panel on Improving Care for Elders with Diabetes. Guidelines for improving the care of the older person with diabetes mellitus. JAGS. 2003;51(5):S265–80.
23. International Expert Committee Report on the Role of the A1C Assay in the Diagnosis of Diabetes. Diabetes Care. 2009;32(7):1–8.
24. Pandya N, Thompson S, Sambamurthi U. The prevalence and persistence of sliding scale insulin use among newly admitted elderly nursing home residents with diabetes. JAMDA. 2008;9(9):663–9.
25. McNabney M, Pandya N, Iwuagwu C, et al. Differences in diabetes management of nursing home patients based on functional and cognitive status. J Am Med Dir Assoc. 2005;6:375–82.
26. Feldman SM, Rosen R, DeStasio J. Status of Diabetes Management in the Nursing Home Setting in 2008: A Retrospective Chart Review and Epidemiology Study of diabetic nursing home residents and nursing home initiatives in diabetes management. J Am Med Dir Assoc. 2009;10(5):354–60.
27. Intensive Glycemic Control and the Prevention of Cardiovascular Events: Implications of the ACCORD, ADVANCE, and VA Diabetes Trials: A position statement of the American Diabetes Association and a scientific statement of the American College of Cardiology Foundation and the American Heart Association. Diabetes Care. 2009;32:187–92.
28. Ladenson PW, et al. American thyroid association guidelines for detection of thyroid dysfunction. Arch Intern Med. 2000;160:1573–5.
29. Canaris GJ, Manowitz NR, Mayor G, Ridgway EC. The Colorado Thyroid Disease Prevalence Study. Arch Intern Med. 2000;160:526–34.
30. Finucane P, et al. Thyroid function tests in elderly patients with and without an acute llness. Age Ageing. 1989;18:398–402.
31. Mohandas R. Managing thyroid dysfunction in the elderly. Postgrad Med. 2003;113(5):54–6; 65–8; 100.
32. Surks MI, et al. Subclinical thyroid disease: scientific review and guidelines for diagnosis and management. JAMA. 2004;291:228–38.
33. Malouf R, Evans GJ. Folic acid with or without vitamin B12 for the prevention and treatment of healthy elderly and demented people [update

of Cochrane Database Syst Rev. 2003;(4):CD004514; PMID: 14584018] [Review] [121 refs]. Cochrane Database Syst Rev. 2008;(4):CD004514.
34. Smith RL. Evaluation of vitamin B12 and folate status in the nursing home. J Am Med Direct Assoc. 2001;2(5):230–8.
35. Hvas AM, Nexo E. Diagnosis and treatment of vitamin B12 deficiency – an update. Haematologica. 2006;91:1506–12.
36. Cahill CK, et al. Scabies surveillance, prevention, and control. Ann Long Term Care Clin Care Aging. 2009;17(4):31–5.
37. Dworkin RH, Johnson RW, Breuer J, Gnann JW. Recommendations for the management of herpes zoster. Clin Infect Dis. 2007;1(44 Suppl 1):S1–26.
38. Harpaz R, Ortega-Sanchez IR, Seward JF; Advisory Committee on Immunization Practices (ACIP) Centers for Disease Control and Prevention (CDC). Prevention of herpes zoster. recommendations of the advisory committee on immunization practices (ACIP). MMWR. 2008;57(RR-5):1–30.
39. Drinka PJ. How should nursing homes use vaccine to prevent zoster? J Am Med Direct Assoc. 2007;8(7):419–20.
40. Nathan DM, Buse JB, Davidson MB, Ferrannini E, Holman RR, Sherwin R, Zinman B; American Diabetes Association; European Association for Study of Diabetes. Medical management of hyperglycemia in type 2 diabetes: a consensus algorithm for the initiation and adjustment of therapy: a consensus statement of the american diabetes association and the European Association for the Study of Diabetes. Diabetes Care. 2009;32:193–203.
41. Jeffrey Halter B, Joseph Ouslander G, Mary Tinetti E, Stephanie Studenski, Kevin High P, Sanjay Asthana. Hazzard's Geriatric Medicine and Gerontology, 6e. Chapter 81. New York: McGraw Hill; 2009.
42. Weiss G, Goodnough L. Anemia of chronic disease. NEJM. 2005;352:1011–23.
43. Chelliah A, Burge MR. Hypoglycaemia in elderly patients with diabetes mellitus: causes and strategies for prevention. Drugs Aging. 2004;21(8):511–30.

# Chapter 6
# Acute Change in Condition

J. Kenneth Brubaker

**Keywords:** Asymptomatic bacteriuria • Urinary tract infections • Pneumonia • Nursing home-acquired pneumonia • Transition of care

## INTRODUCTION

This chapter will cover three common occurrences associated with an acute change of condition in frail older adults residing in nursing or assisted living facilities: (1) asymptomatic bacteriuria and urinary tract infections (UTIs), (2) pneumonia, and (3) the interface with acute care.

One of the most challenging responsibilities the long-term care (LTC) clinician experiences is receiving a call at 2 AM from the nursing facility. The nurse is very concerned by the sudden change in mental status of a resident who has recently been transferred from the hospital to the nursing home. Since the on-call clinician is covering for his colleague who had admitted this resident, he is totally dependent upon the supervisor's assessment of the recently admitted resident. While still trying to awaken from his stage IV sleep, he has a litany of possibilities running through his mind as a cause for the change in the resident's mental status. Is the resident receiving too much opioid pain medication? Maybe there is an electrolyte imbalance? Has there been an inappropriate drug ordered in the hospital that has a long half-life and is now causing delirium? Or, maybe the resident is developing an infection and may have a low-grade fever.

The supervisor gives a very quick history of the resident including the list of medications and completes the summary by stating that the vital signs are normal and the oxygen saturation is 94% on room air. The supervisor dismisses the 99.5°F oral temperature as normal and does not immediately reveal it, since her small children often have low-grade temperatures that usually do not indicate any serious problems. What is the most appropriate next step for the clinician? Should the resident be sent to the emergency room (ER)? If the resident can make medical decisions, what does the resident want done at 2 AM? Since the resident likely has delirium, the resident's Power of Attorney (POA) will need to be called to assist in decision making. Later in the conversation with the supervisor, the clinician learns that the resident does have a low-grade oral temperature. The clinician immediately expands his differential to include an underlying infectious process as the cause of the change in the resident's mental status.

Most LTC clinicians have had similar experiences while covering a colleague's residents over night. What may have sounded like a very straightforward problem to the supervisor is much more complex to the clinician on-call.

Numerous studies consistently report that the two most common infections in LTC residents occur in the urinary tract and lower respiratory system. A recent study indicated that the most frequent reasons for the use of antibiotics in nursing homes were respiratory (33%) and UTIs (32%) [1]. The literature is very clear and consistent in reporting that pneumonia and UTIs should be suspected when there is a change in mental status and no obvious cause of a low-grade fever.

## ASYMPTOMATIC BACTERIURIA AND URINARY TRACT INFECTIONS

### Guidelines for Diagnosing a Urinary Tract Infection or Urosepsis

Whether to treat or not to treat an abnormal urinalysis is a common dilemma faced when caring for frail older adults. However, the greater challenge for the clinician is understanding when to order a urinalysis. Most nursing staff has learned that whenever a cognitively impaired resident demonstrates disruptive behavior, the clinician should be notified to order a urinalysis. However, over 50% of all urine specimens of frail older adult females residing in nursing facilities will be positive for bacteriuria. If a resident solely has a mental status change and no other evidence to suggest a UTI, Nicolle found that only 11% of residents had a UTI [2]. Unless a resident is running a fever, has tenderness over the bladder, and/or has frequency of urination, the clinician should be looking for other contributing factors that may cause a sudden onset of disruptive behavior, rather than immediately suspecting a UTI. It is not uncommon for disruptive behavior to occur as a result of a new nursing assistant caring for the resident, loud or disturbing noise, other aggressive residents, or upsetting family news.

When managing an acute change in a resident and treating a UTI as the possible cause, there are several important diagnostic findings that play a critical role in making an accurate diagnosis. A recent update by the Infection Disease Society of America (IDSA) recommends that a urinalysis and urine culture in *uncatheterized* residents should be reserved for those with the following UTI-associated symptoms and signs [3]:

- Fever
- Dysuria
- Gross hematuria
- New onset or worsening of urinary incontinence
  Suspected bacteremia (A-II) (see Table 6.1)

In the state of Pennsylvania, a recently enacted law (ACT 52) requires all nursing facilities to report UTIs to the state department of health (DOH). All UTIs must meet McGeer's criteria for a UTI. McGeer's

TABLE 6.1. Infectious Disease Society of America – U.S. Public Health Service grading system for ranking recommendations in clinical guidelines

| Category/grade | Definition |
| --- | --- |
| Strength of recommendation | |
| A | Good evidence to support a recommendation for use |
| B | Moderate evidence to support a recommendation for use |
| C | Poor evidence to support a recommendation |
| Quality of evidence | |
| I | Evidence from ≥1 properly randomized, controlled trial |
| II | Evidence from ≥1 well-designed clinical trial, without randomization from cohort or case-controlled analytical studies (preferably from >1 center); from multiple time-series; or from dramatic results from uncontrolled experiments |
| III | Evidence from opinions of respected authorities, based on clinical experience, descriptive studies, or reports of expert committees |

criteria for a UTI *without the presence of a catheter* require at least THREE of the following signs or symptoms:

- Fever or chills (fever is defined as 2°F above the average normal temperature or 100.4°F taken orally or an oral equivalent)
- New or increased burning pain on urination, frequency, or urgency
- New flank or suprapubic pain or tenderness
- Change in character of urine or gross hematuria
- Change in mental and/or functional status (including incontinence) from the daily baseline

*If the resident has an indwelling catheter*, the IDSA recommends changing the urinary catheter before collecting a urine specimen for a culture and sensitivity (C&S). However, even with a catheter change, it is common to culture two or three organisms from a urine specimen. The clinician must then decide whether any of these organisms are significant in the resident's illness. When identifying an organism(s) in a *catheterized resident with urosepsis* (fever, shaking chills, hypotension, and/or delirium), a good case could be made for obtaining a urine culture. But, will this help the clinician decide what organism(s) are significant in the illness? Instead, a more specific test that the clinician should obtain in a catheterized resident is paired blood cultures. While waiting for an organism(s) to be revealed in blood culture results, aggressive treatment with a broad-spectrum antibiotic is also recommended. In these residents *with indwelling catheters*, McGeer requires at least two of the following signs or symptoms to diagnose UTI/urosepsis:

- Fever (oral temp 100.4 F) and/or chills with no other source
- New flank or suprapubic pain or tenderness
- Change in character of urine or gross hematuria
- Change in mental and/or functional status from the daily baseline

A helpful rule of thumb to know is the risk of bacteriuria with various catheter types. Within a month, an indwelling Foley will cause a resident to have bacteriuria from 75 to 95% of the time. A suprapubic catheter will reduce the risk of that bacteriuria to between 18 and 40% in 1 month, whereas a condom catheter reduces the risk of bacteriuria to as low as 12% in that same time period. Finally, the risk of bacteriuria is lowest with proper hygiene and self-catheterization, having a risk reduction to 1–3% in a month [4].

## Urinalysis and Urine Culture

When suspecting a UTI, the minimum laboratory evaluation starts with a urinalysis. While a midstream catch is the usual standard for men and women in the community, at the Masonic Village in Elizabethtown, PA we consistently have found between 40 and 80% of our midstream clean catch urine specimens from nursing facility residents were contaminated. Because of this problem, the IDSA recommends that in most situations one should obtain urine via straight catheterization (B-III). Unless a male resident can do a midstream clean catch properly, a straight catheterization will be the best and most accurate method for culturing an adequate urine collection in them as well.

In determining whether a urine C&S should be done, a dipstick check for leukocyte esterase and nitrite level and a microscopic examination for WBCs (B-II) should be performed. If there are >10 WBCs/HPF or a positive leukocyte esterase or nitrite test, a urine culture and sensitivities should then be ordered (B-III). Blood cultures are rarely helpful for the early diagnosis of UTIs. One exception to this rule is residents who have a Foley catheter and have a temperature consistently over 100°F; they are highly suspected of having bacteremia. As mentioned earlier, blood cultures in these individuals may reveal the infecting organism. The IDSA then recommends getting a urine culture and unspun urine for gram stain in *catheterized residents* (B-III). However, more evidence-based studies are needed to validate this approach, since most residents with Foley catheters culture an average of three to four different organisms. If the culture demonstrates two-gram negative organisms and one-gram positive organism, they recommended that a broad-spectrum antibiotic should be initiated.

## Fever

While it is true that typical signs and symptoms in the frail elderly are often absent or less obvious, nursing facility residents frequently do not have temperature and fever recognized, checked, or documented properly. Too often, many residents have standing orders that include acetaminophen for an elevated temperature and instructions about when to contact the PCP for a fever are rarely written. Treatment of an elevated temperature without notification of the PCP can put the patient into a potentially serious life-threatening situation. For example, a resident may be developing an early pneumonia or a UTI, but has no obvious symptoms. Acetaminophen is given for a low-grade fever as indicated by the PRN order. Two days later, the clinician is called and informed the patient's blood pressure is 80/30, is nonresponsive, and running an oral equivalent temp of 101.8°F. The resident is then transferred to the hospital and found to have urosepsis. Since these situations do occur in the nursing facility setting, one should advocate against nursing facilities having standing orders for an elevated temperature without notifying the PCP (an exception could be for residents who are receiving hospice care).

Then what criteria should LTC clinicians use to define a fever in the frail older adult population? Castle et al. [5] have published helpful data that have been used in developing nursing facility standards for defining a fever. He found that a single temperature reading of 100°F or greater (37.8°C) has a sensitivity of 70% for predicting infection and a specificity of 90% with a positive predictive value of 55% in LTC residents. There are other published data suggesting that an elevated temperature of 99.0 (37.2) or greater on repeated occasions is indicative of a possible infection in a LTC resident or an increase in temperature of at least 2°F (1.1°C) over the baseline is suggestive of a possible underlying infection, especially if the 2° elevation is sustained over a 24 h period [6]. The following are helpful guidelines when assessing residents for possible infection.

- Do not administer acetaminophen for a possible elevated temperature without first notifying the practitioner.
- If a change in mental status occurs or a fever is suspected, check temperatures at least every nursing shift for a minimum of 3 days.
- If the temperature is at least 99°F (37.2°C) or greater but less than 100°F (37.8°C), continue checking temperatures and notify the practitioner in 24 h of any persistent low-grade temperatures.
- If the temperatures are 100 F or greater, the practitioner should be contacted as soon as possible.
- Do not depend solely on elevated temperatures for a possible infection. A significant change in a patient's mental status or functional decline (defined as new or increasing confusion, incontinence, falling, deteriorating mobility, reduced food intake, or failure to cooperate with staff consistently on all shifts) can indicate infection.
- Whatever system is used in determining temperatures, make sure the system is reported as its oral equivalent.
- When determining if a patient has an elevated temperature, it is appropriate to consider 2°F (1.1°C) over the baseline as a significant increased temperature.

## Treatment of Urinary Tract Infections

When the practitioner determines that a patient meets the criteria for a UTI, initiation of antibiotic should be started promptly. When determining which antibiotic to use, several factors should be considered.

- Does the resident with a UTI have a fever or a significant change in mental status?
- Can the patient communicate adequately how she/he feels as it relates to the UTI symptoms?
- Is there a history of recurrent UTIs?
- If so, is it the same organism?
- What were the past sensitivities of the organisms cultured?

If your nursing facility has an infection control staff person, it can be helpful to keep records on the site of the infection, types of organism involved, organism sensitivities, and antibiotics used. This information enables the clinician to make more appropriate antibiotic choices while awaiting the results of the urine C&S. For example, if a resident has classic symptoms of a UTI with a positive urinalysis, the clinician can start an oral antibiotic that has consistently demonstrated good sensitivities to the most commonly cultured organism during the past 1 or 2 months in the facility. If the resident is running a fever over 100°F and has a significant change in mental status but is medically stable, the clinician may consider more aggressive treatment. This could include intramuscular injections of a broad-spectrum antibiotic like ceftriaxone or gentamicin if the facility sensitivities reveal that a broad-spectrum antibiotic would cover over 95% of the identified organisms. If a resident has a Foley catheter, a significantly elevated temperature, and a recurrent history of urosepsis associated with enterococcus that is resistant to all oral antibiotics but sensitive to IV vancomycin, the clinician may consider starting the resident on i.v. gentamicin and vancomycin while awaiting the urine C&S and/or blood culture result. Some facilities may not be able to administer i.v. antibiotics, and if i.v. treatment is desired, their residents will need to be transferred to a hospital.

While there are very limited data relating to the length of treatment of UTIs in residents of nursing facilities, most clinicians treat for 7–10 days. For urosepsis, treatment is recommended for 14–21 days.

By applying the above guidelines and approaches to its LTC resident population, the Masonic Village has been very successful in reducing the number of UTIs from 1 infection/1,000 resident days to 0.5 infections/1,000 resident days (or using the UTI Quality

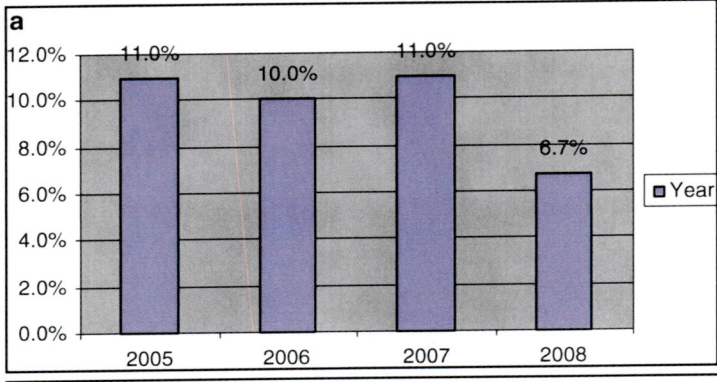

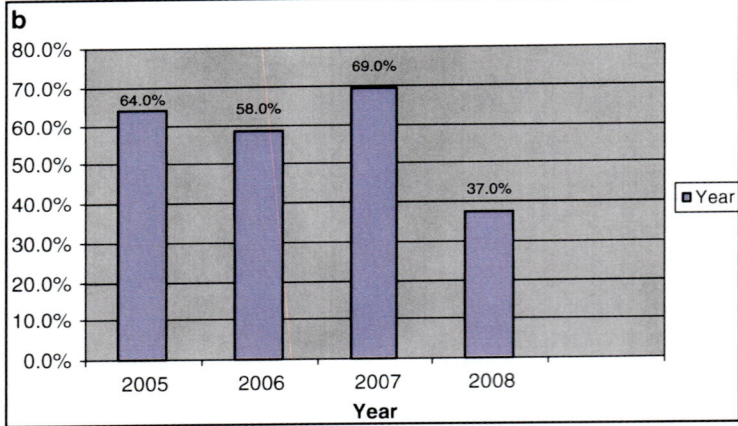

FIGURE 6.1. (**a**) Percent of residents with UTI/year; (**b**) CMS quality indicator percentile.

Indicator, which decreased from the 64th to the 37th percentile) (see Figure 6.1).

Instituting such guidelines can reduce the number of inappropriately treated abnormal urine cultures by preventing the overdiagnosis of UTIs and inappropriate treatment of asymptomatic bacteriuria, while reducing both antibiotic use in the LTC and hopefully the emergence of resistant organisms.

## PNEUMONIA

Pneumonia is a common infection seen in the frail elderly residents of LTC. Some studies have shown that lower respiratory infections are more common than UTIs, since many so-called UTIs are really treated cases of asymptomatic bacteriuria. The incidence rates of pneumonia in the nursing facility setting range from 0.3 to 2.5 infections/1,000 resident care-days [7]. These numbers may vary depending upon the availability and quality of chest X-rays to make an accurate diagnosis of pneumonia. In addition, a number of residents may be inappropriately diagnosed with pneumonia, when in fact the resident has aspiration (chemical) pneumonitis.

There is a tenfold increased incidence of pneumonia in LTC residents compared to age-matched persons living in the community [8]. What factors make the difference? LTC residents are predisposed to lower respiratory infection by their decreased ability to clear mucus from the airways. Many LTC residents have swallowing difficulties with a decreased oral pharyngeal reflex and thus are more prone to aspiration. Residents with dementia are often not cooperative with oral care, and recent data have correlated aspiration pneumonia with poor oral care as well [9]. Underlying diseases such as chronic obstructive pulmonary disease and heart disease seen more frequently in nursing facility residents also increase the risk of pneumonia.

## Diagnosing Pneumonia

*Again, our clinician receives a call from the nurse who is concerned about a resident who has become more confused and has fever.* Does this patient have urosepsis, pneumonia, or some other cause for the fever? The clinical presentation of pneumonia in the elderly is often atypical – a fever only 70% of the time, a new or increased cough 61% of the time, a change in mental status 38% of the time, and an increased respiratory rate over 30 breaths/min only 23% of the time.

If pneumonia or a lower respiratory infection is clinically suspected, the following diagnostic studies should be performed (B-II):

- Pulse oximetry for residents with a respiratory rates of >25 breaths/min
- A pulse oximetry of <90% is suggestive of a pulmonary compromise in a resident who normally has a pulse oximetry 90% or greater
- A chest X-ray if hypoxemia is either documented or suspected (in order to identify a new infiltrate compatible with acute pneumonia)

While obtaining sputum for Gram-stain and C&S has been classically recommended for diagnosing pneumonia, studies show that sputum is obtained in less than 10% of residents in nursing facilities suspected of pneumonia. When sputum has been collected, more than 50% of samples examined have more than 25 squamous epithelial cells/low power field (LPF) and are thus deemed inadequate. In the absence of an available respiratory therapist who can collect adequate sputum samples or is being able to get the collected sputum samples to a laboratory in a timely manner, there is limited value in attempting sputum collection at nursing facilities.

In addition to pulse oximetry, a chest X-ray, and a complete blood count (CBC), a basic metabolic profile (BMP) is generally recommended to assess the hydration status of the resident with pneumonia. Dehydration is a common problem seen in frail elderly residents, especially during any acute illness. Hydration should be assessed early in the evaluation and treatment process, especially if the resident with pneumonia is stable and treatment is to be provided in the nursing facility.

Studies have shown that blood cultures have a low yield and rarely influence therapy in nursing home residents with a lower respiratory infection (B-II). Bacteremia is documented infrequently and has an incidence rate of 5–40 cases/100,000 resident days. Thus, blood cultures are not recommended in most cases of lower respiratory infection.

### Where to Treat Patients with Pneumonia

When the clinician makes the diagnosis of pneumonia, the next most important decision is to determine if the patient should be hospitalized or treated at the nursing facility. Many factors contribute to this decision. If there is some uncertainty about the diagnosis, it is prudent to hospitalize the patient for an additional diagnostic work-up. For example, it is not uncommon to get an X-ray report that suggests that the resident may have either pneumonia and/or congestive heart failure. Or, if the chest X-ray does not validate a suspected pneumonia but oximetry has suddenly dropped below 90%, the clinician must consider other causes for significant decline in pulmonary function such as pulmonary emboli. The only way the clinician can quickly sort out the differential is to do a more aggressive work-up in the acute care setting. It is wise to hospitalize a clinically unstable resident unless the resident and/or the family indicate that they do not want aggressive evaluation and hospitalization.

Dosa reviewed the literature for criteria regarding treating LTC residents in place vs. having them hospitalized [10]. Dosa concluded that those patients with a respiratory rate over 40/min benefit most from hospitalization. Several studies have suggested that mortality rates were similar or even reduced when residents were treated in place as compared to those who were hospitalized. Cost savings were significant when treatment was provided in the nursing facility. Other factors that can assist the clinician in deciding where to treat residents with pneumonia include:

- Ease of making the diagnosis of pneumonia
- Availability and use of antibiotics
- Relevant cost issues
- Barriers to providing adequate supportive care in the facility

When thinking about hospitalizing a resident, it is important to consider the increased risk of developing pressure sores, being colonized with highly virulent or drug-resistant bacteria, and developing delirium at the hospital. This risk is especially increased in residents with dementia. As long as the clinician has the support of the resident and family, a good and reliable nursing facility staff, and a stable resident (with or without supplemental oxygen), it is reasonable to attempt treating the resident at the nursing facility.

### *Pneumonia vs. Pneumonitis*
Another clinically challenging diagnostic problem is determining whether the resident has pneumonia vs. pneumonitis. These situations occur commonly in residents who have a known history of aspiration. *Aspiration pneumonitis is a noninfectious process* that results from aspirating particles of food matter and/or gastric acid that refluxed into the oral pharyngeal area and then into the airway. While there is limited published evidence as to how to appropriately approach this occurrence, clinicians need to be judicious with the use of antibiotics. The following can be helpful in diagnosing pneumonitis:

- Residents with pneumonitis experience a sudden onset of respiratory symptoms that are frequently related to a specific event consistent with aspiration [11].
- Oxygen saturations are frequently normal and stable.
- Examination of the chest reveals coarse rhonchi, but the X-ray is negative for pneumonia.
- Patients may have a sudden elevated temp (>100°F) but don't appear as toxic as one would expect associated with pneumonia.
- Patients improve very quickly, usually in 1–2 days.

The clinician's challenge is to decide if one should begin treatment with antibiotics or wait for the development of new signs and symptoms. With a fever and significant physical findings consistent with early pneumonia, it is very reasonable to initiate antibiotic treatment for aspiration, but the antibiotic can be discontinued if the resident has a negative chest X-ray and clinically has returned to their normal baseline within 1–2 days [12].

### Treatment of Nursing Home-Acquired Pneumonia

The three most common organisms recovered from the nasopharynx in 75% of adults include *Streptococcus pneumoniae*, *Haemophilus influenzae*, and *Moraxella catarrhalis*. But, the nursing facility resident's oropharynx is commonly colonized with anaerobic organisms, *Staphylococcus aureus*, *Enterobacteriaceae*, and *Pseudomonas aeruginosa*. These organisms are commonly found in nursing facility residents because of their many risk factors for colonization, including their decreased ability to clear secretions from the oropharynx that has gram-negative rods, *S. aureus*, or yeast. The decreased saliva found in LTC residents leads to decreased clearance of these organisms and is often exacerbated by anticholinergic drugs, while the presence of periodontal disease frequently found in this population is associated with an exponential increase of anaerobic organisms in their oropharynx. Acid-suppressing medications frequently given to LTC residents, such as a proton pump inhibitors, will increase gastric pH and subsequent bacterial colonization of the gastric mucosa as well. These risk factors for increased bacterial colonization along with an increased risk for aspiration make aspiration pneumonia common in nursing facility residents.

Other less common causes of pneumonia include influenza, legionella, and tuberculosis. More than likely, these pneumonias will be diagnosed in the hospital setting. With influenza pneumonia, one will normally consider the diagnosis during the flu season with a positive nasal swab for influenza, a chest X-ray that confirms pneumonia, and a poor response to the use of broad-spectrum antibiotics. When considering legionella, a urine antigen screen should be done because the urine antigen screen for legionella has a sensitivity of 75% and a specificity of 90%. Finally, active pulmonary tuberculosis should never be forgotten in the differential diagnosis of pneumonia in the LTC setting. If the clinician suspects active TB, the resident should be sent to the hospital for a more thorough evaluation unless a negative pressurized room is available at the facility to house the resident while awaiting sputum for AFB smears and TB culture reports. It is always safer to overreact when suspecting active respiratory TB, as an active case in LTC can significantly impact staff and residents who have had close contact with the infected resident.

Good evidence-based information suggests that greater accuracy in identifying the organism causing pneumonia decreases the need to use broad-spectrum antibiotics. Using less broad-spectrum antibiotics can reduce antibiotic-resistant bacteria in a facility. With increased antibiotic-resistant bacteria in either a hospital or nursing facility, one can frequently observe the spread of resistant organisms to other residents. This is often described as the "herd effect." The reality is that unless one chooses to refer all expected pneumonias to the hospital for a more aggressive work-up, one is left with empirically initiating a broad-spectrum antibiotic for a new diagnosis of pneumonia. A consensus statement recommending minimum criteria for initiating antimicrobial therapy for residents with respiratory infections has been developed [13]. The criteria are as follows:

- New infiltrate on chest X-ray and any one of the following:
  1. Respiratory rate >25
  2. Temperature of 100°F or greater
  3. Productive cough

Or

- Fever of 100°F, cough, and at least one of the following:
  1. Pulse >100
  2. Delirium
  3. Rigors
  4. Respiratory rate >25 breaths/min

Or

- Febrile resident, without chronic obstructive pulmonary disease with new cough and purulent sputum and:
  1. Respiratory rate >25 breaths/min
  2. Delirium

Or

- Afebrile resident with COPD, over 65 years old, and with a new or increased cough with purulent sputum

Guidelines for treating nursing home-acquired pneumonia do change. Since many residents come from the hospital setting at the time of admission to the LTC setting, it may be helpful to know the commonly identified organisms and antibiotic sensitivities observed in the hospital where the residents have last been. If that information is not readily available, a commonly used combination antibiotic for the treatment of nursing facility-acquired pneumonia is amoxicillin-clavulanate plus an advanced generation macrolide or a respiratory fluoroquinolone. A third-generation cephalosporin plus an advanced macrolide can also be used.

If considering MRSA pneumonia, especially in a MRSA colonized resident, consider vancomycin or linezolid in combination with a broad-spectrum gram-negative antibiotic.

Since the nursing facility clinician deals with many terminal patients, aspiration pneumonia is one of the most commonly diagnosed respiratory infections at end-of-life. Often the resident and/or POA may want comfort measures only for end-of-life pneumonia, while other residents and/or POAs desire aggressive antibiotic treatment. If treating aspiration pneumonia, remember to cover for the multiple anaerobic organisms when choosing an antibiotic.

While the above antibiotics suggestions are general guidelines to the empiric treatment of commonly acquired pneumonia in the nursing facility setting, it is extremely important to have staff monitor these ill patients closely. If the patient/POA desires aggressive treatment of the pneumonia and the resident is declining with your empiric antibiotic treatment, it is important to recognize the need to transfer the ill resident to the hospital where additional work-up and treatment can be done.

## INTERFACE WITH ACUTE CARE

Recently, the attention of policymakers in Washington has been focused on the high rates of rehospitalization of patients from the community and community institutions. Jencks et al. [14] analyzed Medicare claims data from 2003 to 2004 and found that 40% of the 11,855,702 Medicare beneficiaries who were discharged from the hospital were rehospitalized within 30 days. He also found that 34% were rehospitalized in 90 days, while 67% of those patients with a medical discharge and 51.5% with a surgical discharge were rehospitalized or died within the first year after discharge. Unplanned rehospitalizations of Medicare patients accounted for about $17.4 billion of the $102.6 billion spent in hospital payments in 2004.

When specifically looking at nursing home readmissions to the hospital, one finds even more interesting data. According to Evercare data, the average admission rate from the nursing home to the hospital is approximately 800 admissions/1,000 residents/year with some nursing facilities as high as 1,100 admissions/1,000 residents/year or as low as less than 200 admissions/1,000 residents/year (see Table 6.2).

So why are there so many variations in readmissions from the nursing facilities to the hospital? In a literature review, Grabowski looked at the association between the decision to hospitalize and factors related to resident welfare and preference, provider

TABLE 6.2. Admissions/1,000 residents/year – Masonic Village (MV) at Elizabethtown

| Indicator | 2008 | 2007 | 2006 | 2005 |
|---|---|---|---|---|
| Total census days | 160,681 | 160,910 | 161,846 | 161,002 |
| Total hospital admissions/year | 139 | 192 | 166 | 208 |
| MV Nonevercare Hospital admits/ 1,000 residents/year | 125 | 172 | 147 | 186 |
| MV Evercare Hospital admits/ 1,000 residents/year | 106 | 144 | – | – |
| Evercare target | 275 | 275 | – | – |

attitudes, and the financial implications of hospitalization [15]. Studies found in the literature suggest that there are multiple factors that determine whether or not a nursing facility resident is rehospitalized, but these studies had selection bias in their research design. Loeb et al. [16] demonstrated that treating residents diagnosed with pneumonia and other lower respiratory tract infections using a clinical pathway can result in a reduction of hospitalizations. Others have demonstrated that the employment of nurse practitioners/physician assistants in nursing facilities, the availability of intravenous therapy, and the presence of certified nurse assistant training programs in facilities appear to also reduce hospitalizations.

As an example, maintaining a significant reduction in hospitalizations at the Masonic Village likely depends on multiple factors. These include:

- Four physicians caring for 450 residents
- One provider rounding all weekends and holidays
- Strong support by ancillary staff for end-of-life care (i.e., chaplains, thanatologist, support groups)
- Providers who are intentional about obtaining orders for DNR, no hospitalizations, and no emergency rooms visits (when appropriate)
- Nurse practitioners Monday through Friday
- Monthly provider staff meetings for educational presentations that include common end-of-life problems
- An active ethics committee
- Supportive administration

### Barriers to Effective Transitions

Clinicians who care for patients who have been hospitalized and then returned to the community or nursing facility for rehabilitation often feel frustrated by the lack of information received from the hospitals.

The issues surrounding transition of care are complex and multiple. These multiple barriers are summed up in the American Medical Director Association's (AMDA) White Paper CO9 [17] on care transitions and include:

- Not identifying and communicating with a patient's primary care physician upon discharge
- Patients not having a primary care physician upon discharge
- Inadequate reimbursement incentives to support adequate care transitions
- Lack of accurate, pertinent, and timely information about the patient sent to receiving facility provider or community-based care setting
- Inadequate instructions for follow-up care, including monitoring the patient and identifying and managing risk factors
- Lack of appropriate measures to determine good quality care
- Need to determine the extent of patient and family understanding of the resident's condition, prognosis, and treatment

### Opportunities to Improve the Interface in Acute Care

The AMDA White Paper CO9 does list items that can play a critical role in the discharge planning of hospitalized patients or to those patients who are being discharged from a nursing facility or from assisted living (AL) back into the community. The essential information that should be collected near or at the time of the patient's discharge or transfer includes the following:

- Whether there is a primary care physician, medical home, or clinic that will assume the care of the patient
- The identity of the receiving entity, and the contact person to receive information
- The best way to communicate information to the receiving facility
- The identity of family or other individuals acting on the patient's behalf
- Whether the discharged patient can afford discharge medications
- Whether the patient has the means (e.g., transportation, delivery, family) to obtain medications

- Whether there are caregivers to appropriately support the patient after discharge
- Whether the patient has responsibilities to care for someone else upon returning home
- Pertinent laboratory and X-ray test results
- Recommended follow-up tests to be preformed, why and when
- Copy of any Advanced Directives
- The identity of other significant high-risk issues at the time of discharge such as non-English-speaking, low-income, social isolation, multiple chronic conditions, and cognitive impairment

In addition to the frequent absence of timely hospital discharge summaries, there is often a lack of medication reconciliation at all health care settings. Residents and their family members often have frequent questions about medications that were discontinued or unintentionally omitted during the hospital stay.

If a nursing facility or hospital is committed to assuring high patient and family satisfaction, a postdischarge contact with the patient and/or family is recommended several days after the discharge:

- To inquire about whether a home health visit had been scheduled, and if so, was it made as scheduled
- To reinforce medication adherence until the community-based PCP has been seen
- To reinforce the need to follow up on diagnostic tests
- To review whether supplemental resources have yet started (e.g., meals on wheels)
- To check whether the patient or family member understands the plan of future care

**Transition of Care from the Nursing Facility to the Hospital**

It is equally important for the nursing facility to send accurate and relevant information to the hospital. Most transfers from the nursing facility to the hospital occur as a result of an acute change in mental status and/or an unstable condition. It is very helpful for the attending to call the ER physician and communicate why the resident is being transported to the ER. There are times when the nursing supervisor should call and report to the ER staff regarding the reasons for sending a resident to the ER. For example, the following items include information important to send with a resident transfer to the hospital (Figure. 6.2).

| Last Name | First Name | Middle Initial | Age | Sex<br>☐ Male<br>☐ Female |
|---|---|---|---|---|
| Address | City | State | Zip | Telephone |
| Attending Physician Name & Contact No.: | | Transferred to | | Social Security # |
| 1. Hearing: ☐ Normal ☐ Impaired ☐ Deaf<br>Hearing Aids: ☐ L ☐ R | | 10. Ambulatory Status: ☐ Independent ☐ Walks with Assistance ☐ Wheelchair bound ☐ Falls Risk | | |
| 2. Sight: ☐ Normal ☐ Impaired ☐ Blind ☐ Glasses | | 11. Assistive Devices: ☐ Crutches ☐ Wheelchair ☐ Cane ☐ Walker | | |
| 3. Memory Loss: ☐ Mild ☐ Moderate ☐ Severe | | 12. Wounds / Dressings: ☐ Yes ☐ No<br><br>☐ Wound Sheet attached | | |
| 4. Speech: ☐ Normal ☐ Impaired ☐ Unable to Speak | | 13. Level of Care: ☐ Nursing Facility ☐ Secure Unit<br>☐ Assisted Living | | |
| 5. Feeding: ☐ Independent ☐ Needs Assistance<br>☐ Total Assist<br>Dentures: ☐ Upper ☐ Lower<br>Partials: ☐ Upper ☐ Lower<br>☐ Aspiration Precautions<br>Diet:<br><br>☐ Tube Feed ☐ NPO | | 14. Oxygen @<br><br>☐ Continuous ☐ PRN<br><br>CPAP ☐ Yes ☐ No | | |
| 6. Bathing & Dressing: ☐ Independent ☐ Needs Help<br>☐ Fully Dependent | | 15. Drug Resistant Organism: ☐ Yes ☐ No<br>(See attached dx list) | | |
| 7. Elimination: ☐ Independent ☐ Needs help to bathroom ☐ Incontinent | | ☐ Immunization Record attached<br>☐ Face Sheet/POA/Insurance Information attached<br>☐ Most recent Medication Record attached<br>☐ Most recent Treatment Record attached<br>☐ Diagnosis List attached<br>☐ Allergy List attached | | |
| 8. Foley Catheter: ☐ Yes ☐ No; if yes, date of last change: _____ ☐ Urostomy | | | | |
| 9. Date of Last BM: _____ ☐ Colostomy | | | | |
| Reason for transfer: | | | | |

FIGURE 6.2. Transfer to hospital record – Masonic Village at Elizabethtown.

## SUMMARY

Caring for residents in LTC can be very challenging and at the same time very rewarding. Of the many complex issues and medical problems the clinician will encounter, it is important to remember that most noncontagious acute facility-acquired infections will likely be pneumonia or a UTI. It is essential that the LTC clinician appreciates the importance of utilizing evidence-based criteria for ordering a urinalysis and avoiding the temptation to routinely collect urine because a cognitively impaired resident had a restless night. It is equally important to decide when an acute respiratory infection requires aggressive evaluation and timely initiation of antibiotic treatment vs. waiting and monitoring as the best course of care.

There is a growing body of literature supporting that many LTC residents can be effectively treated in the nursing facility rather than transferred to the hospital. But, in order to reduce the hospital admission rate, their needs to be strong clinical staff and management support at any facility. Clinicians must be available to assess and treat acutely ill residents in a timely manner.

Finally, the interface between the nursing facility, the hospital, or the resident's home continues to be a significant challenge for health care providers. While there is a need for additional research to determine the most important factors for successful transfers between health care settings, effective communication is essential and foremost.

## PEARLS FOR THE PRACTITIONER

- An elevated temperature of 99° on repeated occasions, but less than 100°, is indicative of a possible infection that requires further evaluation.
- If a resident has a temperature of 100° or greater, the clinician should be notified as soon as possible since there is a high likelihood that the resident has an infection.
- When a LTC resident has a temperature of 100°F or greater, consider either a lower respiratory infection and/or a UTI as the most likely cause for the fever.
- When a resident experiences a change in mental status without any other evidence to suggest a UTI, only 11% will have a true UTI.
- A change in behavior among residents who have significant cognitive impairment is not likely to be due to a UTI *unless* the resident has three of the five findings: fever, dysuria, gross hematuria, new or worsening of urinary incontinence, or suspected bacteremia.
- Due to the presence of multiple organisms colonized in the urine when a resident has a *urinary catheter*, a urine culture and sensitivity has limited value. If the clinician suspects bacteremia in such a resident, blood cultures would be more appropriate before initiating treatment with a broad-spectrum antibiotic for a UTI/urosepsis.
- Pneumonitis usually presents the same as a lower respiratory infection, but does not require antibiotic treatment. The sudden onset of lower respiratory symptoms often related to a specific aspiration event, and clearing of symptoms in 1–2 days, is suggestive of pneumonitis [18].

- Avoid standing orders for treatment of fever in LTC residents, unless evaluation and treatment has already been initiated or the resident is at end-of-life on comfort measures.
- The most essential factor for successful transfers between health care settings is effective communication.

## WEBSITES
- Annals of Long-Term Care www.annalsoflongtermcare.com
- Caring for the Ages http://journals.elsevierhealth.com/periodicals/carage
- Centers for Disease Control and Prevention, Infection Control in Long-Term Care Facilities www.cdc.gov/ncidod/dhqp/gl_longterm_care.html
- Journal of the American Medical Directors Association www.jamda.com
- The American Geriatrics Society www.americangeriatrics.org
- The American Medical Directors Association www.amda.com

## REFERENCES
1. Benoit SR, et al. Factors associated with antimicrobial use in nursing homes. J Am Geriatr Soc 2008; 56: 2039–2044.
2. Niolle LE. Urinary tract infection in long-term care facilities. Infect Control Hosp Epidemiol 2001; 22: 167–175.
3. High KP, et al. Clinical practice guidelines for the evaluation of fever and infections in older adult residents of long-term care facilities: 2008 update by the Infectious Disease Society of America. J Am Geriatr Soc 2009; 57: 375–394.
4. Saint S, Lipsky BA. Preventing catheter-related bacteriuria: should we? Can we? How? Arch Intern Med 1999; 159: 800–8008.
5. Castle SC, Yeh M, et al. Lowering the temperature criterion improves detection of infections in nursing home residents. Aging Immunol Infect Dis 1993; 4: 67–76.
6. Norman DC, Yoshikawa TT. Fever in the elderly. Infect Dis Clin North Am 1996; 10: 93–99.
7. Loeb M, McGeer A, et al. Risk factors for pneumonia and other lower respiratory tract infections in elderly residents of long-term care facilities. Arch Intern Med 1999; 159: 2058–2064.
8. Muder RR. Pneumonia in residents of long-term care facilities: epidemiology, etiology, management, and prevention. Am J Med 1998; 105: 319–330.
9. Yoneyama T, Yoshida M, et al. Oral care reduces pneumonia in older patients in nursing homes. J Am Geriatr Soc 2002; 50: 430–433.
10. Dosa D. Should I hospitalize my resident with nursing home-acquired pneumonia? J Am Med Dir Assoc 2005; 6: 327–333.
11. Marik PE. Aspiration pneumonitis and aspiration pneumonia. N Engl J Med 2001; 344: 665–671.

12. Loeb M, Bentley DW, Bradley S, et al. Development of minimal criteria for the initiation of antibiotics in residents of long-term care facilities: results of a consensus conference. Infect Control Hosp Epidemiol 2001; 22: 120–124.
13. Naughton BJ, Mylotte JM. Tayara A. Outcome of nursing home-acquired pneumonia: derivation and application of a practical model to predict 30-day mortality. J Am Geriatr Soc 2000; 48: 1292–1299.
14. Jencks SF, Williams MV, Coleman EA. Rehospitalization among patients in the Medicare fee-for-service program. N Engl J Med 2009; 360: 1418–1428.
15. Grabowski DC, Stewart KA, Broderick SM, Coots LA. Predictors of nursing home hospitalizations: a review of the literature. Med Care Res Rev 2008; 65: 3–39.
16. Loeb M, et al. Effects of a clinical pathway to reduce hospitalizations in nursing home residents with pneumonia: a randomized controlled trial. J Am Med Dir Assoc 2006; 295: 2503–2510.
17. AMDA White Paper CO9, Columbia, MD. Available at www.amda.com
18. Mylotte JM, Goodnough S, Naughton BJ. Pneumonia versus aspiration pneumonitis in nursing home residents: diagnosis and management. J Am Geriatr Soc 2003; 51: 17–23.

# Chapter 7
# Health Maintenance and Prevention

Ross H. Albert

**Keywords:** Preventive care • Physical activity • Fall prevention • Osteoporosis • Vitamin D deficiency • Vaccinations • Tuberculosis screening • Cancer screening

## INTRODUCTION

With the proportion of older patients in the United States rising, and the average life expectancy increasing as well, decisions regarding health maintenance and preventive care in older patients have become a critical component of long-term care medicine. Over 30 million Americans (10%) are currently over the age of 65, and this number is expected to rise to over 70 million (20%) by the year 2030. Average life expectancy has risen to nearly 75 years of age for men and 80 years for women [1].

Preventive care in older residents requires an understanding of the competing benefits/burdens of medical interventions and screening tests. Certain critical elements are necessary for an effective medical screening test and intervention:

- The target disease being screened should be common and should cause significant mortality and morbidity.
- The screening test should be accurate as well as reasonably tolerable.
- A positive result should allow for beneficial intervention during the asymptomatic phase of the disease.
- The test and curative treatment should be cost effective.

The relative importance of these elements is different in older residents than in younger ones. With a shorter life expectancy of older persons, interventions must have a more immediate onset of benefit to yield a relevant and cost-effective outcome:

- Tests may be less tolerable in older patients with more comorbidities and physical limitations.
- Patients may have different priorities at different ages, electing to forgo medical tests and interventions in exchange for improved quality of life at an older age.

This chapter will address preventive care in long-term care settings, with a focus on physical activity and fall prevention, osteoporosis management, Vitamin D deficiency, vaccinations, and screening for tuberculosis and cancer in residents residing there.

## PHYSICAL ACTIVITY AND FALL PREVENTION

Two critical components of preventive care in older persons are physical activity and fall prevention. Regular exercise has been shown to decrease mortality and morbidity in older adults. Exercise also helps to prevent falls in the elderly that is critical in this population. Two key guidelines have been created to direct physicians on exercise goals for patients. The US Department of Health and Human Services released its 2008 Physical Activity Recommendations for Americans and the Centers for Disease Control and Prevention President's Council on Physical Fitness and Sports created Healthy People 2010. Healthy People 2010 focuses on increasing physical activity in daily life, encouraging more walking, bicycling, and organized exercise. The report notes that over half of Americans over the age of 65 participate in no physical activity in their leisure time [2, 3].

The 2008 Physical Activity Recommendations suggest exercise guidelines for all ages and identify specific details for older people as well. Recommendations for all ages include:

- Avoiding inactivity
- Exercising at moderate intensity for at least 150 min per week
- Or at vigorous intensity for 75 min per week

For older adults who are unable to perform 150 min of exercise, recommendations state:

- They should be as active as able, including exercises that improve strength and balance.

- Exercise intensity and duration may be increased gradually in those who have been inactive in the past.

Regularly exercising and remaining active helps older adults maintain their strength and balance, which usually declines as people age. If an older adult is unwilling or unable to exercise or have a physically active lifestyle, they are placing themselves at ever-increasing risk for falls. Falls result in disability, functional decline, reduced quality of life, and may result in a need for a change in the location of the patient's care as well. Fear of falling can cause further loss of function, depression, feelings of helplessness, and social isolation.

Many older patients in LTC fall each year because they are frail and have many chronic conditions, including problems with thinking and memory from dementia. These underlying problems frequently cause difficulty with walking and activities of daily living. In the nursing facility, as many as 75% of residents fall each year and about 10–20% of nursing facility falls cause serious injuries; 2–6% cause fractures.

Fall prevention is a critical component to health maintenance in these older populations. Interventions to prevent falls should be multifaceted and address the common causes of falling: environmental hazards, muscle weakness and gait problems, and medications. Modalities should therefore include: improving safety of the environment, physical and occupational therapy and exercising, and decreasing medications and monitoring for medication side effects.

Environmental changes in the older person's home that improve safety and reduce fall risk include removing loose items from floors such as small rugs and electrical cords, as well as improving lighting. Home care agencies have expertise in evaluating for these hazards and are able to recommend safety measures appropriate for the older person a risk for falls, like grab bars for the bathroom (see Chap 1). Although in the nursing or assisted living facility environment, the use of low beds and railings in hallways has been shown to help reduce resident falls; the use of bedrails and restraints, hip padding, and softer floors has not been shown to reduce falls or morbidity from falls same.

Physical and occupational therapy given to frail elderly living in the community and in LTC facilities have been shown to not only improve function but also reduce falls. This is especially true following acute illnesses or injury. After participating in these therapies, the elderly may be able to "graduate" to an exercise routine. Exercises may include specific balance and strength modalities, but alternative methods such as yoga and tai chi have been shown to help reduce falls as well.

Finally, a critical component to fall prevention is optimizing the treatment of comorbidities, while reducing the number of medications. Careful attention should be paid to those medications that may have significant side effects and lead to increased falls in the LTC population. These include a large array of medicines (see Chapters 5 and 15 for further details):

- The most frequent offenders are psychotropic medications (antipsychotics and benzodiazepines).
- Antihypertensives cause orthostatic hypotension (diuretics).
- Pain medications cause confusion or instability (opioids).
- Anticholinergics cause sedation, orthostatic hypotension, and confusion (allergy, antispasmodics for bladder or bowel).

## OSTEOPOROSIS MANAGEMENT AND PREVENTION

Osteoporosis affects eight million women and almost two million men in the United States. Studies show that half of all Caucasian women will experience at least one osteoporosis-related fracture. One-year mortality following a hip fracture is almost 20%, and nearly a quarter of those who have a hip fracture will require skilled nursing care [4]. Appropriate screening and treatment of osteoporosis is necessary to prevent the significant morbidity and mortality associated with osteoporosis and osteoporotic fractures. The United States Preventive Services Task Force (USPSTF) and National Osteoporosis Foundation have created guidelines for screening for osteoporosis [4, 5]. The USPSTF states that screening should be carried out with a DEXA scan in all women over the age of 65 and in high-risk women over the age of 60. Though there is no large body of evidence to support this, general consensus is that men over the age of 70 should also be considered for screening. Tools such as the FRAX score may be utilized to identify those at high risk [6]. The FRAX website is http://www.shef.ac.uk/FRAX/. There are no recommendations for when screening for osteoporosis should end, although this is frequently determined by clinical circumstances such as a shortened life expectancy or advanced dementia.

Not only should elderly who have had a positive screening test be treated for osteoporosis but also any patient that has had a "fragility fracture" should be considered for treatment. A fragility fracture occurs when a fall happens from a standing height or less. Besides weight-bearing exercise, treatment of osteoporosis includes adequate calcium and vitamin D intake, bisphosphonates, and other agents in specific clinical situations. A minimum of 1,200 mg of calcium intake is recommended each day.

Minimum vitamin D intake should be 800 IU daily; the treatment of vitamin D deficiency is discussed below.

Bisphosphonates are FDA-approved for the treatment of osteoporosis. Newer formulations with weekly and monthly dosing schedules may improve adherence in the outpatient setting. Caution must be used with bisphosphonates in frail elderly nursing facility residents who might have, among other things, swallowing dysfunction, decreased renal function, multiple chronic illnesses, or poor intake resulting in a contraindication of these drugs. These drugs are difficult to use in the LTC population because these side effects (esophagitis, renal failure) and difficulty of usage. Bisphosphonates can have decreased efficacy because of poor absorption and must be given on an empty stomach with at least 8 oz of liquid, before other medicines or food are ingested. Administering bisphosphonates may be difficult for some less well-staffed assisted living facilities or for patients who are receiving home care. While there is no guideline recommending a specific duration of treatment with bisphosphonates, there is some data that beneficial effects are noted even after cessation of the medicine after 5 years.

Other agents such as Calcitonin, Raloxifene, and hormone therapy may be considered as well for the treatment of osteoporosis. Calcitonin is approved for the treatment of recurrent vertebral fractures in women because it has been shown to increase vertebral bone mineral density as well as reduce the pain of these fractures. Raloxifene may be appropriate for women with osteoporosis and a high risk for breast cancer; hormone therapy may be considered for postmenopausal women with osteoporosis and significant vasomotor symptoms, but should be used with caution in frail elderly because of this population's frequent cardiovascular comorbidities.

## VITAMIN D DEFICIENCY

Vitamin D deficiency and its management is a controversial medical topic. Data clearly show that Vitamin D deficiency is seen in residents with osteoporosis and fractures, as well as in those with certain cancers, cardiovascular disease, and renal failure. It is unclear if the vitamin D deficiency is functionally related to these diseases or is simply a disease marker for chronic illness. It is also unclear if correction of vitamin D deficiency will have any meaningful long-term positive (or negative) outcomes (7).

The USPSTF has not issued a recommendation for screening for vitamin D deficiency. For those who do advocate screening, the general consensus is that it should be carried out in perimenopausal and menopausal women, dark-skinned individuals, those with inadequate sun exposure (*such as long-term care residents*), and those with malabsorption syndromes. Vitamin D deficiency is seen in approximately one third of nursing facility residents. Though the active form of vitamin D is the 1,25-hydroxy-vitamin, the 25-hydroxy-vitamin D level is the most accurate and reproducible for measurement. Currently, a goal level of 40 ng/mL and above is cited as ideal, with a level between 20 and 40 ng/mL noted as vitamin D *insufficiency* and a level below 20 ng/mL as frank *deficiency*.

For those who advocate supplementation, different doses are typically recommended based on a resident's baseline level. For those who are at a normal level, supplementation of 1,000–2,000 IU per day of vitamin $D_3$ is recommended; for vitamin D insufficiency, up to 3,000 IU per day of vitamin $D_3$ is recommended; and for vitamin D deficiency, 50,000 IU once per week of vitamin $D_2$ for 8–12 weeks, then begin 1,000–2,000 IU per day of vitamin $D_3$.

There have been few large trials, to have shown that vitamin D supplementation convincingly reduces morbidity and mortality from chronic illness. But, a multitude of smaller trials, coupled with the strong associations of vitamin D deficiency with various chronic disease states and the relatively low risk of supplementation itself, appear to suggest that screening and supplementing for vitamin D deficiency would be a prudent approach in long-term care settings.

## VACCINATIONS

Vaccinations of older persons in LTC settings are a critical component of health maintenance strategies. Immunizations to consider in residents older than 65 include those targeted at Pneumococcal disease, Influenza, and Herpes Zoster. Few side effects have been associated with adult vaccinations. Benefits include decreased morbidity and pain with the Zoster vaccine and decreased morbidity and mortality with the Pneumococcal and Influenza vaccines. Multiple studies have shown that community vaccination rates remain lower than hoped, with ranges from over 30% receiving annual flu vaccines to over 60% receiving Pneumococcal vaccination. Note that while influenza immunization of LTC residents is important, clinical trials have also shown that programs aimed at immunization of LTC staff are also very effective at reducing influenza morbidity, healthcare utilization, and death.

### Pneumococcal Vaccine

The Pneumococcal vaccine targets the pathogen, *Streptococcus pneumonia,* one of the most common causes of serious bacterial infections in the United States. Pneumococcal disease causes over 3,000 deaths each year in senior citizens over the age of 65. The purified polysaccharide vaccine (PPV23) targets 23 types of pneumococcal bacteria, which cause 88% of invasive pneumococcal disease. The vaccine is 60–70% effective overall in the prevention of invasive pneumococcal disease and is indicated for all residents over 65, as a single vaccination. It is also indicated as a second dose at age 65 for residents who had received a prior dose due to certain chronic disease states or immunosuppression [8].

### Influenza Vaccine
Influenza and pneumonia together are the sixth leading cause of death overall in the United States and the number one cause of death from infectious disease. The influenza vaccine is the best preventive measure for complications from influenza infection; overall efficacy is 70–90% in those younger than 65 and 30–40% in frail elderly persons; however, the vaccine is 80% effective in reducing death from complications of influenza among elderly residents.

The vaccine is indicated for all patients over the age of 50 and is specifically recommended for all long-term care facility residents and healthcare workers. The vaccine is contraindicated in residents with egg allergy or Guillain–Barré syndrome [9].

### Herpes Zoster Vaccine
Approximately 25% of people develop zoster during their lifetime, and there are about one million cases of shingles per year, predominantly in people older than 50 years of age. Shingles is associated with significant morbidity due to acute pain during episodes as well as chronic pain due to postherpetic neuralgia. The vaccine, approved in 2006, has been shown to reduce postherpetic neuralgia by over 50% over the next 3 years; it does not prevent episodes of shingles. The vaccine is a live attenuated varicella virus, with the concentration of virus more than ten times that of the traditional varicella vaccine. The vaccine is approved for residents over the age of 60 as a one-time vaccination. It is contraindicated in those with immunodeficiency [10].

## TUBERCULOSIS SCREENING
Tuberculosis screening in LTC settings is essential to decrease the risk of tuberculosis transmission between residents and staff. One in three people in the world has been exposed to tuberculosis, and those with latent tuberculosis have approximately a 10% lifetime risk of developing active TB. Given that the elderly are at greater

risk for conversion from latent to active TB, effective screening is critical to prevent the spread of active disease.

Prior to the current guidelines from the Center for Disease Control (CDC), older patients were not to be screened for latent TB, as the CDC recommended against treatment for latent TB in the elderly due to concerns of medicine regimen toxicity. Current data support the use and safety of these regimens in older patients who do not have underlying liver disease, and this is reflected in the most recent CDC guidelines, which do not cite a maximum age for treatment [11].

Following baseline two-step purified protein derivative (PPD) testing, the AGS (American Geriatric Society) used to recommend that all nursing home residents should be screened annually for TB. More recent recommendations suggest that the periodicity of routine follow-up single-step PPD testing in nursing facility residents must be defined by each institution considering local issues and prevalence. They also suggest that retesting of the nursing facility population is required when a TB exposure situation or potential outbreak of tuberculosis is identified [12].

A tuberculin skin test (TST) should be done with the PPD, which elicits a delayed-type hypersensitivity reaction to demonstrate past exposure to TB. All residents and staff should initially receive a two-step PPD, with tests done 2–3 weeks apart, to differentiate between anergic responses to old exposures and to new acquisition of infection. Thresholds for treatment are not different for older residents compared to other residents. Treatment should be initiated in the lowest risk residents with a PPD induration greater than 15 mm, in those with certain chronic diseases at 10 mm, and in immunosuppressed residents and those with HIV at 5 mm.

## CANCER SCREENING

Cancer screening in older populations highlights the complexity of health maintenance decision-making. While cancer is more common in older patients, screening and interventions may not have a meaningful benefit, given the shorter life expectancy in this population. Cancers diagnosed by screening may never have become clinically apparent; in fact, quality of life may be worse after diagnosis, due to the effects of further testing and interventions, as well as the adoption by the patient and family of the "sick role." The data and recommendations for screening for cervical cancer, breast cancer, colon cancer, and prostate cancer are reviewed below, but must be taken in the context of the person's overall prognosis and healthcare preferences.

## Cervical Cancer Screening

The primary tool for cervical cancer screening is the Pap smear. Studies have shown that women who have had normal prior screening are more likely to have normal results in the future, and those with abnormal screening results or lack of screening are more likely to have abnormal results in the future. The Pap smear may be technically difficult and uncomfortable for older patients due to vaginal dryness and hip or back pain.

The American Academy of Family Practice (AAFP) the USPSTF, American College of Obstetrics and Gynecology (ACOG), American Cancer Society (ACS), and AGS have released guidelines for cessation of cervical cancer screening in older patients [13–16]. The AAFP and USPSTF state that women may discontinue Pap smears at age 65 "if they have had adequate recent screening with normal Pap smears and are not otherwise at high risk." ACOG recommends that Pap smears may be discontinued over 65 years of age if the woman has had three or more normal test results in a row, no abnormal test results in 10 years, no history of cervical cancer, and no other high-risk characteristics. Unique to the ACOG guideline is the recommendation that annual pelvic exam be continued in women over 65, after Pap smears have been discontinued, despite a lack of evidence supporting this screening modality. ACOG does note that exams may be discontinued if a patient would chose not to pursue treatment for abnormalities found during screening, such as vulvar cancer. ACS also cites a requirement of three normal Pap test results and no abnormal results in 10 years, but recommends that screening be discontinued at age 70. Finally, the AGS supports an age of 70 for the cessation of cervical cancer screening if a patient has had regular screening prior to this age.

## Breast Cancer Screening

Mammography is the most effective modality for breast cancer screening in women. Clinical and self breast exam are often recommended by clinicians, but have far less compelling data supporting its use. Guidelines addressing the cessation of mammograms include those from the ACS, AGS, and USPSTF [17–19]. The ACS and USPSTF do not provide an age at which to stop breast cancer screening, but note that resident comorbidities and life expectancy should be considered on an individual patient basis. The AGS cites a life expectancy of 4 or more years as a threshold to perform breast cancer screening. This 4-year time span is based on two large longitudinal studies assessing the benefits of mammography; both studies showed that screening decreased mortality, though the beneficial effect only appeared in 4–5 years after screeening.

### Colon Cancer Screening

Colon cancer screening may be carried out with the use of fecal occult blood testing and sigmoidoscopy, or colonoscopy. The USPSTF recommends against routine screening in adults 76–85 years of age and against all colon cancer screening in adults older than 85 years. Life expectancy and comorbidities should contribute to decision-making related to colon cancer screening [20]. As one would expect, colon cancer screening is far less effective in residents with a shorter life expectancy and more comorbidities.

### Prostate Cancer Screening

Prostate cancer screening is controversial. As recently as early 2009, two large trials were simultaneously published reporting the effects of prostate screening and mortality – while one trial of over 150,000 men showed a modest benefit (1,410 men would need to be screened to prevent prostate cancer-related death), the other which included over 75,000 men showed no mortality benefit of screening [21, 22]. Various other trials have shown similar results, with modest benefits in some trials, no mortality benefit in the majority of trials, and at least one trial showing increased mortality in residents screened for prostate cancer. The AAFP and the USPSTF state that there is insufficient evidence to assess the balance of benefits and harms of screening for prostate cancer in men younger than 75 years [23]. With regard to screening in older residents, the AAFP and USPSTF recommend against prostate cancer screening in men 75 years of age and older. The American Urological Association (AUA) and ACS recommend continuing screening until residents have a life expectancy of less than 10 years [24, 25].

## PEARLS FOR THE PRACTITIONER

- If possible, residents should increase physical activity to a goal of 150 min per week. Those who have significant comorbidities or a low baseline activity level may benefit by beginning with therapy and should gradually build to this goal.
- Fall prevention efforts should be carried out in all settings. This should include physical and occupational therapy, exercise and balance programs, reduction of fall risks in residents' environment, and reduction of medications and medication side effects.

- Osteoporosis screening should be done in all women over 65 and in high-risk women over 60 years old with a DEXA scan. Men over 70 should also be considered for osteoporosis screening. Treatment of osteoporosis should include intake of over 1,200 mg calcium, over 800 IU vitamin D and bisphosphonates, and may include medications such as Calcitonin, and Raloxifene in select residents.
- Vitamin D deficiency screening should be considered in LTC residents and those at risk because of low sun exposure or malabsorption. There are some experts who advocate screening and treating all residents for this deficiency, though this still remains controversial.
- Vaccinations for Pneumococcal disease, Influenza, and Herpes Zoster should be considered in all older residents. Pneumococcal vaccine should be given once to all residents over 65 years old; Herpes Zoster vaccine should be given once for those over 60; and Influenza vaccine should be given annually for all residents over 50, unless contraindicated.
- Initial TST screening of new residents and newly hired employees should be done with the two-step TST. All employees of the LTC facility should be screened annually for TB by a symptom questionnaire, and if positive, then receive a TST, and if this is positive, then a chest x ray.
- Cessation of cancer screening should be considered in older residents with significant comorbidities.
- Pap smears data and guidelines suggest that it may be appropriate to stop Pap smears at 65–70 years of age if the resident has had prior regular screening.
- Mammograms may be stopped at approximately 75–85 years of age depending on resident comorbidities.
- Colonoscopy may be stopped after 75 years of age.
- Prostate cancer screening may be discontinued at 75 years of age if it is done at all.
- Any decision to stop cancer screening should be made after careful discussion with residents and families to establish resident goals and expectations.

## WEBSITES
- FRAX osteoporosis risk calculator http://www.shef.ac.uk/FRAX/
- Adult immunization schedule http://www.cdc.gov/vaccines/recs/schedules/adult-schedule.htm
- Physical activity guidelines http://www.health.gov/PAGuidelines/guidelines/default.aspx

## REFERENCES

1. He W, Sengupta M, Velkoff VA, DeBarros KA. 65+ in the United States: 2005. Current population reports: special studies. Washington, DC: U.S. Census Bureau (P23–209), U.S. Government Printing Office; 2005. http://www.census.gov/prod/2006pubs/p23-209.pdf. Accessed June 30, 2009.
2. U.S. Department of Health and Human Services. Physical activity guidelines for Americans. Chapter 5: Active older adults. 2008. http://www.health.gov/PAGuidelines/guidelines/Chapter5.aspx. Accessed June 30, 2009.
3. Centers for Disease Control and Prevention and President's Council on Physical Fitness and Sports. Healthy People 2010: Objectives for Improving Health. http://www.healthypeople.gov/document/HTML/Volume2/22Physical.htm#_Toc490380801. Accessed June 30, 2009.
4. National Osteoporosis Foundation. Physician's guide to prevention and treatment of osteoporosis. http://www.nof.org/professionals/Clinicians_Guide.htm. Accessed June 30, 2009.
5. U.S. Preventive Services Task Force. Screening for osteoporosis in postmenopausal women: recommendations and rationale. Rockville, MD: Agency for Healthcare Research and Quality; September 2002. http://www.ahrq.gov/clinic/3rduspstf/osteoporosis/osteorr.htm. Accessed June 30, 2009.
6. World Health Organization Collaborating Centre for Metabolic Bone Diseases. FRAX – WHO fracture risk assessment tool. 2007. http://www.shef.ac.uk/FRAX/tool.jsp. Accessed June 30, 2009.
7. Holick MF. Vitamin D deficiency. *N Engl J Med*, 2007:357;266–81.
8. Prevention of Pneumococcal Disease: Recommendations of the Advisory Committee on Immunization Practices (ACIP). *MMWR*. 1997:46(RR-08);1–24.
9. Prevention and Control of Influenza :Recommendations of the Advisory Committee on Immunization Practices (ACIP). *MMWR*. 2006:55(RR10);1–42.
10. Oxman MN, Levin MJ, Johnson GR, et al. A vaccine to prevent herpes zoster and postherpetic neuralgia in older adults. *N Engl J Med*, 2005:352;2271–2284.
11. Centers for Disease Control and Prevention. Controlling tuberculosis in the United States: recommendations from the American Thoracic Society, CDC, and the Infectious Diseases Society of America. *MMWR*, 2005;54(No. RR-12).
12. AGS Position Statement: Two-step PPD testing for nursing home residents on admission. *Annals of Long-Term Care*, 2006:14(2).
13. U.S. Preventive Services Task Force. Screening for cervical cancer. http://www.ahrq.gov/clinic/uspstf/uspscerv.htm. Accessed June 30, 2009.
14. ACOG Committee on Practice Bulletins. ACOG Practice Bulletin: clinical management guidelines for obstetrician- gynecologists. Number 45, August 2003. Cervical cytology screening (replaces committee opinion 152, March 1995). *Obstet Gynecol.*, 2003:102(2);417–427.

15. Saslow D, Runowicz CD, Solomon D, et al. American Cancer Society guideline for the early detection of cervical neoplasia and cancer. *CA Cancer J Clin.*, 2002:52(6);342–362.
16. American Geriatrics Society. AGS position statement: screening for cervical carcinoma in older women. http://www.americangeriatrics.org/products/positionpapers/cer_carc_2000.shtml. Accessed June 30, 2009.
17. Eyre H, Kahn R, Robertson RM. Preventing cancer, cardiovascular disease, and diabetes: a common agenda for the American Cancer Society, the American Diabetes Association, and the American Heart Association. *CA Cancer J Clin.*, 2004:54(4);190–207.
18. Breast cancer screening in older women. American Geriatrics Society Clinical Practice Committee. *J Am Geriatr Soc.*, 2000:48(7);842–844.
19. U.S. Preventive Services Task Force. Screening for breast cancer: recommendations and rationale. *Ann Intern Med.*, 2002:137(5 part 1); 344–346.
20. U.S. Preventive Services Task Force. Screening for colorectal cancer: U.S. Preventive Services Task Force Recommendation Statement. *Ann Intern Med.*, 2008:149(9);627–637.
21. Schroder FH et al. Screening and Prostate-Cancer Mortality in a Randomized European Study. *N Engl J Med.*, 2009:360;1320–1328.
22. Andriole GL et al. Mortality Results from a Randomized Prostate-Cancer Screening Trial. *N Engl J Med.*, 2009:360;1310–1319.
23. U.S. Preventive Services Task Force. Screening for prostate cancer: recommendation statement. *Ann Intern Med.*, 2008:149(3);185–191.
24. Smith RA, von Eschenbach AC, Wender R, et al., for the ACS Prostate Cancer Advisory Committee, ACS Colorectal Cancer Advisory Committee, ACS Endometrial Cancer Advisory Committee. American Cancer Society guidelines for the early detection of cancer: update of early detection guidelines for prostate, colorectal, and endometrial cancers. Also: update 2001 – testing for early lung cancer detection [Published correction appears in *CA Cancer J Clin.*, 2001:51(3);150]. *CA Cancer J Clin.*, 2001:51(1);38–75.
25. Prostate-specific antigen (PSA) best practice policy. American Urological Association (AUA). *Oncology (Williston Park).* 2000:14(2);267–272, 277–278, 280.

# Chapter 8
# Integrating Palliative Care into Practice

Peter Winn

**Keywords:** Anorexia • Constipation • Delirium • Dyspnea • End-of-life care • Hospice • Illness trajectories • Nausea • Pain management • Palliative care • Symptom assessment • Vomiting

## INTRODUCTION

Practitioners in long-term care medicine are seeing an ever-increasing number of persons with chronic progressive illness who reside either at home or in a LTC setting (nursing facility, SNF, assisted living or residential care). As of 2001, 46% of all deaths in the United States occur in these settings. Accordingly, clinicians have advocated that palliative care practice can be generalized and applied to such patient populations [1]. A multidimensional model of successful aging despite chronic illness where disease and its physiological and functional limitations are offset by compensatory psycho-emotional and social interventions that result in emotional vitality, well-being, and engagement with life and spirituality has been set forth by some [2]. Such an approach to care embodies the true philosophy of palliative care. Palliative care can and should be integrated alongside the traditional treatment of disease, where disease-modifying treatments are not necessarily avoided if appropriate and congruent with patients' goals of care. Such "total care" should be safe, effective, patient-centered, timely, efficient, and equitable, all consistent with the six aims of the Institute of Medicine 2001 report to improve health care in the United States.

## ILLNESS TRAJECTORIES

Generally, illness trajectories that lead to subsequent death can manifest in one of three ways:

- A short period of rapid decline (usually a few weeks or months) as often seen in cancer
- Prolonged dwindling over 6–8 years as seen in dementia, frailty, and generalized debility or
- Long-term functional decline over 2–5 years, with intermittent serious episodes of illness, often associated with multiple ER visits and hospitalizations, with only partial recovery after each episode, and eventual death. This is most often seen in heart and respiratory failure.
- Timely recognition of a patient's illness trajectory and poor prognosis can serve as a springboard to advance care planning, to review *goals of life,* and to establish appropriate goals of care for patients and their families.
- For persons who reside in nursing facilities, common causes of death are [3, 4]:
  - 30–60% cardiovascular (includes sudden cardiac death, myocardial infarction, heart failure, and stroke)
  - 1–23% pulmonary (COPD, pneumonia, lung cancer)
  - 36% Alzheimer's disease and other dementia
  - 7–9% cancer
  - 2–3% end-stage renal disease.

Irrespective of the place of residence, heart disease, cancer, stroke, lung disease, Alzheimer's, influenza and pneumonia, and kidney disease are all in the top 10 leading causes of death in the US (in addition to unintentional injuries, diabetes, and septicemia). These diseases commonly afflict patients/residents in the LTC continuum who can thus benefit from the integration of effective palliative care with traditional medical treatment, whether it is during the early, middle, late, or terminal phase of their illness trajectory.

## PRINCIPLES OF PALLIATIVE CARE

Irrespective of the age of the patient, the clinical setting, place of residence/care, or whether the person is suffering from chronic progressive illness or an acute life-threatening illness, the core principles of palliative care are the same:

- Reduce the symptom burden from pain and other distressful symptoms, including the relief of suffering.

- Recognize and address the physical, psycho-emotional, social, and spiritual needs and dimensions of pain and other symptoms experienced by both the patient and family.
- Provide medical treatment congruent with the wishes, values, preferences, beliefs, and concerns of the patient and family.
- Provide care that is both interdisciplinary and interprofessional.
- Practitioners should be committed to the highest quality (palliative) care that is both timely and comprehensive. To do so, regular clinical assessment, diagnosis, care planning, interventions, monitoring (response to interventions and the natural course of the disease), follow-up, and, if possible, anticipation and prevention of distressful symptoms and suffering are required. Care should be *patient-centered* and *family-focused*. Effective communication skills are essential. Practitioners and the interdisciplinary team (IDT) are challenged to provide seamless transitions in care between institutional, hospital, and home care settings.

For the patient and family, the primary goals of palliative care include:

- Striving for the highest practical quality of life, despite late stage illness
- Being in control (autonomy) and maintaining dignity
- Relief of distressful symptoms and suffering (social, spiritual)
- Alleviate family burden (can be psycho-emotional, financial, practical)
- Coming to peace with spiritual issues and relationships

In LTC medicine, the goals of palliative care are similar to those of patients already under the care of practitioners. Also, medical care should be delivered in accordance with the ethical and legal framework of health care and the practitioner's scope of practice and provided with cultural sensitivity and competency (see chapters on Ethical and Legal Issues and Working with Families and Healthcare Providers).

## SYMPTOM ASSESSMENT AND MANAGEMENT

In persons with advanced illness, appropriate assessment is often challenging due to patient cognitive impairment, fatigue, and comorbidities. Nonpain symptoms are prevalent, often greater than pain, even in persons diagnosed with cancer (see Table 8.1). For *any* symptom experienced by patients, a stepped approach enables practitioners to intervene in a timely and effective manner.

TABLE 8.1. Symptoms in advanced illness

| Symptom | Cancer (%) [17, 20] | Noncancer (%) [19] | Cancer, AIDS, COPD, heart and renal disease (%) [18] |
|---|---|---|---|
| Fatigue | 72–74 | 76 | 32–90 |
| Pain | 71–74 | 67 | 34–96 |
| Lack of energy | 69 | | |
| Weakness | 60 | | |
| Appetite loss | 53–70 | 55 | |
| Breathlessness | 36 | 36 | 60–95% |
| Anxiety/depression | 40 | 57 | |

First, recognize each symptom and its sequelae.

- Establish its intensity, temporal pattern, any exacerbating/relieving factors, location, and effect on function and cognition.
- Determine whether the symptom is acute, chronic, or intermittent.
- Identify any associated symptoms.
- Review previous and current treatment for the symptom.
- Perform an appropriate, timely, and symptom-focused physical exam.
- Ascertain, if possible, the likely pathophysiology underlying the symptom.
- Consider whether any medication could be causing or aggravating the symptom.
- Identify potentially reversible causes.
- If necessary, use the least invasive diagnostic testing to minimize patient pain, discomfort, or suffering.
- Determine the most likely diagnosis, if possible.
- Always evaluate for the presence of any psycho-emotional, spiritual, social, or practical factors to the symptom.
- Initiate treatment based upon the primary illness, phase of illness, prognosis, comorbidities, patient/family preferences for care and care setting.
- Consider complementary and alternative therapies especially if requested by patients and families.

Any symptom can be complex and multifaceted, thus an *interdisciplinary* and *transdisciplinary* approach and treatment plan is more likely to be successful. First, try practical interventions in an attempt to alleviate each symptom, i.e., change in body position, room temperature or ventilation, or patient/family education. Second and foremost, consider pharmacologic interventions to alleviate each symptom. Finally, consider secondary medical and/or pharmacologic treatments directed at the underlying cause of the symptoms. Responses and outcomes, benefits, and burdens must be carefully monitored and treatments adjusted accordingly, acknowledging that the *goals of care can change over time.*

At times, distressful symptoms may inadvertently occur subsequent to interventions, but their overall benefits should outweigh their harm (the concept of *double effect*). In such a situation, it is reasonable to continue the treatment while adding another treatment to alleviate the adverse effects. In a critical situation, characterized by severe and intractable symptoms, use of palliative sedation may be the most humane and ethical option.

At the practitioner and systems level, use of uni- or multidimensional tools may be helpful to assess a variety of symptoms (Table 8.2) dependent upon ease of use and evidence-based palliative care.

TABLE 8.2. Symptom assessment scales

| Symptom | Assessment scales to consider |
|---|---|
| Anorexia | Functional assessment anorexia/cachexia therapy scale |
| Anxiety | Hamilton anxiety rating scale (HAM-A) |
| Cognition | Folstein MMSE, COGNISTAT |
| Constipation | Modified constipation assessment scale, Patient assessment of constipation tool |
| Delirium | Confusion assessment method (CAM), Delirium rating scale |
| Depression | Beck depression inventory, Short form geriatric depression scale, Zung depression scale, Cornell scale for depression in dementia, CES-D Boston short form |
| Dyspnea | Numerical analog scale (i e, 1-10) Visual analog scale (VAS) |
| Fatigue | NAS, VAS, Fatigue symptom inventory |
| Nausea | VAS |
| Pain | Numerical analog scales (NAS), visual analog scales (VAS), verbal descriptive scale, Wong-Baker FACE scale, FLACC scale, brief pain inventory (BPI) |
| Spiritual pain | FICA spiritual assessment tool. |

Resources:
City of Hope Pain and Palliative Care Resource Center http.//www.cityofhope.org/prc
UNIPAC Series. American Academy of Hospice and Palliative Medicine. Third Edition. 2008.
BMJ Group. Putting Evidence into Practice: Palliative Care. United Health Foundation. 2008

These suggested scales are not all inclusive. The Edmonton Symptom Assessment Survey (ESAS) assesses for the presence and intensity of multiple symptoms.

Several reviews have more thoroughly detailed the management of pain and other symptoms that occur in patients with advanced illness who reside in long-term care facilities [5, 6] and in general practice [7]. Other excellent resources include the "UNIPAC" Series, a publication of the American Academy of Hospice and Palliative Medicine [8], the American Medical Directors Association Clinical Practice Guideline (CPG) on "Pain Management in the Long-Term Care Setting" [9], and references [10] and [11].

### Anorexia

Anorexia is defined as a loss of appetite and may be associated with cachexia; the latter is a catabolic state characterized by severe weight loss. Either may occur in the late stages of any severe progressive illness.

Its management includes the following:

- Assess anorexigenic effects of medications such as chemotherapy, antidepressants, NSAIDs, opioids.
- Evaluate whether it could be caused by or related to other symptoms such as nausea, constipation, or pain.
- Assess for any potentially reversible medical condition such as rectal fecal impaction, urinary retention, oral candidiasis, or other treatable causes such as GER, gastritis, or gastroparesis.
- Initiate practical interventions: small, frequent meals; administer medications separate from or with meals; encourage good mouth care; try a variety of foods; improve the social and environmental aspects of eating.

Treat the primary symptom (i.e., anorexia) with an appetite stimulant such as:

- A corticosteroid: prednisone 5–20 mg/day; dexamethasone 4–8 mg/day.
- A progestin: megestrol 400–800 mg/day (trial 4–8 weeks).

Note that the appetite stimulant effect of corticosteroids often decreases after several weeks. Megestrol is associated with lower limb edema and an increased risk of DVT. Consider oral nutritional supplements, though subsequent decreased intake at meals can occur as a result of their use. If used, it is preferable to use nutritional supplements that are lactose free, especially in the elderly or African Americans who have a higher prevalence of lactose intolerance. There is insufficient evidence to recommend the use of cannaboids (dronabinol), cyproheptadine, an androgenic steroid (oxandrolone), or thalidomide, though a therapeutic trial may be worthwhile in individual cases. A patient's advance directive for health care may either request or preclude artificially administered nutrition and hydration. (See the Weight and Nutrition chapter for further discussion.)

**Dyspnea**

Dyspnea is defined as discomfort in breathing that includes the sensation of breathlessness, shortness of breath, or an increased work of breathing. Often it is not associated with tachypnea or hypoxemia. Its management includes the following:

- Initiate practical interventions such as the use of a fan, ensure a comfortable ambient temperature, eliminate respiratory irritants, reposition the person.
- Assess for potentially reversible causes: pneumonia, pleural effusion, pulmonary embolus, heart failure, anemia, bronchospasm.
- Identify any associated symptoms such as aspiration, excessive respiratory secretions, anxiety, social or financial problems, spiritual suffering.
- First-line pharmacotherapy for palliation of dyspnea is an opioid administered every 3–4 h. For mild dyspnea in an *opioid-naïve* patient, start with morphine sulfate 2.5–5 mg PO or the oral morphine equivalent (OME) of another opioid, (refer to OME interconversion Table 8.12 later in this chapter). Titrate the opioid dose upward 25–50% every 12–24 h to attain sufficient relief of dyspnea.
- Optimize medical treatment of the primary respiratory or cardiac condition (i.e., COPD, heart failure).
- Consider addition of a low-dose benzodiazepine for breakthrough or refractory dyspnea as anxiety can be a major contributing factor.
- Consider other medical treatments based upon their benefits and burdens, phase of illness, patient preferences, and advance healthcare directives.
- Remember that patients with dyspnea often do better with a scheduled dose of an opioid (and an anxiolytic) rather than received as needed (PRN). Opioids are effective in treating dyspnea in patients with COPD, though less effective in patients with cancer or heart failure. Use of nebulized opioids is questionable, though they may warrant a therapeutic trial in a more refractory

patient. Though the use of oxygen may reverse hypoxemia, dyspnea may not improve. Beware of the potential for oxygen therapy to cause hypercapnia and subsequent obtundation or respiratory arrest.

Not infrequently a family member may request that the dyspneic patient receive oxygen. Despite it being of no benefit to the patient, it may alleviate the distress families experience while observing their dyspneic family member. When using an opioid for dyspnea, it is prudent to aim for a respiratory rate no less than 14–20 breaths per minute.

### Nausea and Vomiting

The most rational approach to managing nausea and/or vomiting is to understand its four main pathophysiologic mechanisms and the neurotransmitters that mediate the emetic reflex in the brain (Table 8.3). This will allow for a much more rational and effective choice of antiemetic drugs.

TABLE 8.3. Major mechanisms of nausea/vomiting

| Cause | Pharmacologic management |
|---|---|
| **Cortical** | |
| Tumor, increased intracranial pressure | Dexamethasone |
| Anxiety, situational stressors | Benzodiazepine |
| Pain response | Opioid, other pain medication/adjuvants |
| **Vestibular** | |
| | Meclizine |
| | Scopolamine |
| | Dimenhydrinate |
| **Chemoreceptor trigger zone** | |
| Medications | Decrease dose or discontinue, if possible |
| Metabolic (e.g., kidney/liver failure) | Haloperidol, olanzapine |
| Hyponatremia | Sodium chloride, demeclocycline |
| Hypercalcemia | Bisphosphonate, dexamethasone |
| **Gastrointestinal** | |
| Drug related | Stop drug, consider PPI |
| Tumor | Promethazine, metoclopramide, octreotide |
| Constipation | Bowel regimen |
| Cough-induced | Opioid, anticholinergic |

Adapted from UNIPAC Four, 3rd edition, 2008, AAHPM

Management of nausea/vomiting includes:

- Determine whether any medications are emetogenic such as chemotherapeutic agents, some antibiotics, bowel stimulants, opioids, NSAIDs.
- Identify potentially reversible causes such as GER, gastroparesis, constipation, urinary retention, adynamic ileus, UTI.
- Consider emotional and spiritual factors, including *anticipatory anxiety* related to medical treatments.
- Initiate practical, nonpharmacologic interventions such as offering smaller, more frequent meals of blander food, relaxation techniques, appropriate body positioning while eating or when being fed either orally or by PEG tube.
- Prescribe pharmacologic treatment based on the major cause(s) of nausea/vomiting (Table 8.3).
- Combination pharmacotherapy based on each medication's different antiemetic physiologic mechanism may be required especially if nausea/vomiting has multiple etiologies or is refractory. Dexamethasone, metoclopramide, and low-dose antipsychotics have central antiemetic effects. Low-dose haloperidol (0.5–2 mg) or olanzapine (2.5–7.5 mg) may be useful in alleviating nausea/vomiting through several of the four common pathophysiologic mechanisms. But, beware of the likely side effects of serotonin receptor antagonists (headache, constipation, fatigue, xerostomia) and of anticholinergics and antihistamines (drowsiness, fatigue, confusion, dry mouth, constipation, urinary retention, blurred vision). Metoclopramide, like the antipsychotics, can also induce the EPS of dystonia and tardive dyskinesia.

Dronabinol has an antiemetic effect as well (start at 2.5 mg twice a day to a maximum of 20 mg/day). Common adverse reactions of dronabinol can include somnolescence, asthenia, paranoia, nausea, and vomiting. If nausea/vomiting is induced from an opioid, it may require either a dose reduction of the opioid or rotation to another opioid.

### Constipation

Many patients who reside in a long-term care setting experience constipation, especially if terminally ill. Constipation can occur because of a combination of poor fluid intake, low dietary fiber, impaired mobility, and constipating drugs such as opioids, anticholinergics, iron, and calcium preparations and antihypertensives such as calcium channel blockers, diuretics, and clonidine.

Management of constipation includes the following:

*Prevention* is paramount.
- Identify potentially reversible causes, including medication-induced and medical conditions such as a fecal impaction, metabolic disturbances (hypercalcemia, hypothyroidism), GI causes (especially be aware if obstruction is present), and neurologic causes (such as nerve root or spinal cord compression or the visceral neuropathy that may occur in Parkinson's disease).
- Be aware of life-threatening causes such as a bowel obstruction or narcotic bowel syndrome.
- Practical interventions include making toilets accessible, establishing a bowel routine, and encouraging increased fluid intake (if tolerated).
- Reduce the anticholinergic medication load if possible.
- Establish an individualized bowel regimen according to each laxative's mechanism of action (Table 8.4). Combination therapy is often required.
- Monitor for side effects of laxatives that can include bloating, cramping, nausea, and diarrhea.
- Bulk-forming laxatives are usually *not* recommended because they can exacerbate constipation in underhydrated and less mobile patients and often cause or worsen bloating, nausea, or vomiting.

Remember to prevent opioid-induced constipation; as the dose of the opioid is increased, so must the laxative dose be increased. Stimulant laxatives such as senna are most effective for opioid-induced constipation.

TABLE 8.4. Stepwise regimen to prevent or treat constipation, "The sixth vital sign"

| Begin with | Senna with/without docusate | 1–2 tabs/cap qd-bid |
|---|---|---|
| Titrate up to: | Senna | 3–4 tabs bid |
| If needed *add*: | Sorbitol or lactulose or Polyethylene glycol | 30 cc qd-bid 17 g in 8 oz water qd-bid |
| Consider, *in addition* | Glycerin rectal suppository with/without Bisacodyl rectal suppository | Scheduled qd-qod |
| If needed | Mineral oil or soap suds enema | |
| If rectal impaction | May need digital disimpaction | |

Stool softeners have poor effectiveness, but can be considered initially in some patients upon initiating a bowel regimen, i.e., the "laxative ladder". Remember that some patients may also require use of a rectally administered lubricating agent (glycerin) and/or stimulant (bisacodyl) in combination with the oral agents to ensure adequate defecation. Be aware that rectal fecal impaction can cause "paradoxical" diarrhea or urinary retention, either of which may or may not be evident.

**Delirium**
Delirium is an acute confusional state that is characterized by a fluctuating course through the day/night, inattention, and disorganized thinking and speech. Delirium can be either hyperactive or hypoactive. A good caveat to consider is that any acute illness or any medication (either recently prescribed or its dose increased or possibly decreased) can precipitate delirium especially in frail patients with advanced illness.

Management of delirium includes the following:

- Identify potentially reversible causes, especially whether it may be medication-induced.
- Discontinue nonessential medications and reduce anticholinergic load.
- Practical interventions include: familiarize the patient to the environment, improve sleep and the sleep–wake cycle, reduce environmental stimuli and optimize hearing and eyesight (i.e., hearing aides "in," eyeglasses "on"), and adequate hydration.
- Increase mobility by removing/minimizing use of any physical restraints, including Foley catheters.
- Determine whether pain could be contributing to the delirium, and if so, treat it appropriately.
- First-line medication therapy is with low-dose haloperidol (no more than 2–3 mg/day), often in divided doses.
- Second-line medication may include a low-dose benzodiazepine, usually lorazepam 0.5–1 mg PO/SL every 6–8 h, more frequent if necessary; or valproic acid 125–250 mg every 12 h or upon awaking in the morning and at bedtime.

Remember that opioids and steroid medications can cause delirium. Both haloperidol and lorazepam can cause paradoxical agitation or restlessness in which case their dose should be decreased (not increased) or discontinued. It is not uncommon to use combination therapy with both haloperidol and lorazepam. Beware that patients with dementia are more sensitive to the antipsychotic medications' adverse effects of sedation and EPS, and that these medications have been associated with an increased risk of sudden death and cerebrovascular events. Overall, judicious medication management as well as social, environmental, and practical interventions must all be implemented in an attempt to prevent and treat delirium.

## PAIN MANAGEMENT

Effective pain management is the cornerstone of high-quality palliative care in LTC medicine. There is a high prevalence of potentially pain producing medical conditions in this patient population. The goals of pain control include:

- Relief of pain
- Relief of suffering
- Prevent/minimize disability and maximize mobility
- Preserve decision-making capacity

It is always necessary for practitioners to assess each patient for the presence of pain and for "total pain", that is the physical, psychoemotional, social, and spiritual components of pain and how each can affect the other. Successful pain management entails evaluation and interventions that address each component of a patient's total pain. As with any distressful symptom, pain is more optimally managed if its cause and pathophysiologic mechanisms can be understood, together with an interdisciplinary approach and use of multiple treatment modalities, both nonpharmacologic and pharmacologic. The most recent AMDA Clinical Practice Guideline on pain management [12] and the AGS publication, *Geriatrics at Your Fingertips* [13] are excellent up-to-date resources that provide more in-depth content than this chapter permits. Also, the recently updated AGS guidelines (2009) on the pharmacologic management of persistent pain in older persons are another noteworthy resource [14].

Key components to the *evaluation* of pain include the following:

If possible, *prevent* the occurrence of pain or a painful condition. For example, advanced osteoarthritis of one knee may result in contra-lateral hip pain: a total knee arthroplasty may prevent this happening. Another example is prescribing medication in an attempt to prevent the occurrence of postherpetic neuralgia.

*Anticipate* the occurrence of pain. For example, postsurgical incision pain, the pain associated with the onset of peripheral neuropathy in diabetics, or onset of bone pain in cancer patients with known bone metastases.

*Identify* the presence of pain or a painful condition. Remember to look for nonverbal cues of pain such as guarding on movement or on transfers, rubbing and grimacing, or other behaviors such as agitation, restlessness, and insomnia.

*Establish* its location, intensity, temporal pattern, any exacerbating and relieving factors, and effect on (loss of) function and cognition. Consider using a pain assessment scale.

*Determine* whether the pain is acute, chronic (duration of 1 month or more), new onset, intermittent, incidental (i.e., related to movement), or breakthrough pain, and whether multiple sources of pain are present.

- Try to determine whether the pain is nociceptive (either somatic or visceral), neuropathic, or inflammatory, according to the patient's description of the pain (see Table 8.5).
- Identify associated signs and/or symptoms such as headache, dizziness, nausea/vomiting, constipation, decreased urination, a swollen joint, or extremity.
- Review previous and current treatments and their effectiveness, including pain medications, therapies, including nonpharmacologic, and any complementary and alternative medicine interventions.
- Assess "total pain" by elucidating any psycho-emotional, social, and spiritual dimensions to the physical pain, as well as the person's cultural beliefs as to the meaning of pain and manner of expressing pain.
- Perform a detailed physical exam, with particular attention to those body regions or organs systems that appear to be related to or contributing to the pain.
- Assess the need for diagnostic testing, if likely to be helpful in determining a diagnosis, always considering the potential pain or discomfort these tests may cause.

TABLE 8.5. Classification of Pain

| Type of pain | Descriptors |
| --- | --- |
| **Nociceptive** | |
| Somatic pain | Sharp, tender |
| Visceral pain | Dull, cramping |
| Bone pain | Throbbing, aching |
| **Neuropathic** | Burning, tingling, stabbing, shooting |
| **Inflammatory** | e.g., Pleuritic, abdominal rebound, inflamed joints |

Von Roenn JH et al. Current Diagnosis and Treatment of Pain, Lange Series, McGraw Hill 2006.

- Determine the probable cause of the pain. Remember persons may have multiple and different types of pain. Always evaluate for reversible causes of pain. For example, abdominal pain may be due to urinary retention, constipation, rectal/fecal impaction, or caused by medications such as stimulant or bulk-forming laxatives.
- Remember that other conditions such as bladder spasms, contractures, improper positioning, pressure ulcers, muscle strain, oral thrush, urinary retention, fecal impaction, or DVT can all cause pain.
- Key components to the *treatment* of pain include the following:
- Treatment options should take into account the patient's health status, prognosis, known advance directives for health care as well as preferences for care, and thorough discussions to ensure informed choices by the patient and family or proxy decision-maker.
- Promote an interdisciplinary treatment plan, part of which will be determined by the disciplines available at the patient's care setting (i.e., nursing facility, SNF, residential/assisted living, home, or hospital).
- Set goals for pain relief. For example, the desired or accepted level of pain reduction that promotes the achievement of positive functional outcomes in self-care, participation in desired personal and recreational activities, and improved sleep, mood, or cognition.

In up to 90% of persons with pain, practitioners can adequately control pain through orally administered medications guided by the World Health Organization's (WHO) three-step analgesic ladder (see Table 8.6). The WHO recommends administering analgesic and coanalgesic (i.e., adjuvant) medications as follows:

*By mouth*: whenever possible, prescribe an oral analgesic. Avoid IM injections as they can be painful; subcutaneous injections are less painful. Opioids in a concentrated liquid form can be administered sublingually or transbuccally.

TABLE 8.6. The WHO 3-step analgesic ladder

| 1. Mild | 2. Moderate | 3. Severe |
|---|---|---|
| ASA | A/Codeine | Morphine |
| Acetaminophen | A/Hydrocodone | Hydromorphone |
| NSAIDs | A/Oxycodone | Methadone |
|  | A/Dihydrocodeine | Levorphanol |
|  | Tramadol/apap | Fentanyl |
|  |  | Oxycodone |
| ± Adjuvants | ± Adjuvants | ± Adjuvants |

Adapted from: Technical Report Series 804: Geneva WHO. 1990

*Around-the-clock*: scheduled dosing for continuous pain and to minimize breakthrough pain

*According to the ladder*: the initial choice of analgesic and use of adjuvants is based on the severity of the pain. Using the numerical pain scale, 1 through 3 can be considered mild pain, 4 through 6 moderate pain, 7 through 9 severe pain, and 10 excruciating pain.

*Adapted to the individual*: the choice of analgesic should be based upon the patient's condition, comorbidities (such as liver and kidney failure; coexistent dementia or delirium), drug safety and toxicity profile, ease of administration, and goals of both pain relief and the overall desired outcome.

*With attention to detail*: ensure correct dosing, consider drug pharmokinetics and pharmacodynamics, make appropriate dose adjustments in timely manner, always monitor benefit verses potential harm and adverse effects.

Optimal pain management entails the choice of the most appropriate analgesic(s) based upon the primary and secondary diagnoses, the physiologic mechanism underlying the pain (see Table 8.7), pain severity, diagnosis, the potential adverse effects of each medication and/or treatment modality, and the patient's individual characteristics that can alter each drug's pharmokinetics and pharmacodynamics.

Several caveats for pain management include:

- In most patients, prescribe at least one analgesic as scheduled, i.e., administered routinely, rather than just as needed (i.e., PRN).
- Choose an appropriate analgesic and dose for breakthrough pain.
- Most types of pain respond, at least partially, to an opioid.
- The maximum dose of acetaminophen is now 2000–3000 mg/day, but 2,000 mg/day if renal or hepatic insufficiency is present.

TABLE 8.7. Select first- and second-line analgesics based on type of pain

| Type of Pain | Consider First-line | Second-line |
| --- | --- | --- |
| Nociceptive pain | WHO Step 1 or 2 drug | WHO Step 3 drug |
| Neuropathic pain | TCAs, anticonvulsants | WHO Step 2 or 3 drug |
| Bone pain | NSAIDs, corticosteroids | WHO Step 2 or 3 drug |
| Intracranial pain | Corticosteroids | WHO Step 2 or 3 drug |
| Visceral pain | Anticholinergic, opioid | Steroids, opioids |

Source: UNIPAC Three. AAHPM 2008

- The maximum dose of tramadol is 300 mg/24 h; may precipitate confusion, seizures, serotonin syndrome.
- Conventional nonselective NSAIDs (e.g., ibuprofen, naproxen) should be used only short term – that is, a few days to 3–4 weeks; precautions include risk for gastrointestinal bleeding, renal impairment, platelet dysfunction, and exacerbation of edema, blood pressure, and heart failure.
- Selective COX-2 inhibitors (e.g., celecoxib) still have a significant risk of GI bleeding and renal insufficiency.
- Consider holding or discontinuing ASA chemoprophylaxis when administering a conventional or COX-2 NSAID.
- Consider concomitant proton pump inhibitor therapy in patients at increased risk for GI bleeding when prescribing a NSAID.
- Never prescribe a NSAID if the patient is taking warfarin as the risk for GI bleeding is too high.
- Consider use of a topical analgesic such as capsaicin cream, diclofenac gel, or a lidocaine patch for persons with one or two localized areas of musculoskeletal, arthritic, or neuropathic pain.
- Remember that use of the lidocaine patch is noncontinuous, that it is to be applied for only 12 h each 24-h period, off the remaining 12 h, applying no more than three patches at a time.
- Avoid use of propoxyphene and meperidine due to their potential for causing undesirable CNS side effects such as confusion or seizures.
- Partial opioid agents such as butorphanol, pentazocine, buprenorphine, and nalbuphine are not recommended either because of their analgesic ceiling effects or ability to counteract the analgesic effect of pure agonist opioids; these medications can precipitate an opioid withdrawal pain crisis.

### Opioid Analgesics

Opioids are both appropriate and effective for the treatment of moderate to severe acute or chronic pain not relieved by other analgesics or modalities. Judicious prescribing can provide effective pain management in the various patient populations served by LTC medicine with a low likelihood of psychological dependency or addiction. Scheduled low doses of opioids can be very effective in the treatment of chronic pain associated with various chronic musculoskeletal conditions that afflict the elderly. Be aware that physical dependency, characterized by withdrawal symptoms, can occur when regularly scheduled opioids are abruptly discontinued. Gradual dose reduction can prevent this if an opioid is to be discontinued.

TABLE 8.8. Suggested equianalgesic starting doses for selected oral opioids

**Frail or elderly opioid naïve patients**

The practitioner may choose from the following suggested starting doses:

| | |
|---|---|
| Morphine 2 mg PO or SL | 0.1 cc morphine 20 mg/cc (Roxanol®) |
| Oxycodone liquid 2 mg PO or SL | 0.1 cc oxycodone 20 mg/cc (Oxyfast®) |
| Oxycodone 2.5 mg | ½ tablet 5 mg oxycodone |
| | ½ tablet oxycodone 5 mg/acetaminophen 325 mg (Percocet®) |
| Hydromorphone 0.5 mg PO | 0.5 cc hydromorphone 1 mg/cc (Dilaudid®) |
| Hydrocodone 2.5 mg PO | ½ tablet hydrocodone 5 mg/acetaminophen 500 mg (Vicodin®) |

**Adult opioid tolerant patients**

The practitioner may choose from the following suggested starting doses:

| | |
|---|---|
| Morphine 5 mg PO or SL | 0.25 cc morphine 20 mg/cc (Roxanol®) |
| Oxycodone liquid 5 mg PO or SL | 0.25 cc oxycodone 20 mg/cc (Oxyfast®) |
| Oxycodone 5 mg | 5 mg oxycodone |
| | 1 tablet oxycodone 5 mg/acetaminophen 325 mg (Percocet®) |
| Hydromorphone 1 mg | ½ of 2 mg tablet PO (Dilaudid®) |
| | 1 cc of hydromorphone 1 mg/cc SL |
| Hydrocodone 5 mg | 1 tablet (Vicodin®) 5/500 |

Source: Permission granted by American Medical Directors Association. Palliative Care in the Long-Term Care Setting (LTC Physician Information Tool Kit Series). Columbia, MD: 2007

General guidelines to the use of opioids include:

*For acute pain*: start by prescribing an immediate-release opioid preparation (see Table 8.8 for suggested equianalgesic starting doses).

*For chronic pain*: consider starting a *sustained-released* opioid, with a sufficient dose of an *immediate-release* opioid for breakthrough pain.

Remember that the total dose of a mixed opioid (i.e., an opioid with acetaminophen) is limited by its 24 h dose of acetaminophen.

Once the total daily dose of an opioid has been established to adequately control the patient's pain, consider converting it to an equivalent dose of a sustained-release opioid (see Table 8.9 on

TABLE 8.9. Available formulations of sustained-release oral opioids

| | | |
|---|---|---|
| Morphine sulfate ER (MS Contin®)[a] | q 8–12h | 15,30,60,100,200 mg ER |
| Morphine sulfate ER (Kadian®)[a,b] | q 12–24h | 10,20,30,50,60,80,100,200 ER |
| Morphine sulfate ER (Avinza®)[a,b,c] | q 24h | 30,45,60,75,90,120 ER |
| Oxycodone ER (Oxycontin®)[a] | q 8–12h | 10,15,20,30,40,60,80 ER |
| Oxymorphone (Opana ER®)[a] | q 12h | 5, 7.5, 10, 15, 20, 30, 40 ER |

[a]Formulation not to be crushed
[b]Capsules can be opened and contents administered per PEG
[c]Formulation components: 90% ER and 10% immediate release

TABLE 8.10 Pharmacodynamics of immediate-release morphine

| Administered | Peak analgesic effect (min) | Duration of analgesia (h) |
|---|---|---|
| Oral/sublingual | 45–60 | 3–4 |
| Subcutaneous | 15–30 | 3–4 |
| Intravenous | 5–15 | 3–4 |

the different formulations of sustained-release opioids that are available).

Note that the duration of analgesic action for all immediate-release morphine preparations whether administered PO, SL, SC, or IV is 3–4 h, though their onset of action and peak effect do vary (see Table 8.10).

The opioid dose for breakthrough pain is 10–15% of the total daily opioid dose, administered every 1–2 h as needed.

One can usually and safely titrate up the total 24 h dose of an opioid 25–50% for mild to moderate pain and 50–100% for moderate to severe pain.

When starting a patient on an opioid, *ALWAYS start the patient on a prophylactic bowel regimen to prevent constipation.* A stimulant and/or osmotic agent are preferable.

Adjuvant analgesics can allow use of a lower dose of an opioid and thus decrease the likelihood of opioid adverse effects.

In contrast to nonopioids and NSAIDs, opioids commonly used for the treatment of pain have no analgesic ceiling. However, adverse drug effects may limit further dose increases

TABLE 8.11. Common and less common side effects of opioids

| Common | Less common |
|---|---|
| Constipation (almost always) | Hypotension |
| Somnolescence | Diaphoresis |
| Nausea/vomiting | Urinary retention |
| Dizziness | Confusion, delirium |
| Sweating | Bradycardia |
| Dry mouth | Seizures |
| Asthenia | Respiratory depression, apnea |
| Dysesthesias | Paralytic ileus |
| Pruritus | Paresthesia, hyperesthesia |
|  | Shock, cardiac arrest |

(see Table 8.11) or require "rotating" to another opioid, especially if adequate pain relief is not achieved (see below).

As already noted, propoxyphene and meperidine should be avoided because of their high potential for CNS toxicities. Codeine is too constipating in relation to the dose required for an adequate analgesic effect. Using two or more different opioids together is not recommended because of the potential for adverse drug–drug or opioid–receptor interactions, either unknown or unrecognized by clinicians. Different opioids interact to different degrees at the mu, delta, and kappa opioid receptors. One exception is the patient on the fentanyl patch, where an immediate-release opioid such as morphine or oxycodone needs to be used for breakthrough pain. Transmucosal oral fentanyl (i.e., Actiq®) is only indicated for severe breakthrough cancer pain and its use should be *avoided* in the LTC setting if at all possible.

When changing from one opioid to another, whether because of inadequate pain relief or unmanageable adverse effects of the opioid, use *morphine equivalents* as a common denominator for opioid dose conversion. Morphine equivalents can usually avoid underdosing or overdosing, while maintaining or obtaining effective pain relief (see Table 8.12 on OMEs). When using morphine equivalents, the dose of the new opioid is converted via decreasing its dose by 25–50% in order to adjust for incomplete cross-tolerance. When converting from one opioid to another, it may be prudent to do so over 2 or 3 days: with downward titration of the opioid being discontinued, coupled with the upward titration of the newly prescribed opioid. This is especially important if the patient is on a high dose of opioid in order to avoid a pain withdrawal crisis.

TABLE 8.12. Oral morphine equivalents (mg)

|  | Oral | Parenteral |
|---|---|---|
| Morphine | 30 | 10 (1/3 oral dose) |
| Oxycodone | 20–30 | N/A |
| Oxymorphone | 10 | 1 (1/10 oral dose) |
| Hydromorphone | 7.5 | 1.5 (1/5 oral dose) |
| Meperidine | 300 | 75 (1/4 oral dose) |
| Hydrocodone | 30 | N/A |
| Codeine | 180–200 | N/A |

(25 µg fentanyl patch = 50 mg oral morphine/24 h); N/A = no parenteral formulation available
Source: Adapted from American Pain Society. Principles of Analgesic Use in the Treatment of Acute Pain and Cancer Pain. 6th Edition.2008

Caution is warranted when prescribing opioids in an *opioid-naïve* patient where the dictum "start low and go slow" is advisable. The suggested starting dose of oral morphine is 2–5 mg every 3–4 h or the equianalgesic dose of another opioid. The use of a fentanyl patch when initiating opioid treatment in the frail elderly opioid-naïve patient is not advisable as the lower strength patches of 12 µg/h and 25 µg/h provide an OME approximate dose of 25 mg and 50 mg, respectively, *every 24 h*. Such doses can cause excess fatigue or sedation especially in these opioid-naïve patients. Though expensive, the fentanyl patch has an ease of administration and can provide excellent analgesia in some patients, but is likely ineffective in thin patients and those who weigh less than 105 lbs due to inadequate subcutaneous fat necessary for fentanyl absorption through the skin.

Morphine, oxycodone, and hydromorphone should be used cautiously in patients with moderate to severe renal failure (GFR 30–50 ml/min or less) because of the risk of metabolite accumulation. Methadone and fentanyl are safe to use for patients with advanced renal failure and on dialysis, though neither is dialyzable. Nonopioid medications that are safe to use for patients with renal failure include acetaminophen and tramadol, though the maximal daily dose of tramadol should be reduced from 300 mg a day to no more 100–200 mg, divided twice a day. Morphine and codeine doses may need to be reduced in patients with liver disease, especially those with cirrhosis. Fentanyl may be easier to use in such patients, unless there is inadequate subcutaneous tissue.

Methadone is gaining popularity in the treatment of chronic musculoskeletal pain and clinicians are more frequently prescribing it for the treatment of cancer pain and neuropathic pain. Other indications for its use include refractory pain, intolerance to other opioids, or clinician concern about patient diversion of opioids. Methadone has several mechanisms of action, is extensively metabolized in the liver, and is minimally renally excreted and cheap. However, its prolonged and variable metabolism (half-life may vary from 45 to 180 h) is such that its steady-state plasma concentration is not reached for up to 10 days. It has complex medication interactions and has been associated with prolongation of the QT interval and an increasingly higher cause of opioid-related deaths. Thus, methadone should only be used by (or in consultation with) a clinician who is experienced with its use. When treating frail elders prescribing low-dose methadone 2.5–5 mg, 2 or 3 times a day would be prudent. *Methadone should never be used for the treatment of* acute *or breakthrough pain,* as the risk of respiratory depression is too high. For more complete information on methadone use in long-term care, refer to Appendix 6 of the AMDA Clinical Practice Guideline on Pain Management [12].

For guidelines on the use of patient-controlled analgesia, refer to references [8] (UNIPAC Three) and [15].

### Eligibility Guidelines for Hospice

Practitioners in LTC medicine must consider, offer, and facilitate resident access to hospice care as residents transition into the terminal phase of advanced illness. Hospice is an underutilized benefit with many patients referred too late in their illness and thereby unable to fully benefit from its services. Studies have shown that hospice stays of 7 days or less have increased to 34% of hospice admissions, while long stays greater than 180 days are less than 10% of admissions.

Practitioner awareness of the *general eligibility guidelines* and *disease-specific guidelines* (see Table 8.13) for hospice can help prognosticate whether a resident with advanced illness may have less than 6 months to live. Such a determination can provide the opportunity to open a frank discussion with the resident and family on advance care planning in order to decide upon a more palliative approach to care whether or not the resident and family opt for life-sustaining treatment.

General indicators (i.e., general eligibility guidelines for hospice) that any advanced illness has progressed to its terminal phase include the following:

- Frequent transfers to the ER
- More frequent hospitalizations
- Significant weight loss (5% in 1 month; 10% in the past 6 months)

TABLE 8.13. Disease-specific eligibility criteria/guidelines for hospice

*Cancer*
Widespread metastatic disease
No longer seeking curative care

*Dementia*
Inability to ambulate or dress without assistance
No consistent meaningful speech
Life-threatening infections, multiple stage 3 or 4 skin ulcers
Inability to maintain sufficient fluid and calorie intake

*Failure to thrive*
Mainly in bed, requires assist with all BADLs
Body mass index (BMI) <22
Refusing or not responding to enteral or parenteral nutritional support

*Heart disease*
Poor response or intolerant to optimal medical treatment
NYHA Class IV CHF
EF $\leq$ 20% (helpful, not required)

*HIV/AIDS*
CD 4 count <25
Persistent viral loads >100,000/ml
Major Aids-defining refractory infections or other medical conditions
Significant functional decline in ADLs

*Neurologic diseases*
(PD, ALS, MS, MD, Myasthenia gravis)
Rapid disease progression and critical nutritional state
Life-threatening infections in preceding 12 months
Stage 3, 4 decubitus ulcers
Critically impaired breathing capacity, declines ventilator

*Nonspecific terminal illness*
Rapid decline and disease progression
Weight loss, dysphagia with aspiration
Increase in ER visits, hospitalizations
Worsening pressure ulcers despite optimal care
Decline in blood pressure to below 90 systolic

*Pulmonary disease*
Disabling dyspnea at rest or with minimal exertion
Increasing visits to ER, hospitalizations
Hypoxemia on room air (<88%); hypercapnia of $_pCO_2$ >50 mmHg
FEV 1<30% (helpful, not required)

*Renal failure*
Not seeking dialysis, not a candidate
Calculated creatinine clearance <10 (<15 for diabetics)
Creatinine >8 (>6 for diabetics)

(continued)

TABLE 8.13. (continued)

*Stroke*
Coma (acute phase)
Dysphagia with insufficient intake of fluids and calories
Poststroke dementia (see Dementia criteria)

*Liver disease*
INR >1.5 not on Warfarin
Serum albumin <2.5 g/dl
Refractory ascites
Previous spontaneous bacterial peritonitis
Hepatorenal syndrome
Recurrent variceal bleeding

Adapted from: Prescription for Hospice Services. VistaCare Inc., 2005; National Hospice and Palliative Care Organization

- Multiple stage 3 or 4 decubitus ulcers
- Serum albumin less than 2.5 g/dl
- Recurrent life-threatening infections such as pneumonia, pyelonephritis, or sepsis
- Declining functional status as determined by either a Karnofsky Performance score of <50% or increasing dependency in 3 of 6 Basic Activities of Daily Living

When the *guidelines* for disease-specific eligibility for hospice are not met, the presence and severity of comorbid medical condition(s) and/or psychosocial factors can support eligibility for hospice. For example, advanced COPD or dementia may support eligibility for hospice in a resident with late stage heart failure. Or the recent death of a resident's spouse or a life-threatening illness in a resident's family member may support the resident's eligibility for hospice.

*Certification* for hospice requires that two physicians, the hospice medical director and the attending or referring physician, sign a statement certifying that the patient's medical prognosis suggests a life expectancy of 6 months or less if the individual's illness follows its normal course. Once on hospice, a patient must be *recertified* for each benefit period. Recertification only requires a statement as to continued eligibility by the hospice medical director. The first two hospice certification periods are 90 days each and all subsequent periods are 60 days (with no limit as to the number of 60 day periods). However, continued eligibility for hospice requires that the eligibility parameters present on admission to hospice continue to be met *and* that physical, functional, and/

or nutritional *decline continues* and suggests that life expectancy is 6 months or less if the individual's illness follows its normal course. Every patient on hospice has the right to *revoke* their hospice benefit at any time in order to seek life-sustaining or curative treatment. In such circumstances, if these treatments are of no benefit, patients can be readmitted to hospice if still eligible.

Billing by practitioners for services rendered to patients on hospice can be confusing and dependent upon the Local Medicare Intermediary (now called Medicare Administrative Contractors). It is recommended that practitioners clarify hospice-billing practices with their Medicare Administrative Contractor and refer to Chapter 14 of this text.

### End-of-Life Care

As patients with advanced serious illness enter the last months and weeks of life, practitioners need to both recognize this terminal phase and inform patients and family accordingly. Goals of care need to be reviewed and modified through advanced care planning. Whether the patient and family want to continue to pursue life-prolonging treatments or are amenable to hospice care, palliative care can be integrated into either choice. Irrespective of where the patient resides, interdisciplinary management is essential in maintaining hope, dignity, and the best possible quality of life until the patient dies. Eventually, however, continuing life-sustaining treatments (such as IV fluids, PEG tube feeding, blood transfusions, antibiotics, pacemakers, ICDs, and hemodialysis) during the last weeks and days of life can become overly burdensome and cause more harm, pain, and suffering than benefit to both patient and family.

The physiologic changes of dying, although complex, can be effectively managed if practitioners and the IDT understand the etiologies and underlying pathophysiology of each distressful symptom and use appropriate nonpharmacologic and pharmacologic interventions [16]. Given each patient's terminal illness and their comorbidities, palliative drugs, equipment, and supplies should be available in anticipation of those symptoms that are most likely to occur at the end of life (EOL).

As death approaches, patients and families should be advised that fatigue and weakness will increase while the desire for food and fluid intake is reduced as manifested by the loss of both appetite and thirst. Reduced cardiac output and intravascular volume depletion result in tachycardia, hypotension, peripheral cooling, cyanosis, and mottling. Urine output will diminish with eventual anuria. Neurologic dysfunction will occur, leading to a decreased level of consciousness and eventual coma. Ten percent of patients may experience an agitated delirium during the last days of life.

Practical interventions to maintain patient comfort include periodic repositioning, decreasing food and fluid intake to prevent choking or aspiration, maintaining a moist oral mucosa, and providing moisture and lubricating agents to the conjunctiva and lips. Family members should be encouraged to participate in this care as it can often provide them with a sense of fulfillment in having helped to comfort their loved one at EOL.

Nonessential drugs (e.g., aspirin, multivitamins, calcium supplements, lipid-lowering agents) should be discontinued. Practitioners should also consider the benefits and risks of continuing drugs such as antidepressants, antihypertensives, warfarin, and thyroid replacement. Other drugs, such as diuretics, ACE inhibitors, and hypoglycemic agents (even insulin), may require a dosage reduction or even discontinuation. Reduced hepatic function and renal perfusion can precipitate an opioid-induced terminal delirium. If this occurs, consider reducing the opioid dosage while ensuring that pain is still adequately controlled.

During the last few days of life, medication reconciliation is essential to avoid polypharmacy and its potential sequelae, especially as "comfort medications" are administered to manage pain and distressful symptoms and suffering.

Remember that a peaceful death is just as important to the family as to the patient, perhaps even more so.

General guidelines on the use of comfort-directed pharmacologic interventions include:

- For tachypnea or breathlessness: use low doses of an immediate-release opioid and/or benzodiazepine, administered sublingually or transbuccally.
- For excessive respiratory or oral secretions: consider an anticholinergic agent administered sublingually (e.g., hyoscyamine or an ophthalmic solution of atropine) or topically (e.g., transdermal scopolamine).
- For pain: use a concentrated oral formulation of either morphine (e.g., Roxanol[R] 20 mg/cc) or oxycodone (Oxyfast[R] 20 mg/cc). Either can be administered sublingually or transbuccally. Avoid IM or SC injections if possible as these can be painful.
- For anxiety, agitation, or restlessness: use a benzodiazepine or an opioid, possibly an antipsychotic. Remember any of these can cause a paradoxical agitation.

- For fever: schedule regular doses of acetaminophen administered orally, per rectum or per PEG (if present).
- If excessive sweating: consider an opioid dose reduction.
- If delirium: perform a careful medication review and rule out rectal fecal impaction or urinary bladder retention; treat accordingly with a benzodiazepine and/or antipsychotic; and ensure adequate pain control.

Compounded formulations applied topically on the skin may be effective for EOL restlessness, for example, ABH gel compound that comprises lorazepam, diphenhydramine, and haloperidol. Review of compounded topicals is beyond the scope of this chapter; practitioners are encouraged to contact their local compounding pharmacies and hospice agencies.

## PEARLS FOR THE PRACTITIONER
- Integrate palliative care into traditional care provided to residents and patients throughout the long-term care continuum, irrespective of whether they choose to continue disease-directed or alternative therapies.
- Support informed patient and family decision-making (i.e., advance care planning) that supports their values and preferences for care.
- Determine, if possible, the pathophysiologic and clinical factors underlying each pain and nonpain symptom in order to choose the most appropriate interventions.
- Treat pain through the use of multiple modalities, both nonpharmacologic and pharmacologic as well as complementary and alternative therapies.
- Choose the most appropriate analgesic based on the type of pain, pain severity, potential adverse effects of the medication, and the patient's individual characteristics.
- Always initiate a bowel regimen to prevent constipation when prescribing an opioid and remember to intensify the bowel regimen when the dose of the opioid is increased.
- Anticipate which symptoms are most likely to occur during each patient's illness trajectory, in addition to identifying, assessing, treating, and monitoring distressful symptoms, and if possible, preventing their emergence.
- Consider both the general and disease-specific guidelines when evaluating persons for hospice.
- Consider palliative sedation to alleviate unbearable pain or suffering that persists despite aggressive palliative care.
- Use as resources healthcare professionals in your community who have expertise in palliative care.

## WEBSITES
- City of Hope Pain and Palliative Care Resource Center www.cityofhope.org/patient_care
- American Academy of Hospice and Palliative Medicine www.aahpm.org
- Center to Advance Palliative Care www.capc.org
- Fast Facts and Concepts www.eperc.mcw.edu
- American Pain Society www.ampainsoc.org
- Morphine Equivalent Dose Conversion www.hopweb.org

## REFERENCES
1. Currow DC, Wheeler JL, Glare PA, et al. A framework for generalizeability. in palliative care. J Pain Symptom Manage 2009;37(3): 373–386.
2. Young Y, Frick KD, Phelan EA. Can successful aging and chronic illness co- exist in the same individual? A multidimensional concept of successful aging. J Am Med Directors Assoc 2009;10:87–92.
3. Aronow WS. Clinical causes of death in 2372 older persons in a nursing home during 15-year follow-up. J Am Med Directors Assoc 2000;1: 95–96.
4. Goldberg TH, Botero QA. Causes of death in elderly nursing home residents. J Am Med Directors Assoc 2008;9:565–567.
5. Winn PA, Dentino AN. Quality palliative care in the long-term care setting. J Am Med Directors Assoc 2005;6:589–598.
6. Winn PA, Dentino AN. Effective pain management in the long-term care setting. J Am Med Directors Assoc 2004;5:342–352.
7. Winn PA, Salinas RC, Cook JB. End-of-life Care. FP Essentials, Edition No. 336, AAFP Home Study. Leawood, KS: *American Academy of Family Physicians* May 2007.
8. Storey CP, Levine S, Shega JW, eds. Hospice and Palliative Care Training for Physicians: A Self-Study Program. 3rd Edition. American Academy of Hospice and Palliative Medicine, Glenview, IL. 2008. UNIPAC Three: Bail A and Levine S. Assessment and Treatment of Physical Pain Associated with Life-limiting Illness; UNIPAC Four: Policzer JS and Sobel J. Management of Selected Non-pain Symptoms of Life-limiting Illness; UNIPAC Nine : Curtis JR, Levine S, Rocker G et al. The Hospice and Palliative Medicine Approach to Selected Chronic Illnesses: Dementia, COPD, and CHF.
9. Clinical Practice Guideline: Pain Management in the Long-Term Care Setting. Columbia, MD: American Medical Directors Association, 3rd ed. 2009. Available at http://www.amda.com/tools/cpg/chronic pain.cfm. (last accessed September 2, 2009).
10. ePocrates on Line. End of life care. Available at https://online.epocrates.com/u/29111020/End-of-life+care (last accessed September 2, 2009).
11. Brunnhuber K, Nash S, Meier D, Weissman DE, Woodcock J. Putting Evidence into Practice: Palliative Care. The BMJ Publishing, London. 2008.

12. American Medical Director Association. Pain Management Clinical Practice Guideline. Columbia, MD: AMDA 2009.
13. Reuben DB, Herr KA, Pacala JT, et al. Geriatrics at Your Fingertips: 2009, 11th Edition. New York: The American Geriatrics Society; 2008.
14. American Geriatrics Panel on the Pharmacologic Management of Persistent Pain in Older Persons. Pharmacologic management of persistent pain in older adults. J Am Geriatr Soc 2009;57(8):1331–1346.
15. Principles of Analgesic Use in the Treatment of Acute Pain and Cancer Pain. Fifth Edition. 2003. The American Pain Society: Glenview.
16. Emanuel LL, vonGunten CF, Ferris FD. Education for Physicians on End-of- Life Care. Participant's Handbook. Module 12. Last Hours of Living. Chicago: EPEC;1999
17. Teunissen SCCM, Wesker W, Kruitwagen C, et al. Symptom Prevalence in Patients with Incurable Cancer: A Systematic Review. J Pain Symptom Mange 2007;34:94–104.
18. Solano JP, Gomes B and Higginson IJ. A comparison of symptom prevalence in far advanced cancer, AIDS, heart disease, chronic obstructive pulmonary disease and renal disease. J Pain Symptom Mange 2006; 31(1):58–69.
19. Cantin B, Rothuisen LE and Buclin T. Referrals of cancer versus non-cancer patients to a palliative care consult team. Do they differ? J Pall Care 2009; 25(2):92–99.
20. White C, McMullen D and Doyle J. Now that you mention it, Doctor… symptom reporting and the need for systematic questioning in a specialist palliative care unit. J Pall Med 2009;12(5):447–450.

## SUGGESTED READING

AMDA White Paper on Palliative Care and Hospice in Long Term Care 2007.
UNIPAC Quick Reference: A Quick-Reference Guide to the Hospice and Palliative Care Training for Physicians: UNIPAC Self-Study Program. Storey CP (Editor). AAHPM 2009.
End-of-life care overview–Epocrates Online https.//online.epocrates.com/u/2911102/End-of-life+care
Lynn J, Chaudhry E. Simon LN, Wilkinson AM and Schuster JL. The Common Sense Guide to Improving Palliative Care. Oxford University Press 2007.
Brunnhuber K, Nash S, Meier DE, Weissman DE, Woodcock J. Putting Evidence into Practice. Palliative Care. BMJ Publishing, London; 2008.
Snyder L and Quill TE (Editors). Physician's Guide to End-of-Life Care. American College of Physicians–American Society of Internal Medicine: Philadelphia; 2001.
Kiebler KK, Heidrich DE and Esper P. Palliative and End-of-Life Care. Clinical Practice Guidelines. Second Edition. Saunder/Elsevier. Elsevier Health Sciences, Inc; 2007.
Matzo M. and Sherman D. (Eds.) Palliative Care Nursing Education: Toward Quality Care at the End of Life, Third Edition. Springer: New York; 2010.
Improving Palliative Care in Nursing Homes. Center to Advance Palliative Care. 2007. Available at www.capc.org. (last accessed August 10, 2009)

# Chapter 9
# Weight and Nutrition

Todd H. Goldberg and Joel A. Levine

**Keywords:** Nutritional status • Nutritional status assessment • Weight • Weight management • Nutritional intervention • Feeding tube • Ethical issues

## INTRODUCTION

The nutritional needs of the geriatric patient are influenced by many factors. Changes associated with aging, individual behavior, drugs, and disease augment nutritional risk for older adults. As with persons of all ages, proper nutrition and maintaining a healthy weight are very important in elderly Long-term care (LTC) residents (including subacute care, assisted living, and nursing homes, all herein generically grouped together under the rubric of "LTC"). Optimal nutrition should ideally improve health, functioning, and quality of life and reduce the risk of morbidity, mortality, and complications such as osteoporosis, weakness, pressure sores, impaired immunity, frailty, and sarcopenia. Weight loss is a negative quality indicator and risk factor for poor outcomes – survival is markedly improved with appropriate and adequate nutrition. However, maintaining appropriate nutrition, hydration, oral intake, and weight may be challenging particularly in some elderly LTC residents. Those who have dementia, depression, and gastrointestinal, neurological, musculoskeletal, or psychiatric disorders or indeed any medical condition or drug that may impair appetite, mobility, swallowing, chewing, feeding, digestion, and bowel function are especially at nutritional risk.

Older adults reside in residential care, subacute, or LTC facilities for a variety of reasons, ranging from temporary disability, e.g., due to hip fracture, to severe dementia. Hospitalized and healthy community dwelling elderly persons are not the main focus of this chapter. Every resident has important and individual nutritional needs, but those with chronic illness and disability require extra attention to diet and nutritional assessment and need for assistance. Up to 60% of hospitalized elderly patients and LTC residents with dementia have been reported to have significant eating difficulties and/or nutritional deficiencies. There is a strong correlation between low body mass index (BMI) and serum albumin, and increased mortality that persists for months to years after discharge from a hospital setting. Even when nutritional deficiencies are recognized, therapy is often suboptimal, leading to both poor outcomes and potential ethical and legal concerns [1].

Some general nutritional guidance relevant to the problems of elderly residents in LTC will be offered here with some specific dietary supplement recommendations, but each resident's diet must be individualized. Detailed dietary guidelines and Dietary Reference Intakes for every nutrient are beyond the scope of this brief review and are freely available on many web sites including the web site of the U.S. Department of Agriculture and the Institute of Medicine (Refer to list of web sites at end of chapter.). A summary table of recommendations for a few common key nutrients is included in Table 9.1.

## IMPACT OF AGING, DISEASE, AND MEDICATION

Nutritional status and weight are affected by both aging and disease. Normal aging generally is accompanied by only modest changes if any in appetite, metabolism, intestinal functioning, and absorption of nutrients. It has been demonstrated that older residents will be less hungry than younger residents after a period of underfeeding. In addition to any effects of aging alone, the various physiological functions that assure appropriate nutrition, ingestion, digestion, assimilation, and absorption are indisputably affected by the resident's medical, psychosocial, and functional status. Appropriate elimination of waste products also will affect the resident's well-being, appetite, and nutritional status, thus a good bowel program along with adequate fluid intake is equally important [2]. Inadequate intake of food and fluids may lead to dehydration, constipation, cognitive impairment, slow gastric emptying, regurgitation, aspiration, infection, sepsis, and decubiti.

TABLE 9.1. Recommended intake for key nutrients

| Nutrient | Typical recommended intake/DRI[a] | Comments for geriatrics/LTC |
| --- | --- | --- |
| Calories/energy | 1,800+ calories | Varies by body size and activity level and desired weight loss or gain |
| Protein | 46+ g, 10–35% of calories | Increased protein to 1–1.2 g/kg/day suggested for geriatric LTC residents |
| Fat | 20–35% of calories | |
| Carbohydrate | 100–130 g, 45–65% of calories | |
| Water | 2.7–3.7 L | Includes total water; all beverages, in average temperate climate |
| Vitamin A | 3,000 IU | Higher doses associated with increased toxicity and mortality |
| Vitamin $B_{12}$ | 3–6 mcg. Typical oral supplement dose 1,000 mcg/day | Common deficiency in elderly; measure levels. Often malabsorbed requiring supplements |
| Vitamin C/Zinc | 75–90 mg C/11 mg Zinc | Larger doses often recommended of Vitamin C and Zinc together for pressure sores but not evidence-based |
| Vitamin D | 600 IU (15 mcg) | Older adults often deficient. Consider measuring 25OHD levels and adding supplements ≥800 IU/day, found to reduce falls, fractures, and mortality |
| Vitamin E | 15–30 IU (20 mg) | Supplementation >200 IU no longer recommended due to metaanalysis showing increased mortality [24] |
| Calcium | 1,200 mg | Calcium + vitamin D supplements should be provided to all older adults at risk for osteoporosis |
| Iron | 18 mg | Doses >325 mg/day on Beers list of inappropriate drugs [25], causes constipation |

[a] Adapted from various sources, chiefly "Dietary Reference Intakes" from the Institute of Medicine, National Academy of Sciences, available online at http://www.iom.edu/?id=21381. What were formerly called Recommended Daily Allowances (RDA's) are now called Dietary Reference Intakes (DRI's) [2]. Not all vitamins and minerals are included; for more complete lists see sources cited above

Virtually every resident admitted to a LTC facility or service will have some nutritional risk factors:

- History of weight loss or appetite change
- Oral/dental problems/edentulousness
- Reduced mobility and functional disability
- Skin breakdown or pressure ulcers
- Dementia
- Depression
- Chronic illness or terminal illness
- Fluid retention and edema
- Nausea or vomiting
- Change in bowel habits
- Recent surgery
- Multiple medications

The average LTC resident is on 6–10 or more medications, with 9 or more being considered polypharmacy and a negative quality indicator. Certainly drugs, whether necessary and appropriate or inappropriate, are among the top causes of weight, appetite, and bowel problems in the elderly. Innumerable medications and drugs can cause GI disturbances and anorexia, including but not limited to:

- NSAIDs
- Opioid pain medications
- Anticholinergic drugs including loperamide
- Diabetic drugs such as metformin
- Cardiac drugs such as digoxin
- Antidementia drugs such as cholinesterase inhibitors
- Psychotropic drugs
- Antihypertensives including ACE-inhibitors, calcium channel blockers, and beta blockers
- Antibiotics
- Antacid drugs
- Alcohol
- Over-the-counter drugs

Anticholinergic drugs may reduce salivary and gastric secretions as well as GI motility; antidementia drugs such as cholinesterase inhibitors can commonly cause nausea. Almost any psychotropic drug or prokinetic drugs such as metaclopramide may cause diminished cognition, motor problems, poor oral intake, and constipation, particularly the tricyclic antidepressants. Antacids, ACE inhibitors and antibiotics may distort normal smell and taste. Antacid drugs, especially proton pump inhibitors, may reduce absorption of nutrients such as iron, calcium, and vitamin $B_{12}$. Numerous drugs cause constipation, including analgesics and antihypertensives (especially calcium channel blockers and beta blockers). Opioids or antidiarrheals such as Loperamide may decrease peristalsis even to the point of toxic megacolon, and similarly surgery or trauma may result in postoperative immobility, ileus, and constipation. Indeed almost any drug or illness can cause GI upset or affect bowel function, including over-the-counter preparations and alcohol. Additionally, polypharmacy, common in the elderly, may further compound side effects and interactions that could impact appetite, weight, and nutrition. Some drugs even cause weight gain and they are:

- Antipsychotics
- Antidepressants such as mirtazapine
- Diabetic drugs such as glyburide

Thus when assessing a resident admitted to LTC, one of the most critical tasks of the admitting clinician is to review and verify the list of medications they are on and eliminate all which are not necessary or appropriate to continue.

Difficulty with weight, appetite, swallowing, esophageal, gastric, and intestinal functioning may be related to numerous specific disease-related factors in addition to normal aging and medications. Among the many disorders, which could be important in this regard include:

- Endocrine disorders such as hyper-or hypothyroidism and diabetes
- Neurologic and psychiatric disorders such as Parkinson's disease or disorder, dementia, or depression
- Alcohol and other substance abuse
- Oral/dental problems
- GI disorders such as achalasia, malabsorption, peptic ulcers, and irritable or inflammatory bowel diseases
- Systemic conditions such as Sjogrens, scleroderma, heart failure, AIDS, malignancies, and infections
- Physiologic stress from acute or chronic illness

Physiologic stress resulting from almost any acute or chronic illness will increase protein and energy requirements. If the intake of nutrition is too limited for the resident's needs, unhealthy weight loss will occur and the resident will eventually succumb to acute and chronic illness. The community dwelling elderly person's ability to obtain and prepare and eat food, even in the setting of facility care, may be impeded by:

- Psychosocial and functional problems
- Sensory deficits
- Limited mobility
- Inadequate income

Although community dwelling elderly receiving home care may become nutritionally impaired because an adequate diet is unavailable, this should not be issue in LTC facilities. Simply entering and remaining in a LTC institution where three good meals a day are offered may improve nutrition and reverse weight loss in many previously undernourished elderly. Identification and modification of whatever underlying conditions remain which are modifiable may further improve nutritional status. Transition of residents between health care settings needs to be improved across the health care system so that the risk factors for weight loss can be more easily discovered. Improving communication between facilities and clinicians involved in the care of these frail elderly residents is essential for this to happen.

### Assessment of Nutritional Status

Assuming the average older adult is offered an appropriate and healthful diet in their care setting, evaluation of problems with nutrition and weight begins with a medical history, physical examination, and nutritional/laboratory assessment. Often problems with eating or weight loss will be reported by staff, family, or by the resident themselves. Body weight is the easiest screen for the nutritional status of a resident on admission to the LTC facility, and subsequently serial weights are the simplest tool for recognizing a change in the nutritional well-being of the resident. It should be noted that obtaining accurate weights in older residents may be challenging especially with bedridden or immobilized residents; a calibrated bed or chair scale can be used for residents who cannot freely stand on a standard scale.

Weight monitoring along with other vital signs is required regularly in all nursing facility residents and becomes part of the MDS (Minimum Data Set), which in turn forms the basis of various Quality Indicators. Nursing or dietary staff must, according to OBRA regulations, report 5% weight loss over the past 30 days, >10% weight loss over the past 180 days, or any observation that the resident is not eating, feeling, or swallowing well to the primary care provider in this setting [3].

TABLE 9.2. Instant nutritional assessment (INA)

| Laboratory result | Abnormal |
| --- | --- |
| Serum albumin | Less than 3.5 mg/dL |
| Total lymphocyte count | Less than 1,500/mm$^3$ |

On examining the resident, general medical history questions may be asked of the resident or caregiver such as "is there any difficulty with eating, swallowing, elimination, or with maintaining weight?" Additionally, though no single test exists that accurately identifies all residents at risk, many formal tools are available for nutritional assessment such as the VA Nutritional Risk Index and Geriatric Nutritional Index (NRI/GNRI) [4], Subjective Global Assessment (http://www.hospitalmedicine.org/geriresource/toolbox/subjective_global_assessmen.htm), and the Mini Nutritional Assessment (http://www.mna-elderly.com). But again simple weight loss itself is one of the best indicators of nutritional problems and is a proven risk factor for increased morbidity and mortality.

Another one of the simplest and most rapid tests for nutritional assessment is the Instant Nutritional Assessment (INA) (Table 9.2) [5]. The INA consists of the two laboratory parameters listed in Table 9.2, and allows one to recognize a resident at risk quickly so that early intervention can occur. It is not supposed to replace a more extensive evaluation.

### Additional Laboratory Assessment and Monitoring

In addition to a medical history and physical examination, several laboratory parameters should also be monitored in residents with weight loss, fatigue, or other symptoms of undernutrition or inadequate hydration. These include:

- CBC
- Comprehensive Metabolic Profile (which includes electrolytes, renal function, glucose, and albumin and liver functions)
- Lipids
- Thyroid functions
- Also consider vitamin $B_{12}$, and 25-hydroxy-vitamin D

Serum albumin is the single most commonly used indicator of protein undernutrition and the level is correlated with mortality in older persons [6]. Levels may also be obtained of several vitamins particularly vitamin $B_{12}$ and 25-hydroxy-vitamin D, which are common deficiencies in the elderly. These laboratory tests should be ordered not only when problems are reported but perhaps considered periodically in all elderly residents at risk for poor nutrition, and are often abnormal in the elderly requiring changes in medications or supplements. In addition to monitoring weight, laboratory values and nutritional parameters, swallowing and food intake; psychological health and physical mobility are also significantly related to nutrition and weight as residents may have physical difficulty getting out of bed, getting to the dining room, and feeding themselves.

Nursing facility residents should be evaluated for depression and dementia because they strongly impact oral intake and weight and may be the most common causes of weight loss in this population. Weight loss may be an unavoidable symptom of generalized deterioration in dementia, either in the advanced stages when the resident cannot eat, or sometimes even in early stages or preceding clinically obvious dementia. Depression was one of the most common causes of weight loss (30% of older residents) followed only by malignancies in one study [7]. Thus, a dementia and depression interview or scale is an appropriate component of the algorithm for management of undernutrition in LTC [8].

AMDA's Clinical Practice Guideline on Altered Nutritional Status ([4]; available from http://www.amda.com) recommends a process of over 20 steps to evaluate and treat nutritional issues in long-term care, beginning with a baseline evaluation of the resident's nutritional status, weight, height and BMI, and dietary preferences. The AMDA guideline recommends that risk factors for altered nutritional status including a history of recent weight or appetite change and impaired functional status, and related medical complications such as pressure ulcers should be documented. Presence of terminal illness, depression, or medications affecting taste or appetite should be noted according to this guideline. Several additional steps are listed as part of the evaluation of residents in whom weight or nutritional alterations are observed.

## WEIGHT MANAGEMENT

Achieving a healthy weight in LTC residents is controversial and may be difficult. A resident should be counseled and provided such menus and nutrition as to maintain a healthy weight neither too high nor too low. Obese residents should be put on a healthy diet with perhaps some mild caloric restriction, but dramatic weight loss should not be expected in impaired elderly residents, especially those who cannot exercise. A too-restrictive diet may be both disadvantageous to the resident's quality of life in their few remaining years, and unhealthy leading to nutritional deficiencies. The optimal weight range for nursing facility residents has not been clearly defined but is presumably the same as the general population. In agreement with generally used definitions of obesity, a recent article in the Lancet reported that overall mortality rates were lowest with a normal BMI in the range of 22.5–25 kg/m$^2$ [9]. Another recent longitudinal study of Canadian adults [10] indicated that mortality was lowest in moderately overweight individuals (BMI up to 30), perhaps because older adults need a reserve of body fat and protein stores in case of illness, while being underweight suggests illness and increased mortality risk.

Accordingly more common and concerning problems than overweight in the nursing facility are undernutrition and anorexia. Undernutrition and anorexia leads to excessive weight loss and frailty and are associated with failure to thrive, depression, low energy and activity, and poor skin integrity. Residents with weight loss over 5% during 1 month period or 10% over a 6 month period are reported as an Incident and negative Quality Indicator in the nursing facility. They need to be evaluated by the practitioner and documented not only because of their importance, but also because of the federal survey guideline requirement [4]. Nursing facility residents who lose at least 5% of their body weight have been reported to be 5–10 more times likely to die [11]; even those who regain weight still have increased mortality.

A workup for reversible causes of weight loss should be done, and identified conditions treated appropriately. GI and other diseases, medication side effects, and depression should be included in the workup. Depression and dementia commonly entail decreased appetite and food intake, and as previously discussed, medications used for these conditions (antidepressants, cholinesterase inhibitors) may affect food intake. Certain specific antidepressants such as mirtazapine and nortriptyline tend to increase appetite or weight more than others as a side effect, and may be taken advantage of therapeutically [12].

If no specific cause is found, one may reasonably call it anorexia of aging, dementia, or failure to thrive, which may be preterminal, natural, and unavoidable. It is often difficult to determine how aggressive to be with LTC residents who have a limited quantity and quality of life, as will be further discussed. Ample enjoyable food should be provided by the institution and family, with a liberalized diet and appropriate supplements.

AMDA's aforementioned Clinical Practice Guideline on Altered Nutritional Status [4] recommends that treatment should address underlying issues identified, tailoring meals/food to individual preferences and function, limiting unnecessary dietary restrictions, adding supplements, and considering appetite stimulants, and as a last resort, tube feedings on an individual basis. Individuals at facilities must further be continually monitored for maintenance and improvement of nutrition.

## NUTRITIONAL INTERVENTION

### Fluids

Adequate fluid intake for the average adult males is 3.7 L/day and 2.7 L/day for adult females. This assumes a typical temperate climate and includes total water and all beverages, plus water content of solid foods. Residents with illnesses or fever or experiencing unusual environmental conditions may require extra fluids. Oral intake is preferred; IV therapy is often not available in LTC. An interesting alternative means of hydration when the resident cannot take adequate fluids orally but is otherwise not quite ill enough to require hospitalization for i.v. therapy is hypodermoclysis (subcutaneous infusion of isotonic fluids). Note that not all lab abnormalities of electrolytes or renal function are true "dehydration" [13]. A diagnosis of dehydration may be judged, appropriately or inappropriately, as an indicator of inadequate care and a sentinel event, which is reported to regulatory agencies, so should be made only with certainty and caution in the LTC facility.

### Supplements

Food is always preferable to any artificial formulas or supplements. In addition to offering and providing sufficient fruits, vegetables, starches, healthy fats, dairy products, and fluids, a recent paper in the *Journal of the American Geriatrics Society* also suggested that increased protein intake should be generally beneficial in the elderly. Increased protein intake in the elderly is thought to maximize muscle and bone health and minimize sarcopenia and osteoporosis; increasing the RDA for protein in older individuals to 1–1.2 g/kg/day was recommended [14].

General nutritional supplements such as Ensure are tasty, safe, and beneficial for those who can eat and drink but cannot consume sufficient quantities of calories and nutrients via "normal" meals. While "real" food is preferable, one can of Ensure is approximately equal in calories (250/6 oz) and nutrition to half of an average modest meal. So based on quantity of intake, when extra calories and nutrients are needed, such supplements can be a valuable addition/alternative. Various brands/products exist with slightly different ingredients/properties, e.g., with fiber, low glucose for diabetics, or higher in fat for residents with chronic pulmonary disease. For detailed ingredients and available products in your local institution, refer to a dietitian who should be available in all health care settings. It should be noted that caloric supplements optimally might need to be given between meals to minimize appetite suppression.

Specific vitamin and mineral supplements are generally reserved only for those noted to have specific deficiencies or conditions which require or suggest the need for extra nutrients. However, it is reasonable to provide a broad-spectrum multivitamin or "senior" multivitamin for virtually all LTC residents, as most will have inadequate dietary intake of one or more nutrients. Particularly, all elderly residents at risk of osteoporosis or being treated for osteoporosis should be on calcium and vitamin D supplements. This group includes mostly women and even many men residing in LTC facilities. Recent studies have also shown that even those elderly residents on multivitamins and calcium/vitamin D supplements are often still vitamin D deficient [15]. Emerging literature correlates vitamin D deficiency with numerous health problems, not only bone health. Hypovitaminosis D is very common in elderly residents especially those in nursing facilities, due to low intake, low production and absorption, and lack of exposure to sunshine. Thus consideration should be given to supplementing all elderly LTC residents specifically with vitamin D (800+ IU/day), or at least measuring 25-OH-vitamin D levels and supplementing those who do not have sufficient levels (defined as approximately 32 ng/mL) [16], see Chapter 7 for further discussion.

**Appetite Stimulating Medicines**
All problems with eating should be evaluated not only by the physician, NP, or PA, but also by the dietitian and speech pathologist [17], in order to evaluate for swallowing problems and optimal dietary content and consistency. Adequate feeding assistance should be provided, and appealing "mealtime ambience" is also important [18]. Additionally one must make sure that dentures are worn and fitted properly.

If residents are still unable to take in adequate nutrition, cautious use of "appetite stimulant" or orexigenic medications may be considered. But, appetite stimulants like megestrol acetate (Megace®, MA) and Oxandrolone (Oxandrin®) are expensive and of questionable efficacy, and may have safety concerns [19]. All orexigenic agents are officially FDA approved only for AIDS and cancer and are used off-label in elderly residents with illnesses like dementia and failure to thrive. They have some evidence-based support in the approved indications but little in the elderly. However, in residents who cannot eat adequately they are often tried. MA is a progestational hormone, which tends to stimulate appetite and put on weight, though it is said to mostly put on fat, and beneficial outcomes on health and mortality have not been documented in the elderly. In AIDS and cancer residents, MA is officially indicated and shown to increase weight and quality of life. MA is usually well tolerated but significant side effects can occur including GI upset, diarrhea, and most significantly DVTs, which have been reported in up to 4–32%. The usual dose of 400–800 mg/day of MA (pills or oral suspension) is also expensive, up to $4,750 per year. Other agents sometimes used to increase appetite include the antidepressant mirtazapine (Remeron®) that has been noted to cause weight gain (1–6 lb) in depressed and demented residents. Dronabinol (Marinol®) is a cannabinoid derivative also approved for anorexia and nausea in cancer and AIDS patients. It has been used and tested in the elderly, with little evidence of efficacy, and can cause somnolence and seizures [20]. Particularly in the hospice or palliative care setting, steroids including prednisone (5–10 mg) and dexamethasone (4 mg twice a day) have been used to stimulate appetite in residents with diseases such as COPD.

## INDICATIONS AND USE OF FEEDING TUBES

Artificial feeding through a feeding tube may be considered if the resident presents with prolonged protein/calorie deprivation, moderate to severe weight loss, hypermetabolic or hypercatabolic state, cannot swallow adequately, and does not or cannot improve sufficiently through oral intake. Nasogastric (NG) or oroenteric tubes are the first means of access to the GI tract. A more permanent access; i.e., gastrostomy or jejunostomy tube, placed by a gastroenterologist or surgeon, may be considered if enteral support is required for more than a few weeks. Feeding tube placement should especially be considered in a LTC facility that often may not be able to manage an NG tube. The only absolute contraindication to a feeding tube is a mechanical obstruction or a resident's advance directive or stated wishes preclude artificial feeding. However problems such as aspiration and diarrhea are common, thus tube feedings should be approached and offered only with great caution as a "last resort" in a limited number of suitable residents.

Recent literature argues that tube feedings are ethically debatable and not proven effective in preventing complications such as aspiration, pressure sores, and death in elderly demented residents [21]. A recent article in *JAMDA* [22] further supported not inserting feeding tubes; approximately 5% of demented nursing facility residents that had feedings tubes inserted over a 1 year period in the hopes of preventing pneumonia, dehydration, and dysphagia had a median survival of only 56 days. The 1-year postinsertion, mortality of these residents with feeding tubes was 64%, with many residents requiring multiple hospital transfers for hospitalizations and tube replacements. Thus feeding tubes are associated with poor survival and quality of life, and should generally not be supported except when there is reasonable expectation or hope of recovery from a temporary condition such as an acute stroke. Not eating is a natural and inevitable sign of impending death; considering or needing a feeding tube should trigger recognition that the resident is likely to die within the next 2–12 months, and perhaps is more appropriate for palliative care rather than invasive and expensive procedures.

If tube feedings are decided upon, there are many different formulas that are used for enteral feedings. When they are used appropriately with the proper indication, adequate nutrition can usually be attained. Standard formulas have low residue, supply 1 kcal/mL with 13–17% of calories as protein (Ensure HN and Osmolite HN are examples). A high fiber formula, such as Jevity, contains 10–14 g of fiber per liter, 1 kcal/mL, and about 14–18% kcal as protein. High protein formulas, such as Replete or Promote, contain 20–25% as protein. Some products have added fiber, vitamins, and minerals. Residents with the problem of increased gastric residual require a lower volume. Formulas such as Two-Cal HN or Magnacal are then appropriate. They have up to 2 kcal/mL of which 14–17% is protein and 68–78% water. Vivonex Plus or Vital HN are examples of some of the hydrolyzed formulas that are available for postpyloric or jejunal feeding. In hydrolyzed formulas, medium chain triglycerides are used to replace long chain triglycerides with some formulas adding glutamine and arginine as well, which are important for bowel integrity. Renal and hepatic formulas are necessary in the face of renal and hepatic impairment respectively. On one hand, Suplena and Nepro are examples of the renal formulas which are restricted in water and sodium, potassium, magnesium, and vitamin A. On the other hand, hepatic formulas have limited aromatic amino acids and methionine, as well as are higher in branched chain amino acids.

Immune formulas such as Immune-Aid are recommended in residents who suffered great physiologic stress and those who are on ventilators in LTC ventilator facilities. They contain increased amounts of omega-3 and decreased omega-6 compounds. Immune formulas are also enriched with arginine and glutamine. A number of modular additives are available including glucose polymers, protein powder, vegetable oil, or medium chain triglyceride oil.

### Ethical and Legal Issues

The consensus of the ethical literature appears to be that withholding or withdrawing feedings when unsuccessful is no different than initiating or not initiating feeding or other medical treatment based on appropriateness and resident preferences. Again, not eating is an expected and natural part of advanced dementia and the dying process. Tube feedings unfortunately do not reduce aspiration, pneumonia, pressure sores or infections, and decrease rather than increase quality of life due to tube-related complications, mobility restrictions, and discomfort. Thus, while provision of food and fluids in the usual sense is considered basic caring and can never be withheld, artificial tube feeding should be considered as a medical intervention which has risks and benefits and may be refused or withdrawn, or even not offered when not appropriate. However, residents and families should generally be given a choice and informed consent. When residents, due to advanced illness or dementia, cannot eat or swallow safely or sufficiently, careful hand feeding as tolerated and appropriate comfort care should be offered. Palliative care and hospice are very appropriate for residents nearing the end of life due to advanced dementia or other illnesses.

Further and finally, it should be understood that undernutrition and weight loss, though sometimes judged as signs of poor care or neglect, may in some cases be natural and unavoidable despite the best efforts of clinicians, due to the resident's underlying age, functioning, and medical comorbidities. To avoid unjustified/inappropriate claims of negligence or liability, an appropriate evaluation and attempted interventions should be performed and documented, consistent with the resident's condition and wishes, the family or POA notified, and if weight loss or other nutritional complications continue and truly prove to be unavoidable, this fact and all discernable reasons for it should be clearly documented in the chart. OBRA regulations which are federal requirements for nursing facilities (F-Tags 325–327; CFR 483.25, 483.35), while quite specific and strict, form a common legal and medical standard of care with which all practitioners in LTC must be very familiar (Figure 9.1) [23].

---

**CFR 483.25**

(i) *Nutrition.* Based on a resident's comprehensive assessment, the facility must ensure that a resident Maintains acceptable parameters of nutritional status, such as body weight and protein levels, unless the resident's clinical condition demonstrates that this is not possible; and receives a therapeutic diet when there is a nutritional problem.

(j) *Hydration.* The facility must provide each resident with sufficient fluid intake to maintain proper hydration and health.

**CFR 483.35**

*Dietary services.*

    The facility must provide each resident with a nourishing, palatable, well-balanced diet that meets the daily nutritional and special dietary needs of each resident....

    The facility must employ a qualified dietitian either full-time, part-time, or on a consultant basis....

    Menus must—Meet the nutritional needs of residents in accordance with the recommended dietary allowances of the Food and Nutrition Board of the National Research Council, National Academy of Sciences

    Be prepared in advance; and

    Be followed.

(d) *Food.* Each resident receives and the facility provides—

    Food prepared by methods that conserve nutritive value, flavor, and appearance;

    Food that is palatable, attractive, and at the proper temperature;

    Food prepared in a form designed to meet individual needs; and

    Substitutes offered of similar nutritive value to residents who refuse food served.

(e) *Therapeutic diets.* Therapeutic diets must be prescribed by the attending physician.

(f) *Frequency of meals.*

- Each resident receives and the facility provides at least three meals daily, at regular times comparable to normal mealtimes in the community.
- There must be no more than 14 hours between a substantial evening meal and breakfast the following day.
- The facility must offer snacks at bedtime daily.
- When a nourishing snack is provided at bedtime, up to 16 hours may elapse between a substantial evening meal and breakfast the following day if a resident group agrees to this meal span, and a nourishing snack is served.

(g) *Assistive devices.* The facility must provide special eating equipment and utensils for residents who need them.

---

FIGURE 9.1. OBRA federal requirements related to nutrition.

## PEARLS FOR THE PRACTITIONER

- All adults in LTC require careful attention to nutrition and hydration, which are a clinical, quality of life, and legal-ethical issue and should be well documented.
- The top five causes of weight loss in elderly LTC residents (not necessarily in order) include dementia, depression, drug effects/side effects, malignancies, and GI problems.
- Optimal health and longevity is achieved at a BMI of about 22.5–30.
- Innumerable drugs and diseases affect nutritional status and weight.
- Weight and laboratory monitoring for causes of weight loss should be performed regularly in all LTC residents.

- Almost all elderly LTC residents should receive a multivitamin, calcium and vitamin D, and $B_{12}$ supplements if blood levels indicate deficiency.
- Nutritional supplements such as Ensure can supplement inadequate calorie and protein intake.
- Hypodermoclysis may be used to augment fluid intake and avoid dehydration in the short-term situation.
- Restricted diets are generally not advisable or tolerable in LTC residents and should be avoided when not absolutely necessary.
- Tube feedings are ineffective in reducing morbidity and mortality in demented residents and should preferably be limited to carefully selected and willing residents needing temporary nutritional support during a potentially reversible illness such as stroke.
- OBRA regulations and good medical care require adequate nutrition and hydration unless the resident's clinical condition or advance directive makes this impossible.
- Incorporate directives regarding nutrition and hydration in advance directives and advance care planning.

## WEBSITES
- Official OBRA Nursing Home Regulations http://www.access.gpo.gov/nara/cfr/waisidx_02/42cfr483_02.html
- Food and Nutrition Information Center of the US Department of Agriculture http://fnic.nal.usda.gov
- Institute of Medicine http://www.iom.edu
- American Medical Directors Association http://www.amda.com
- American Geriatrics Society http://www.americangeriatrics.org
- American Psychiatric Association http://psychiatryonline.com

## REFERENCES
1. Morley JE, Silver AJ. Nutritional issues in nursing home care. Ann Intern Med 1995;123:850–859.
2. American Medical Directors Association. Dehydration and Fluid Maintenance. Clinical Practice Guideline, 2001, Rev. 2009.
3. American Medical Directors Association. Altered Nutritional Status. Clinical Practice Guideline, 2001.
4. Bouillanne O, Morineau G, Dupont C, et al. Geriatric nutritional risk index: a new index for evaluating at-risk elderly medical patients. Am J Clin Nutr 2005;82(4):777–783.
5. Seltzer MH, Bastidas A, Cooper DM, et al. Instant nutritional assessment. JPEN J Parenter Enteral Nutr 1979;3:157–159.
6. Corti MC, Guralnik JM, Salive ME, Sorkin JD. Serum albumin level and physical disability as predictors of mortality in older patients. JAMA 1994;272:1036–1042.
7. Wilson MM, Vaswani S, Liu D, et al. Prevalence and causes of undernutrition in medical. Am J Med 1998;104:56.

8. Thomas DR, Ashmen W, Morley JE, et al. Nutritional management in long-term care: development of a clinical guideline. J Gerontol Med Sci 2000;55A:M725–M734.
9. Prospective Studies Collaboration. Body mass index and cause specific mortality in 900000 adults: collaborative analysis of 57 prospective studies. Lancet 2009;373:1083–1096.
10. Orpana HM, Berthelot JM, Kaplan MS, et al. BMI and mortality: results from a national longitudinal study of Canadian adults. Obesity 2010;18(1):214–218.
11. Thomas DR. But is it malnutrition? JAMDA 2009;10(5):295–297.
12. American Psychiatric Association Practice Guideline for the Treatment of Patient Residents with Major Depressive Disorder, 2nd Edition. Available online at http://www.psychiatryonline.com/pracGuide/pracGuideTopic_7.aspx. Accessed 26 June, 2009.
13. Thomas DR, Tariq SH, et al. Physician misdiagnosis of dehydration in older adults. JAMDA 2003;4:251–254.
14. Gaffney-Stomberg E, Insogna KL, Rodriguez NR, Kerstetter JE. Increasing dietary protein requirements for elderly people for optimal muscle and bone health. JAGS 2009;57:1073–1079.
15. Goldberg TH, Hassan T, Grant R. High prevalence of vitamin D deficiency in elderly nursing home patients despite vitamin supplements (abstract). JAMDA 2008;9(3):B15.
16. Morley JE. Should all long-term care residents receive vitamin D? JAMDA 2007;8:69–70.
17. Vitale CA, Monteleoni C, et al. Strategies for improving care for patients with advanced dementia and eating problems: optimizing care through physician and speech pathologist collaboration. Ann LTC 2009;17(5):32–39.
18. Nijs K, Graaf C, Staveren W, et al. Malnutrition and mealtime ambience in nursing homes. JAMDA 2009;10:226–229.
19. Yeh S, Lovitt S, Schuster MW. Pharmacological treatment of geriatric cachexia: evidence and safety in perspective. JAMDA 2007;8(6):363–377.
20. Miller LJ, et al. Pharmacological treatment of undernutrition in the geriatric patient. Consult Pharm 2002;17:739–747.
21. Finucane TE, Christmas C, Travis K. Tube feeding in patients with advanced dementia: a review of the evidence. JAMA 1999;282:1365–1370.
22. Kuo S, Rhodes R, Mitchell SL, et al. Natural history of feeding tube use in nursing home residents with advanced dementia. JAMDA 2009;10:264–270.
23. American Medical Directors Association. Synopsis of Federal Regulations in the Nursing Facility: Implications for Attending Physicians and Medical Directors, Rev. 2007. Available online at http://www.amda.com.
24. Miller ER, Pastor-Barriuso R, Dalal D, et al. Meta-analysis: high dosage vitamin E supplementation may increase all cause mortality. Ann Intern Med 2005;142(1):37–46.
25. Fick DM, Cooper JW, Wade WE, Waller JL, Maclean JR, Beers MH. Updating the Beers criteria for potentially inappropriate medication use in older adults: results of a US consensus panel of experts. Arch Intern Med 2003;163:2716–2724.

# Chapter 10
# Wound Care

Andrew Rosenzweig and Mary Lee

**Keywords:** Wound development • Wound types • Wound prevention • Wound management • Pressure ulcers

## INTRODUCTION

The growing medical and psychosocial implications of wound care reflect the increasing complexities facing practitioners in long-term care (LTC). Wounds are classified as a medical problem, a geriatric syndrome, or part of a larger systems-based problem. Understanding wound formation and healing is critical to preventing and treating wounds. Treatment plans for wound care need to address not only the wound itself, but also complexities ranging from comorbidities and medications that may hinder healing or predispose patients to wounds. The psychosocial and ethical principles of caring for patients who may no longer be able to participate in their own care also play critical roles in treatment success or failure. Although wounds may have more than one etiology, the four common types of wounds will be discussed: pressure, diabetic, ischemic or arterial, and venous. Pressure ulcers will be emphasized due to their implications in the LTC environment.

More than 20% of residents living in a nursing facility for 2 or more years will develop at least one pressure ulcer [1]. The estimated prevalence of pressure ulcers among patients residing in these facilities has been reported as 2.3–28% and has been an increasingly common reason for litigation [2]. The annual risk of pressure ulceration in patients with neurologic impairment is 5–8%, with a lifetime risk of approximately 85% and a mortality rate of 8% [3]. For hospitalized patients, the presence of a pressure ulcer increases nursing workload for that patient by 50% and adds approximately $20,000 in costs. The treatment of pressure ulcers in the United States is estimated to cost more than $1 billion annually [4].

The Centers for Medicare and Medicaid Services (CMS) implemented a new payment system, effective October 1, 2008, that would cease paying hospitals for "preventable complications," including stage III and IV pressure ulcers [5]. In fiscal year 2006, pressure ulcers had the highest prevalence of the preventable complications, with 322,946 Medicare cases that had an added average cost of $40,381 to each admission [6]. However, in the November 2004 "Guidance to Surveyors for Long Term Care Facilities," CMS acknowledged that *some* pressure ulcers are "unavoidable" [7]. The LTC facility is required to follow strict guidelines for evaluating pressure ulcer risk factors and implementing preventive interventions consistent with each resident's needs and goals. If a pressure ulcer develops despite the facility's best efforts to prevent it, the pressure ulcer is determined to be unavoidable. CMS has not applied this standard in other health care settings [8].

## RISK FACTORS FOR WOUND DEVELOPMENT

Wounds develop when causative factors increase a patient's susceptibility to developing a wound or persist when prolonging factors impair the healing of an existing wound [9–12]. These risk factors for wound development and prolongation are seen in Table 10.1. Managing pressure on the wound area is a cornerstone of both wound prevention and care. Because pressure is a primary causal factor in pressure ulcer development, a plan for repositioning needs to be tailored to the needs of the individual at risk.

- Seats should be padded with air, foam, or gel cushioning while avoiding donut-shaped devices [9].
- Patients at risk of pressure ulcer development or delayed healing should have a static support surface such as a foam overlay or gel mattress placed on their standard mattress.
- Residents at highest risk of pressure ulcer development, who completely compress a static surface or who fail to heal, should be placed on a dynamic surface [7, 9].
- A person should never be placed directly on their greater trochanter for more than momentary positioning. Padding (i.e., heel or "bunny" boots, egg crates, heel lifts, suspension devices, etc.) or off-loading may be required to redistribute pressure on heels and elbows because of their small surface area [7, 9].

TABLE 10.1. Risk factors

| Risk factor | Examples | Notes |
| --- | --- | --- |
| Comorbid conditions | Diabetes, end-stage renal disease, thyroid disease | Conditions that increase risk of wounds by affecting patient's immune response, skin integrity, or environment risks |
| Drugs | Steroids, antimetabolites | Drugs that hinder proliferation of fibroblasts and collagen synthesis |
| History of healed ulcer | History of stage III or IV ulcer | Patient may still have the risk factors that predisposed to these ulcers |
| Impaired blood flow | Atherosclerosis, lower-extremity arterial insufficiency | Decrease blood flow to wounds for healing |
| Impaired or decreased mobility and functional ability | Bed bound, decreased lower extremity use, altered mental status (e.g., dementia) | Environmental risk of developing wounds due to increased pressure on skin, friction, or shear from transfer by others |
| Malnutrition and hydration deficit | | Protein–calorie malnutrition and deficiencies of vitamins A, C, and zinc impair normal wound-healing mechanisms |

Adapted from American Medical Directors Association [9]

Because wounded skin has only about 80% of the tensile properties of intact skin, it is at increased risk of breakdown. Because of this and other factors, people with a history of pressure ulcers are five times more likely to develop another pressure ulcer as compared to others [13]. Dermatologic conditions and contractures can also increase wound formation.

The lack of blood supply seen in atherosclerosis, especially when it affects the peripheral vasculature, hinders healing by dampening the recruitment process needed for new skin formation as well as depriving the injured area of oxygen and nutrition. Diabetes not only causes atherosclerosis, but also a peripheral neuropathy related to long-standing and/or poorly controlled diabetes. This peripheral neuropathy is the primary pathologic process responsible for the increased risk of foot wounds seen in diabetes. Microvascular disease and suboptimal glycemic control found in diabetes also increase the risk of foot wounds. All of these pathologic processes combine to make diabetes an independent risk factor for wound formation. It is estimated that among patients with diabetes, 15% will develop a foot wound and 12–24% of those with a foot wounds will require amputation [2, 14]. Even with successful treatment and wound healing, the recurrence rate of diabetic foot wounds is 66% [14].

End-stage renal disease and thyroid disease are also known to be comorbid medical conditions that are independent risk factors for wound formation. Wound formation may occur when medications such as steroids and antimetabolites hinder proliferation of fibroblasts and collagen synthesis placing an individual at risk [4].

The cognitive impairment which is seen in 45–67% of assisted living residents and 69% of nursing facility residents creates another array of risk factors for skin breakdown [15–17]. Because patients with dementia often have functional disabilities, poor nutritional status, and a higher incidence of skin exposure to pressure, friction, or shear, they are at higher risk for wound development. Exposure of the skin to urinary or fecal incontinence increasing the incidence of wound development, though, is controversial. Although intuitively it makes sense that urinary incontinence would increase the risk for wound development, data thus far showing a causal relationship have been inconclusive [9]. On the other hand, secondary data analysis suggests a possible association between fecal incontinence and pressure ulcer development, likely related to skin exposure to bile acid and gastrointestinal enzymes [18].

The poor nutritional status frequently seen in patients with advanced dementia is another risk factor for wound development. Dehydration, deficiencies of arginine, vitamins A, C, and zinc, and protein–calorie malnutrition have been implicated in impairing wound healing. Skin integrity and wound healing are impaired when decreased tissue perfusion occurs in dehydration as well. Severe protein–calorie malnutrition hinders tissue regeneration, the inflammatory reaction, and immune function. Studies have linked malnutrition to wound development and impaired wound healing [19]. Nutritional supplementation in those at risk or already suffering from a pressure ulcer is a controversial topic. Enteral nutritional support is believed to significantly reduce the risk of developing pressure ulcers in selected patients, by up to 25% in some studies. The benefits of nutritional support in facilitating wound healing are still being debated [20–22]. The benefit of vitamin C supplementation in wound healing is also disputed. For example, two well-designed randomized controlled trials compared high-dose vitamin C with either low-dose vitamin C or placebo and had opposite results [23].

Any discovered wounds should prompt an assessment and a subsequent treatment plan that includes a timeline for future wound reassessment. Wound assessment involves a complete medical evaluation of the patient including careful attention to conditions that may affect wound development and healing. A comprehensive wound history should note the onset and duration of a wound and any previous wound care. Assessment of a person's cognitive status, behavior, financial resources, and access to caregivers are essential when developing a treatment plan.

When determining a person's risk for developing or chance of healing a wound, assessment of their environment is also critical. Frequency of repositioning, surfaces, turning schedules, transferring techniques, and apparatus present (such as assistive devices, trapeze, bed rails, and padding) all impact wound development and repair [9]. Risk assessment scales may increase awareness, but have limited predictive ability and effectiveness in pressure ulcer prevention [24]. A meta-analysis of 33 studies demonstrated a lack of evidence for risk assessment scales in decreasing pressure ulcer incidence, but the scales did increase preventative interventions [25]. The two most commonly used tools are the Braden and Norton Scales. No conclusive evidence exists showing that one is superior to the other.

- The Braden scale (see website below) evaluates six categories: sensory perception, moisture, activity, mobility, nutrition, friction/shear for predicting pressure sore development.
- Research has shown that patients with scores of 18 or less on the Braden scale are at risk for the development of pressure sores [26].
- The Norton Score is another commonly used tool for assessing pressure ulcer risk that evaluates five categories: physical condition, mental condition, activity, mobility, and incontinence.

Most nursing facilities use a pressure ulcer report to document identified wounds: location, stage, measurement, and description. Pressure ulcer reports fulfill standardized documentation as mandated by both state and federal (F314) regulations in the nursing facility. When documenting wounds, the clinician should document the number, location, and size (length, width, and depth) of wounds and assess for the presence of exudates, odor, sinus tracts, necrosis or eschar formation, tunneling/undermining, infection, healing (granulation and epithelialization), and wound margins. If the wound is a pressure ulcer, the clinician should determine the stage of the ulcer according to the National Pressure Ulcer Advisory Panel (NPUAP) Staging System (see Table 10.2).

TABLE 10.2. 2007 NPUAP staging of pressure ulcers

| Stage | Definition | Comment |
|---|---|---|
| Suspected deep tissue injury (SDTI) | Pressure-related necrosis of soft tissue with intact overlying skin | Discoloration (crimson → purple), changes in temperature, texture, tenderness. May progress rapidly |
| Stage I | Localized area of nonblancheable erythema. Skin is intact and sandwiched between a bony prominence and external surface | Clinically similar to SDTI. May be harder to detect as skin pigmentation deepens |
| Stage II | Partial thickness destruction of dermis characterized as either a shallow open ulcer with a crimson wound bed (without slough or bruising) or as an intact or ruptured fluid-filled blister | Do not use to describe skin tears, tape burns, dermatitis, maceration, or excoriation |
| Stage III | Full thickness tissue loss. Subcutaneous fat may be visible, but bone, tendon, or muscle is not exposed | Slough may be present. May include tunneling or undermining. Depth varies by anatomical location |
| Stage IV | Full thickness tissue loss characterized by exposed bone, tendon, or muscle. Extensive destruction, necrosis, or damage to the muscle, bone, or supporting structures | Slough or eschar may be present on some parts of the wound bed. Often include undermining and tunneling |
| Unstageable | Full thickness tissue loss which cannot be staged until slough or eschar in the ulcer bed is remove | Do *not* remove eschar present on heels |

Adapted from the National Pressure Ulcer Advisory Panel. Updated staging system. Available at http://www.npuap.org/pr2.htm. Accessed June 1, 2009

After an initial assessment on admission to a nursing facility, weekly reassessments should occur for the first 4 weeks, followed by quarterly assessments. Reassessments should also occur if there is a change or deterioration in the resident [27]. Various resident assessment instruments exist that can be utilized by nursing staff to monitor daily and/or weekly progress. Every nursing facility is required to develop and implement its own comprehensive wound care plan in accordance with CMS regulations.

## TYPES OF WOUNDS

A wound may not necessarily fit into one of the four general categories of wounds (pressure ulcer, diabetic, arterial, and venous), but may be a mix of two or more etiologies. Usually, the type of wound can be distinguished by its location, combined with inspection of the wound and the patient's clinical history. If the wound type remains uncertain, laboratory and/or radiographic studies may help clarify the wound type. For example, in lower extremity ulcers an ankle–brachial index or Doppler arterial studies can help determine whether a lower extremity ulcer is caused by vascular insufficiency, pressure, or a combination of the two.

### Pressure Ulcers

- Ninety-five percent develop on the lower body, 65% in the pelvic area, and 30% on the lower extremities. Other common pressure ulcer sites include the coccyx, heel, ischium, iliac rest, lateral foot, lateral malleolus, sacrum, and trochanter.
- A pressure ulcer is a localized area of damaged or necrosed tissue that develops when soft tissue is compressed between a bony prominence and an external surface for a prolonged period of time.
- Pressure alone or pressure combined with external forces of shearing, friction, or moisture can cause a pressure ulcer.
- Pressure applied to the skin in excess of arteriolar pressure leads to tissue ischemia.
- Pressure ulcers can range from nonblancheable erythema of intact skin to deep ulcers extending down to the bone.

### Diabetic Wounds

- Commonly occur at metatarsal heads.
- Diabetic wounds are due to vascular complications of diabetes mellitus including decreased healing and peripheral neuropathy.
- Diabetic wounds are typically painless; therefore the wound is usually not noticed until symptoms of infection such as odor, fever, or chills.

- When inspecting diabetic ulcers, providers should probe the depth of the wound with a sterile instrument to help determine if any undermining or osteomyelitis is present [28].

**Ischemic Wounds**
- Typically occur at lower extremities, but can also occur at upper extremities.
- Ischemic wounds are due to decreased arterial blood flow seen in peripheral vascular disease, diabetes mellitus, and smoking.
- Clinical signs of arterial insufficiency that often precede an ischemic wound include: a cold, pale or cyanotic foot, absence of digital hair, and thin atrophic skin.
- Ischemic wounds present as a painful wound with discrete borders, a "punched out" appearance, and wet or dry gangrene.
- The base of the ulcer can be covered with a dry black brown to brown eschar or appear pale pink and fibrous.

**Venous Wounds**
- Commonly seen on the lower extremities.
- Venous wounds are different from ischemic wounds because venous wounds are caused by peripheral edema due to venous insufficiency/stasis, medications, or organ dysfunction (i.e., heart, liver, and kidney disease) [29].
- Venous wounds are less painful than ischemic wounds.
- Venous stasis wounds have irregular borders and can be seen clustered together with associated hyperpigmentation changes.

## PREVENTION

Paramount to wound care management is prevention. The Agency for Health Care Policy and Research (AHCPR) published two companion practice guidelines in 1994 with recommendations for prediction, prevention, and early treatment of pressure ulcers in adults [30, 31]. These guidelines were pioneering in their scope and are still widely utilized today because they are applicable in many LTC settings. The first step recommended for preventing pressure ulcers by the Institute for Healthcare Improvement (IHI) is to identify patients at risk, then implement prevention strategies in these selected patients [26]. The IHI suggests "six essential elements of pressure ulcer prevention" in its guidelines.
The six steps are [26, 32]:

- Conduct a pressure ulcer admission assessment for all patients
- Reassess risk for all patients daily
- Inspect skin daily

- Manage moisture
- Optimize nutrition and hydration
- Minimize pressure

The IHI also recommends that prevention measures include a comprehensive treatment plan with risk factor modification, multidisciplinary interactions, functional and environmental adjustments, and a psychosocial evaluation. Evaluating and optimizing any of the residents' predisposing conditions and comorbidities can help prevent wounds from developing [9]. Daily inspection during any bathing or personal care, as well as schedules for turning and positioning patients, has been shown to help prevent wound appearance. Special attention should also be paid to at-risk areas such as bony prominences so that pressure on these areas is minimized. Frequent repositioning or off-loading may be required in those deemed to be at higher risk for ulcer development. The supine patient should be maintained at the lowest head elevation possible as an elevation ≥30° provides as much pressure as being in a seated position [33]. Repositioning every 4 h has been shown in randomized, controlled trials to be as effective as 2-h intervals in improving wound healing. Care should be taken to minimize shearing or friction during repositioning and lift devices may be necessary to prevent soft tissue injury.

Research suggests that inadequate hydration and nutrition are predisposing conditions strongly associated with pressure ulcer development [34]. The caloric intake of 30–35 kcal/kg and daily protein intake of 1.2–1.5 g/kg of body weight are recommended for nutritionally compromised patients who have or are at risk of pressure ulcers [5]. Adequate hydration is provided by 30–35 mL of fluid per kilogram body weight per day or 1 mL of fluid per calorie feed for persons receiving enteral tube feeding [9]. (For a more in-depth discussion on nutrition please see the Chap. 9.)

In clinical circumstances such as metastatic cancer, multiple organ failure, cachexia, severe vascular compromise, and terminal illness, unavoidable wounds may develop [35]. The clinician should document the reasons why preventive interventions may not be appropriate or feasible, such as frequent repositioning causing intractable pain. In these situations, it is important to inform the caretaker and document relevant issues.

## STAGING

The American Medical Directors Association (AMDA) utilizes the guidelines set forth by the NPUAP to define, classify, and stage pressure ulcers. The last update was published in February 2007 and is summarized in Table 10.2. Staging is based on the extent of observable tissue damage [36]. The latest version of the NPUAP guidelines includes the classically described stages I–IV along with two adjunctive stages ("suspected deep tissue injury" and "unstageable") utilized to more accurately classify pressure ulcers (see website below). Reverse staging does not accurately characterize ulcer healing and should not be used in this manner. For example, a lesion may be referred to as a "healing stage IV," but it cannot be described as progressing from a stage IV to a stage III with therapy. An ulcer covered by eschar should be categorized as a Stage IV until the eschar has been debrided.

Despite the theoretical simplicity of this system, confusion regarding its use and interpretation still exists leading to interpractitioner variability in staging ulcers as seen in a study by Defloor et al. [37] The NPUAP guidelines have been used (at times inappropriately) as quality of care indicators, to document progression or treatment of existing ulcers or to identify mismanagement [36].

## MANAGEMENT

In wound care treatment the burden should be weighed against the benefit. Communication with the patient and family/caregivers is important and their wishes should be identified and respected. But, it is also imperative to establish realistic expectations for wound healing. As with any medical treatment, if a patient with decision-making capacity declines or does not adhere to the recommended treatment, the providers should offer alternatives and document them in the medical record with any patient's deferral.

## TREATMENT

Treatment ensues after risk factor modifications and preventative interventions have been exhausted. Because numerous risk factors present in the LTC population impede healing by a multitude of mechanisms, most often the interdisciplinary approach is required for optimal wound care. Table 10.3 provides some commonly encountered barriers to optimal wound treatment. A team in conjunction with the patient and/or appropriate decision-maker should develop a wound care treatment plan. Potential causal factors should continue to be identified and addressed including systemic factors and comorbidities [9]. This should include optimizing nutritional status, addressing psychosocial issues, and managing pain and infection. Managing pain and infection, both local and systemic, are crucial to effective wound care. If necrotic tissue exists, it should be removed in order to allow viable tissue to granulate and wound healing to occur.

TABLE 10.3. Wound care challenges

| Wound type | Challenge to wound care | Standard medical treatment approach | Treatment |
|---|---|---|---|
| Pressure | Excess pressure and shear/friction forces | Pressure relief | Topical: packing with hydrogel or saline. Devices: pressure reduction mattresses, padding overlying bony prominences |
| Ischemic | Inadequate blood flow | Revascularization or surgical removal/correction | Topical: dry or antimicrobial |
| Venous | Venous insufficiency causing edema | Correct incompetent valves, reduce edema | Topical: moist environment |
| Diabetic | Peripheral neuropathy causing pressure points on feet | Offload pressure, careful routine evaluation of feet | Topical: pack with antimicrobial solution or hydrogel |

Adapted from Takahashi et al. [38]

Wounds should be cleansed and irrigated to remove necrotic debris at each dressing change. Necrotic tissue impedes the healing process and may represent a nidus for infection. Saline should be chosen for wound irrigation over cytotoxic antiseptic agents such as Dakin's solution, iodine, and acid-based and alcohol-based solutions that can retard healing [9]. Be sure to assess for pain and minimize mechanical force applied to the wound during dressing changes. Any dry black eschar on heels should not be debrided as long as it is not tender, fluctuant, erythematous, or suppurative. Wounds with no surrounding local infection can have an occlusive hydrocolloid dressing placed over them allowing the eschar to autodigest itself via autolytic debridement [9]. Enzymatic debridement involves applying a topical debriding agent such as collagenase or papain–urea to devitalized tissue. This may cause some degree of pain, but is more tolerable than surgical debridement. When various dressings are allowed to dry and then extract adherent tissue with dressing removal, mechanical debridement is being used. When a wound is exceptionally large, malodorous, or there is a large degree of necrotic tissue, more aggressive measures may be required. If all other methods of debridement have failed and/or timing is critical because of worsening infection and imminent sepsis, surgical debridement may be necessary. Obviously, the risks of an invasive procedure with sharp debridement, albeit relatively low, must be weighed against the benefits in the context of the individual.

Thousands of different products exist that can cover the wound. But a chosen dressing must be able to maintain a moist wound bed, keep surrounding skin dry, and limit contamination of the wound so that healing can take place [9]. The ideal wound bed is not too moist or dry. The wound characteristics as well as the wound coverings' cost, ease of use, and potential benefit or burden should all be considered when choosing a product [9]. The basic principles of wound care include not only tailoring the care to the individual wound, but also using transparent, impermeable films on wounds that could be contaminated by urinary or fecal incontinence. These dressings need to be attached with waterproof tape while limiting trauma to intact skin when removing the dressing. Deep wounds and wounds where tunneling or undermining is present should be lightly packed with moist gauze or cavity filler. Packing should be changed regularly to avoid contamination with bacteria. Hydrogels are useful for deep wounds with little exudate, whereas alginates, which help absorb fluid, are useful when significant exudate is present. Overly dry intact skin should be protected with moisturizers. Silver-impregnated dressings provide broad-spectrum antimicrobial coverage in lesions that are colonized or particularly susceptible to becoming infected based on location, mechanism, or clinical context. Collagen dressings promote the development of new granulation tissue.

Several novel modalities have recently been developed with mixed results in the LTC population. These include growth factors (fibroblast growth factor, platelet-derived growth factor, and nerve growth factor), electrotherapy, and negative pressure wound therapy. One type of negative pressure therapy is vacuum-assisted closure (VAC). VAC is a closed system that uses negative pressure to drain wound fluid away and approximate wound edges, thereby promoting wound healing. Although this therapy may improve healing, it has not been shown to be cost effective [38]. Hyperbaric oxygen therapy increases oxygen tension at the wound site, but has not demonstrated improved healing rates. Its use has also been limited by high cost and lack of availability. Other novel therapies that have proven successful in research protocols and in published studies are currently being utilized including noncontact normothermic wound therapy, ultrasound/ultrasonic misting, as well as infrared and ultraviolet light therapy.

## COMPLICATIONS

Pressure ulcers in LTC settings are associated with a multitude of short and long-term medical and psychosocial complications [39]. These may have a significant and damaging impact on a person's sense of well-being by worsening quality of life with isolation, increased dependence, pain, and disfigurement [40–42]. Pain occurs when sensory nerve endings are irritated near the lesion during wound care and infection. Infection is a major wound complication that spans the spectrum of scenarios beginning with clinically insignificant bacterial colonization, occasionally advancing to local cellulitis, deep tissue infection, osteomyelitis, and sepsis. Treating wounds for infection locally can be difficult because they may be chronically contaminated and/or colonized and antibiotic agents are often caustic to cells and growth factors required for healing [43]. Osteomyelitis is relatively more common in this population because pressure sores frequently occur over bony prominences [43]. Pressure ulcers in LTC residents have been shown to increase morbidity and mortality. Bone infection is associated with higher levels of morbidity because of the need for long-term antibiotics, extraradiographic imaging, surgical manipulation, and the associated pain and immobility. Because skin breakdown can be a portal for bacteremia, nursing facility residents with wounds have been shown to be at higher risk of sepsis and death as well. Mortality rates as high as 50% have been associated with nursing facility residents with pressure ulcers and sepsis [44]. Nursing facility residents with pressure ulcers have also been shown two to three times more likely to die than their cohort with a mortality rate in one study of 50% at 1 year as compared to 27% [43]. The length of hospitalization for nursing facility residents with pressure ulcers is also approximately two to three times greater than those without [45]. Anyone with a large wound or massive amount of drainage should be monitored for dehydration and metabolic derangements. Any patient with a wound should be monitored for fistula formation, heterotopic calcification, and squamous cell carcinoma.

Wound prevention and management also has financial implications. Some estimates triple the cost of care for a nursing home resident if a pressure ulcer is present [43]. As of October 2008, new CMS guidelines under Federal Tag 314 state that a nursing facility may be cited if they fail to prevent new pressure ulcer development, promote healing of previously identified ulcers, or fail to prevent progression to or development of Stage IV ulcers unless they are deemed unavoidable [5, 46].

## DOCUMENTATION

Accurate and standardized documentation is vital for wound care. The AMDA has recently updated its clinical guidelines for managing wounds (Table 10.4). For optimal wound care, AMDA recommends that timelines for assessment, descriptions, care plans, and treatments of wounds should be standardized. A timeline should include an initial assessment leading to a wound care plan that has the timing of reevaluations based on the severity of the wound. As previously discussed, a thorough skin examination should take place on admission to LTC that identifies and documents any existing wounds. Regularly scheduled 2–3 week reevaluations should be performed by trained staff members who know how to follow a consistent procedure for wound care and its documentation. Multidisciplinary teams integrating the recommendations from the wound care nurse, dietitian, physical and/or occupation therapist, and doctor are recommended in the nursing facility and are optimal in any LTC setting [9]. In home care or in the assisted living environment, this multidisciplinary wound care can be accomplished when the physician or physician and facility staff teams up with members of the home care agency. Documentation should also include characteristics of

TABLE 10.4. Recommended components for documentation of wounds

| Parameter | Description |
| --- | --- |
| Type | Pathology or disease etiology |
|  | Duration of wound |
|  | If applicable, what setting it occurred |
| Size | Measurement in centimeters: length, width, depth |
| Color | Define in percentage, with red indicating amount of granulation tissue, yellow indicating amount of slough present, and black indicating necrotic tissue or eschar |
| Exudates | Describe absence or presence of exudates |
|  | If exudates present, describe if serous, serosanguinous, sanguineous, or purulent |
| Odor | Determine after wound is cleaned, if odor is present or absent |
| Peri-wound tissue | Describe if viable, macerated, inflamed, or hyperkeratotic |
| Undermining | Describe absence or presence of tunneling or sinus tracts |

Adapted from American Medical Directors Association [9]

existing wounds, as listed in Table 10.4. Turning and positioning schedules, as well as any wound and/or pertinent resident complications, should be documented as well.

## SUMMARY

The prevalence of wounds in LTC residents has increased in proportion to the worldwide explosion of the geriatric demographic. Wounds represent a geriatric syndrome with large medical, psychosocial, and economic implications. Given the increase in morbidity, mortality, and costs related to wounds, they have become a top priority in LTC regulation at a national level. LTC residents are more susceptible to developing pressure ulcers due to impaired mobility, nutrition status, and comorbidities including diabetes, cardiovascular disease, and dementia. If prevention through risk factor modification has failed or a resident is found to have a wound on admission, assessment includes thorough and timely evaluation of the resident and their environment in addition to actual wound characteristics and proper NPUAP staging if appropriate. Management requires a multidisciplinary approach based on frequent assessment and use of wound-specific modalities. The functional status of the resident, goals of care, and risk:benefit ratio factor into the treatment plan. In all situations, pain should be assessed and managed. Care should be taken to reduce pressure, friction, shearing forces, moisture, exposure to bacteria, and pain. Preventing and treating wounds can reduce medical and psychosocial complications, decrease morbidity and mortality, and improve quality of life in appropriate LTC residents.

## PEARLS FOR THE PRACTITIONER

- As the complexities of LTC have increased, along with the growth of populations like the frail elderly, the prevalence of wounds has increased as well.
- A multidisciplinary team in conjunction with the patient and their family should ideally develop a holistic wound care treatment plan that considers available resources and incorporates all relevant resident factors into its practical goals of care, as well as appropriate wound-specific care and adequate pain control.
- All wounds are not pressure ulcers. Thus, the NPUAP guidelines *cannot* be applied to traumatic, ischemic, venous, or diabetic wounds.
- Reverse staging does not accurately characterize ulcer healing and should not be used.
- All ulcers covered by eschar should be categorized as a Stage IV until the eschar has been debrided.

- Any dry, black eschar on a heel should *not* be debrided if it is nontender, nonfluctuant, nonerythematous, and nonsuppurative.
- Not all ulcers are preventable. Some pressure ulcers are unavoidable due to overwhelming burden of disease and terminal illness.

## WEBSITES
- Home of the Braden Scale http://www.bradenscale.com
- National Pressure Ulcer Advisory Panel http://www.npuap.org/
- American Medical Directors Association (AMDA) www.amda.com/ http://www.amda.com/tools/library/ref-pressureulcers.cfm
- Institute for Healthcare Improvement http://www.ihi.org/IHI/Programs/Campaign/PressureUlcers.htm
- Centers for Medicare & Medicaid Services. "Guidance to Surveyors for Long Term Care Facilities" http://www.cms.hhs.gov/transmittals/Downloads/R4SOM.pdf
- Wound, Ostomy and Continence Nurses Society http://www.wocn.org/index.php
- Wound Research http://www.woundsresearch.com

## REFERENCES
1. Brandeis GH, Morris JN, Nash DJ, Lipsitz LA. The epidemiology and natural history of pressure ulcers in elderly nursing home residents. JAMA. 1990;264(22):2905–2909.
2. Bergstrom N, Horn SD, Smout RJ, et al. The national pressure ulcer long-term care study: Outcomes of pressure ulcer treatments in long-term care. J Am Geriatr Soc. 2005;53(10):1721–1729.
3. Bergstrom N. Litigation or redesign: Improving pressure ulcer prevention. *J Am Geriatr Soc*. 2005;53(9):1627–1629.
4. Stillman R. Wound care. Available at: http://emedicine.medscape.com/article/194018-overview june 14, 2009.
5. Centers for Medicare and Medicaid Services. Action plan for further improvement of nursing home quality. Available at: www.cms.hhs.gov/quality/nhqi/2009 june 14, 2009.
6. Centers for Medicare and Medicaid Services (CMS), HHS. Medicare program: Changes to the hospital inpatient prospective payment systems and fiscal year 2008 rates. Fed Regist. 2007;72:47379.
7. Centers for Medicare and Medicaid Services. Guidance to surveyors for long term care facilities. CMS manual. Washington, DC: CMS; 2004.
8. WOCN Society. Wound, ostomy, and continence nurses society position statement on avoidable versus unavoidable pressure ulcers. J Wound Ostomy Continence Nurs. 2009;36(4):378–381.
9. American Medical Directors Association. Pressure ulcers in the long-term care setting clinical practice guideline. Columbia, MD: American Medical Directors Association; 2008.

10. Gosnell DJ. An assessment tool to identify pressure sores. Nurs Res. 1973;22(1):55–59.
11. Ayello EA, Braden B. How and why to do pressure ulcer risk assessment. Adv Skin Wound Care. 2002;15(3):125–131.
12. Bergstrom N, Braden B. A prospective study of pressure sore risk among institutionalized elderly. J Am Geriatr Soc. 1992;40(8):747–758.
13. Horn SD, Bender SA, Ferguson ML, et al. The national pressure ulcer long-term care study: Pressure ulcer development in long-term care residents. J Am Geriatr Soc. 2004;52(3):359–367.
14. Singh N, Armstrong DG, Lipsky BA. Preventing foot ulcers in patients with diabetes. JAMA. 2005;293(2):217–228.
15. American Health Care Association. Medical condition – mental status. CMS OSCAR data current surveys. 2007.
16. U.S. Department of Health and Human Services, Centers for Medicare and Medicaid Services. Nursing home data compendium; Baltimore, MD. 2008. https://146.123.140.205/DataCompendium/16_2008DataCompendium.asp TopOf. Page. Accessed June 22, 2009.
17. Hyde J, Perez R, Forester B. Dementia and assisted living. Gerontologist. 2007;47(Spec 3):51–67.
18. Wishin J, Gallagher TJ, McCann E. Emerging options for the management of fecal incontinence in hospitalized patients. J Wound Ostomy Continence Nurs. 2008;35(1):104–110.
19. Young ME. Malnutrition and wound healing. Heart Lung. 1988;17(1):60–67.
20. Stratton RJ, Ek AC, Engfer M, et al. Enteral nutritional support in prevention and treatment of pressure ulcers: A systematic review and meta-analysis. Ageing Res Rev. 2005;4(3):422–450.
21. Heyman H, Van De Looverbosch DE, Meijer EP, Schols JM. Benefits of an oral nutritional supplement on pressure ulcer healing in long-term care residents. J Wound Care. 2008;17(11):476–478.
22. Reddy M, Gill SS, Kalkar SR, Wu W, Anderson PJ, Rochon PA. Treatment of pressure ulcers: A systematic review. JAMA. 2008;300(22):2647–2662.
23. Kosiak M. Etiology of decubitus ulcers. Arch Phys Med Rehabil. 1961;42:19–29.
24. Schoonhoven L, Haalboom JR, Bousema MT, et al. Prospective cohort study of routine use of risk assessment scales for prediction of pressure ulcers. BMJ. 2002;325(7368):797.
25. Pancorbo-Hidalgo PL, Garcia-Fernandez FP, Lopez-Medina IM, Alvarez-Nieto C. Risk assessment scales for pressure ulcer prevention: A systematic review. J Adv Nurs. 2006;54(1):94–110.
26. Ayello E, Lyder C. A new era of pressure ulcer accountability in acute care. Adv Skin Wound Care. 2008;21(3):134.
27. Ratliff CR; WOCN. WOCN's evidence-based pressure ulcer guideline. Adv Skin Wound Care. 2005;18(4):204–208.
28. Grayson ML, Gibbons GW, Balogh K, Levin E, Karchmer AW. Probing to bone in infected pedal ulcers. A clinical sign of underlying osteomyelitis in diabetic patients. JAMA. 1995;273(9):721–723.
29. Takahashi P. Chronic ischemic, venous, and neuropathic ulcers in long-term care. Ann Longterm Care. 2006;14(7):26–31.

30. Bergstrom N, Allman R, Alvaraez O. Treatment of pressure ulcers. Rockville, MD: U.S. Department of Health and Human Services; 1994.
31. Bergstrom N, Allman R, Carlson C. Pressure ulcers in adults: Prediction and prevention. Rockville, MD: Agency for Health Care Policy and Research, Public Health Services, US Department of Health and Human Services; 1992.
32. Ayello EA, Lyder CH. Protecting patients from harm: Preventing pressure ulcers in hospital patients [reprint in *Adv Skin Wound Care.* 2008 Mar;21(3):134–140; quiz 140–142; PMID: 18388668]. Nursing. 2007;37(10):36–40.
33. Wound Ostomy Continence Nurses Society. Guidelines for prevention and management of pressure ulcers. Glenview, IL: Wound, Ostomy, and Continence Nurses Society (WOCN); 2003:12.
34. Ayello EA, Thomas DR, Litchford MA. Nutritional aspects of wound healing. Home Healthc Nurse. 1999;17(11):719–729.
35. Witkowshi J, Parish L. The decubitus ulcer: Skin failure and destructive behavior. Int J Dermatol. 2000;39:894.
36. Black JM; National Pressure Ulcer Advisory Panel. Moving toward consensus on deep tissue injury and pressure ulcer staging. Adv Skin Wound Care. 2005;18(8):415–416.
37. Defloor T, Schoonhoven L. Inter-rater reliability of the EPUAP pressure ulcer classification system using photographs. *J Clin Nurs.* 2004;13(8):952–959.
38. Takahashi P, Chandra A, Kiemele L, Targonski P. Wound care technologies: Emerging evidence for appropriate use in long-term care. Ann Longterm Care. 2008;16(12). Available at: http://www.annalsoflongtermcare.com/content/wound-care-technologies-emerging-evidence-appropriate-use-long-term-care june 22, 2009.
39. Hopkins A, Dealey C, Bale S, Defloor T, Worboys F. Patient stories of living with a pressure ulcer. J Adv Nurs. 2006;56(4):345–353.
40. Moore Z, Cowman S. Reviewing the evidence for selecting cleansing fluids for pressure ulcers. Nurs Times. 2009;105(5):22–24.
41. Bates-Jensen BM, Guihan M, Garber SL, Chin AS, Burns SP. Characteristics of recurrent pressure ulcers in veterans with spinal cord injury. J Spinal Cord Med. 2009;32(1):34–42.
42. Pieper B, Langemo D, Cuddigan J. Pressure ulcer pain: A systematic literature review and national pressure ulcer advisory panel white paper. Ostomy Wound Manage. 2009;55(2):16.
43. Smith DM. Pressure ulcers in the nursing home [see comment]. Ann Intern Med. 1995;123(6):433–442.
44. Bryan CS, Dew CE, Reynolds KL. Bacteremia associated with decubitus ulcers. Arch Intern Med. 1983;143(11):2093–2095.
45. Allman RM, Goode PS, Burst N, Bartolucci AA, Thomas DR. Pressure ulcers, hospital complications, and disease severity: Impact on hospital costs and length of stay. Adv Wound Care. 1999;12(1):22–30.
46. Lyder CH. Implications of pressure ulcers and its relation to federal tag 314. Annals Longterm Care. 2006;14(4):19–24.

# Part 3
Psychosocial Aspects of Long-Term Care

# Chapter 11
# Dementia, Delirium, and Depression

Deborah Way

**Keywords:** Cognitive impairment • Delirium • Dementia • Depression

## INTRODUCTION
Elderly persons are at high risk for cognitive and mood disorders and the risk for these disorders increases even further in the LTC setting. Cognitive disorders can either be chronic, as in dementia, or acute, as seen in delirium [1]. Depression, which can also cause a change in cognition, is the most commonly seen mood disorder in LTC. Understanding the similarities and differences between the behaviors and symptoms of dementia, delirium, and depression is the key to evaluating the resident with a change in mentation. Table 11.1 provides a comparison of these three conditions; Table 11.2 displays the clinical evaluation of depression, delirium, and dementia.

## DEMENTIA IN LONG-TERM CARE
Cognitive impairment and its related dementia is the primary diagnosis for an estimated 39% of residents in LTC [2] and will frequently complicate the evaluation of a resident with a change in mental status [3].

### Definition of Dementia
Dementia is a syndrome of chronic, irreversible, progressive global decline in cognition, including impairment of memory. Dementia occurs in a clear sensorium [4]. It is caused by an abnormal change

TABLE 11.1. Comparison of depression, delirium, and dementia[a]

|  | Depression | Delirium | Dementia |
|---|---|---|---|
| Onset | Gradual, may be recurrent | Sudden | Gradual, progressive |
| Mood | Low | Variable | Variable |
| Course | Chronic | Acute | Chronic |
| Apathy or loss of interest | Present | May be present or absent | Present |
| Self-awareness | Present | May be present or absent | May be present or absent |
| ADLs | Intact or impaired | Intact or impaired | Intact early, impaired later |
| IADLs | Intact or impaired | Intact or impaired | Intact early, impaired before ADLs |
| Memory | Intact or impaired | Usually impaired | Impaired |
| Attention | Intact or impaired | Impaired | Intact early, may become impaired later |
| Hallucinations or Delusions | Absent, except in the case of depression with psychotic features | Present | Variable |
| Other signs of illness | Present | Present | Usually absent |

[a]Table adapted from [1, 17, 20]

in the structure and function of the brain and is sufficient to interfere with daily function. The diagnosis of dementia starts with a patient history, which is often given by a family member or long-term facility staff. It is important to establish if the onset of the condition was insidious and difficult to pinpoint in time or whether it was more acute and if the progression (if any) was gradual or stepwise. Specific neurologic and psychiatric symptoms that have occurred since the onset of the illness also need to be determined [3]. The diagnosis can then be refined on the basis of the neurologic and mental status examinations and the results of neuropsychologic testing, imaging, and laboratory studies if clinically appropriate. Not only may these tests help determine the type of dementia but they will also help to delineate the patient's strengths and weaknesses, to identify likely areas of concern, to suggest compensation strategies, and to aid in behavioral management [5].

TABLE 11.2. Clinical evaluation of depression, delirium, and dementia[a]

| Evaluation | Depression | Delirium | Dementia |
|---|---|---|---|
| History or interval history and physical examination | x | x | x |
| Screening tool | GDS, SIGECAPS Cornell scale for depression in dementia | CAM | Folstein MMSE, SLUMS |
| CBC with differential | x | x | x |
| Complete metabolic panel | x | x | x |
| Vitamin B12 level | x | | x |
| Medication review and medication level | x | x | x |
| Thyroid-stimulating hormone | x | x | x |
| RPR | | | x |
| Lyme titer | | | x |
| Urinalysis with culture | | x | x |
| Chest X-ray | | x | |
| Arterial blood gas | | x | |
| Electrocardiogram | | x | |
| Brain imaging | | x | x |
| Lumbar puncture | | x | x |
| Electroencephalogram | | x | |

[a]The clinical evaluation of dementia, delirium, and depression should *always* be guided by presentation and goals of care

Alzheimer's Disease (Dementia of Alzheimer's Type or DAT), vascular dementia (multi-infarct dementia), dementia with Lewy Bodies (with or without Parkinson's Disease), fronto-temporal dementia, and dementia due to HIV/AIDS are the most commonly seen types of dementia. Alzheimer's Disease is the most frequently seen and is estimated to account for 55–75% of all cases of dementia, the next most frequently seen type of dementia is vascular and accounts for another 13–16% of affected individuals [1, 3, 5]. Dementia can be loosely categorized as cortical or subcortical, with DAT being a classic example of a cortical dementia. Cortical dementias are typically characterized by amnesia, disorientation, and relatively preserved personality, subcortical dementias show relatively preserved memory, but patients have difficulties in executive function, attention, and concentration. Dementia associated with Parkinson's disease is an example of subcortical dementia.

It is important to remember that persons may suffer from more than one type of dementia, which is referred to as *mixed dementia* [6].

## Evaluation of Dementia

When the staff in a long-term care facility is adequately trained and experienced in caring for persons with dementia, residents who develop symptoms associated with dementia are more readily recognized. In facilities that provide any kind of skilled care, evaluation and documentation with the Minimum Data Set (MDS), which tracks cognitive function and symptoms, must be performed on a regular basis. The MDS is a multipage assessment tool completed at admission, quarterly, and at the time of any changes in the resident's condition in the long-term care facility. MDS evaluations can be compared to past evaluations to document even subtle changes in a resident's cognition. Residents with dementia can present with memory loss and changes in behaviors such as:

- Inability to perform activities of daily living or other daily tasks.
- Changes in hygiene habits.
- Changes in interactions with staff and other residents.

## The Importance of Dementia Screening

It is important to evaluate a resident with suspected dementia, as there are many medical conditions that can cause or worsen dementia, some of which can be potentially reversible:

- Delirium
- Developmental disability
- HIV/AIDs
- Hyperglycemia or hypoglycemia
- Hypothyroidism
- Mental retardation (i.e., neuropsychologic impairment)
- Normal pressure hydrocephalus
- Sequelae of traumatic brain injury
- Subdural hematoma
- Tertiary syphilis
- Vasculitides
- Vitamin B12 deficiency

In particular, a patient presenting with new symptoms of memory or cognitive impairment should be evaluated for depression. Depression can cause a form of cognitive impairment referred to as *pseudodementia*, for further discussion, see section on depression.

## Medication Management and Cognitive Impairment

The average nursing facility resident takes seven medications, and nearly a third of residents take nine or more medications [7]. Therefore, when evaluating for cognitive impairment, it is crucial to consider the resident's medications because the variety of medications and the interactions between medications they take can alter cognitive function. Medications that are commonly implicated include antiarrhythmics, hypnotics, psychotropics, sedatives, analgesics, and any medication with significant anticholinergic properties such as those used for urinary urge incontinence. Toxicity from certain medications such as digoxin can also cause changes in cognition. In 1991, Dr. Mark Beers created a list of *potentially* harmful medications used in the geriatric population. The Beers List was reviewed and updated in 2003 [8]. It is used by many in long term care.

## Evaluation of the Resident with Cognitive Impairment

A basic evaluation of the resident with new cognitive impairment includes laboratory tests such as a complete blood count with differential, complete metabolic panel, Vitamin B12 level, thyroid function panel including a TSH, and possibly blood levels of any concerning medication such as digoxin, lithium, theophylline, anticonvulsants such as phenytoin or valproic acid, and tricyclic antidepressants such as amitriptyline. Other tests to consider, if clinically indicated are: an RPR (etc) for syphilis, urinalysis with culture, or perhaps a test for Lyme disease (depending on local prevalence and other risk factors) to rule out an infectious cause for the change in cognition [3, 4].

When performing tests and evaluating a resident with cognitive impairment, it is also necessary to evaluate for any underlying medical conditions that may affect cognitive function and optimize their management. Medical conditions commonly implicated in cognitive dysfunction include recent coronary artery bypass grafting, hypertension, nutritional deficiencies including B vitamins, type II diabetes mellitus, stroke, Parkinson's Disease, and diseases which cause oxygen deprivation such as COPD and obstructive sleep apnea [4].

A simple screening tool to evaluate cognition should be part of the evaluation, such as the Folstein Mini Mental Status Exam (MMSE). The MMSE is a 30-point screening tool for cognitive impairment. Recently, the official form has been copyrighted and must be purchased (www.minimental.com). Because of this expense, some practitioners have chosen instead to use the St. Louis University Mental Status Exam (SLUMS) available at http://medschool.slu.edu/agingsuccessfully/pdfsurveys/slumsexam_05.pdf.

More tools can be found in "Other Resources" at the end of this chapter. Keep in mind that the MDS in skilled nursing facilities will also provide an evaluation of the resident's mental and functional status.

Finally, neuro-imaging of the resident's brain may be performed to rule out structural lesions such as a neoplasm or a reversible condition such as normal pressure hydrocephalus. A neuro-imaging study should be considered especially when the onset of the dementia has occurred within the past 6 months to a year, the dementia is rapidly progressive, or is following an unpredictable course.

If there is a question of diagnosis, or if the resident or their family has difficulty accepting the diagnosis of dementia, further neuropsychiatric testing may be done to more definitively diagnose the resident's change in mental status.

### Implications of a Diagnosis of Dementia

The diagnosis of dementia in a resident will aid in further care of the resident. It is valuable in understanding symptoms and behaviors and also in prognosticating. A diagnosis of dementia will provide a framework for prognostication by the physician and will aid in healthcare decision-making of all those involved, especially the resident and their family. Although dementia is a chronic, progressive, and ultimately terminal illness, this is not well recognized by many individuals – either within or without the LTC community.

### Progression of Dementia

Dementia is a progressive disease. Although different types of dementia have different manifestations at onset, the final common pathway is inability to perform any function. Residents will become unable to care for themselves, incontinent of bowel and bladder, and unable to safely swallow either nutrition or their own secretions. The resident with end stage dementia will become unable to take in sufficient nutrition to sustain life. Even when carefully hand-fed, the resident with end-stage dementia will eventually develop progressive weight loss and be at high risk for developing pressure ulcers. The resident may also develop urinary retention, constipation, and repeated infections of urinary tract or respiratory system (the latter due to unpreventable aspiration of food and secretions) [5]. It is imperative that the resident and their family be educated on the disease process of dementia. This may be difficult for families to accept, as many people do not recognize that dementia is a terminal illness.

## Treatments for Dementia

In Alzheimer's disease (AD), the mainstay of treatment is neurotransmitter modulation. The two major classes of medications are cholinesterase inhibitors and NMDA receptor antagonists. The most widely used cholinesterase inhibitor is donepezil (Aricept), but other medications include rivastigmine (Exelon) and galantamine (Razadyne). Cholinesterase inhibitors are currently indicated for mild (MMSE >19), moderate (MMSE 19–10), or severe (MMSE <10) AD. The only currently available NMDA receptor antagonist is memantine (Namenda). Memantine is currently indicated for moderate to severe AD either in conjunction with a cholinesterase inhibitor or as monotherapy [3, 4].

Other medications and treatments have been studied and not been shown to successfully treat or prevent AD. These include anti-inflammatory medications such as NSAIDs, hormone replacement therapy such as estrogen, gingko biloba, and antioxidants such as Vitamin E. Research in this area continues especially in the prevention of inflammation and beta-amyloid plaques, which are hallmarks of AD [3].

The mainstay of treatment for dementias other than Alzheimer's type is preventing progression of the underlying disease process (as in the case of vascular dementia) and treating the symptoms that arise in the course of the disease (as in the case of hallucinations in Lewy Body dementia). There has been some research hoping to show that these diseases respond to cholinesterase inhibitors and possibly memantine as well.

In residents with coexistent depression, the use of antidepressants with serotoninergic activity may improve both depressive symptoms and cognitive manifestations secondary to the depression [3].

## Challenging Behaviors in Dementia

Challenging behaviors in those with dementia include pacing, wandering, hoarding, agitation, insomnia, aggression, hypersexuality, perseveration, hallucinations, paranoid thinking, and crying [4, 9]. Agitation frequently occurs in "sundowning," which is a syndrome of disorientation, confusion, and agitation that often starts in the middle to late afternoon and progressively worsens through the evening into the night. An environmental and medical evaluation often gives insight into ways in which these behaviors can be mitigated or prevented. Frequently, these behaviors are a manifestation of the dementing process, but they may be exacerbated by a stimulus in the environment or a medical illness. On one hand, commonly seen environmental causes of disruptive behavior include a new routine or new caregiver, an absent family member, or another disruptive resident. On the other hand, commonly seen medical causes of disruptive or changed behaviors include pain, constipation, urinary retention, drug effect(s), dehydration, or infection. It is important to first evaluate the resident for any reversible environmental and/or physical stimuli to their behavior, before initiating any treatment interventions for the behavior [4].

## Treatment of Behaviors in Dementia

Behaviors in dementia may be addressed using pharmacologic and/or nonpharmacologic treatment.

### Nonpharmacologic Treatment

An adjustment of environmental factors (both physical and human) may lessen or resolve distressing behaviors. For example, providing safe areas in the facility with more home-like furnishings and wall decorations has not been shown to reduce wandering and pacing of residents with dementia, but residents who were previously difficult to monitor did prefer to remain in those areas and so were more easily monitored [9].

Other suggested interventions to the environment include:

- Establish a daily routine for personal care and meals while maintaining some flexibility to accommodate the resident's needs and preferences. If a resident initially refuses care or a meal, a caregiver may reapproach the resident a short time later and the resident may then be willing to allow care or eat a meal.
- Reduce isolation; segregate noisier or disruptive residents from quieter ones.
- Maintain adequate and appropriate lighting at all times.
- Provide pleasant experiences including recreational experiences, ethnic food or other culturally oriented activities, pet therapy, or stuffed animals [4].

Other interventions for behaviors include:

- Residents exhibiting inappropriate sexual behavior can be dressed with clothing that reduces access to their own genitalia, can receive care from same-sex caregivers, and can be seated away from residents of the opposite sex [9].
- Residents with other behaviors can be redirected with individual and group activities.

Information about the resident's life before admission may provide opportunities for activities that will satisfy the resident. An example is the resident who was always moving the tables and chairs in the dining area. This resident had worked at a supermarket for years and had been responsible for returning the carts from the parking lot to the store. When staff observed him moving furniture safely, they allowed him to continue this activity with supervision

## Pharmacologic Treatment

If distressing behaviors cannot be eliminated by modifying the environment, an adjustment to medications should be considered. As with other changes to a resident's plan of care, this should not be done without an evaluation of the risks and benefits of a particular medical treatment. The staff and the family of the resident should be advised of any issues and interventions that have been tried before instituting medical therapy for behaviors. There has not been a great deal of consensus on the use of medications to treat challenging behaviors in dementia [9]. One must also take into consideration federal and State regulations and facility policies regarding medications that are considered chemical restraints. The following should be considered:

- Residents who exhibit agitation with psychotic features such as hallucinations, delusions, or perseverative behaviors such as pacing or hoarding may respond to treatment with antipsychotic medications.
- Residents with sundowning behaviors or insomnia may improve with a medication that promotes sleep (trazodone) or reduces confusion (antipsychotic).
- Residents who exhibit behaviors with an anxiety component may benefit from the use of a serotonin reuptake inhibitor or trazodone.
- Residents with hypersexual behaviors may respond to antipsychotic medication or to antiandrogenic hormone therapy such as estrogen. This has been better studied in male residents.
- Residents with expression of anger or aggression may respond to the use of serotonergic agents, mood stabilizing agents such as divalproex, carbamazepine, and gabapentin, or antipsychotic medications such as risperidone and olanzapine [9].
- All medication regimens must be reviewed on a regular basis to evaluate effectiveness. This includes periodic attempts to reduce dosing or discontinue medications used for behaviors. For example, it is not uncommon for a resident to have previously necessary medications reduced or eliminated three to six months after admission. It is possible that benzodiazepines and sometimes antipsychotics to cause *paradoxical agitation* or worsening of confusion.

## DELIRIUM

In contrast to dementia and depression, delirium is a medical condition with either an acute or subacute (and often unrecognized) onset. It is a classic geriatric syndrome in which the symptoms are psychiatric. The delirious patient presents with a disturbance of consciousness and attention. This patient will also experience a change in cognition including perceptual impairments such as illusions, delusions, or hallucinations [10].

The frail elders who comprise many of the residents in postacute and LTC facilities are at particular risk of developing delirium due to the multiple risk factors already present in these individuals. Delirium is likely to occur in a vulnerable resident who develops an acute illness. A good example is the resident with dementia, multiple comorbidities, and a complicated medication list who suddenly develops an infection, becomes dehydrated, or both.

Delirium can be most easily described according to the level of psychomotor activity manifested by the patient. A patient with *hyperactive* delirium experiences increased psychomotor activity and may appear anxious or agitated. In contrast, a patient with *hypoactive* delirium shows reduced psychomotor activity, which may resemble depression. These patients are often described by the staff as quiet and requiring little or no attention. This may lead to the delirium being overlooked and therefore untreated. In the third type of delirium, a mixed delirium, the resident exhibits fluctuating levels of psychomotor activity ranging from immobility to extreme agitation [4, 11].

### Importance of Recognizing Delirium

Delirium is an extremely common condition that affects at least one third of hospitalized elders [12]. It may last for weeks to months and has been associated with poor health outcomes including increased in-hospital mortality, longer length of stay, functional decline, and risk of institutionalization. As pressure increases to discharge individuals sooner from acute inpatient facilities, many of these acutely confused elders transition from hospital to a postacute facility, where they remain delirious and can experience potentially life-threatening complications [11, 13].

In LTC, the identification, evaluation, and management of delirium is urgent because it may signify an underlying medical emergency. Frequently, delirium is the only indication that the resident has had a change in their medical condition. Each resident with delirium should be evaluated for multiple risk factors, especially those that are reversible. Dementia is the leading risk factor for delirium [12]. The following are other risk factors for delirium [14]:

Dementia
Older age
Functional impairment
Multiple comorbidities
Dehydration
Malnutrition
Sensory impairment
History of depression
History of substance abuse

## Assessment of Delirium

One of the simplest ways to evaluate a resident for delirium is the Confusion Assessment Method (CAM). It is a four-item evaluation, developed by Inouye et al. (see Yale website,) as shown below:

Characteristics:

I. Acute onset and fluctuating course
II. Inattention
III. Disorganized thinking
IV. Altered level of consciousness

The diagnosis of delirium requires I and II, and either III or IV in order to be satisfied. The CAM has been shown to have excellent sensitivity and specificity and may be administered by experienced care providers.

As with any other change in mental status, an evaluation of the resident must be done to rule out all potentially reversible causes of the resident's change. This should include a complete interval history to help determine onset and course of the resident's new status. The history must also include questions to elicit a possible withdrawal syndrome. Another integral part of this history is a review of medications, including all current medications but with a special focus on all recent medication changes. Recent changes in medications should include all medications that are new, have had recent dosage changes, or have been recently discontinued. All prescription medications, over-the-counter medications, supplements, and substances with potential for abuse (alcohol and illicit drugs) should be reviewed. These medications may have been provided by the facility, or brought to the facility by the resident or by a family member or friend. It is also important to include topical medications as well, such as eye drops, nasal sprays, or suppositories. One should also determine if delirium could be due to withdrawal from alcohol, analgesics, benzodiazepines, or antidepressants.

Interactions between medications, changes in metabolism with aging (such as decreased renal or liver function), or recently acquired or advancing disease (such as dementia or diabetes) all increase the likelihood that a medication can cause or contribute to a delirium. Medications that were previously necessary or recommended may now be causing unwanted effects and contributing to the delirium, and therefore may need to be discontinued.

A physical exam should include vital signs: temperature, pulse, blood pressure measurements, pulse oxygenation, and blood sugar measurements if appropriate. A careful mental status and neurologic examination should be performed, while the remainder of the physical exam should focus on signs and symptoms that may indicate a new disease process. Diagnostic tests should be guided by findings from the history and physical examination, as well as the suspicions of the clinician. Laboratory tests should include a complete blood count, electrolytes, and renal function, as well as a urinalysis. Other lab tests to consider are: thyroid function tests, B12 level, and serum levels of prescribed medications (such as digoxin, lithium, and valproic acid). If indicated, an arterial blood gas analysis or chest X-ray should be done. Other testing may include neuroimaging to look for a cerebrovascular accident, brain tumor, or normal pressure hydrocephalus, and electrocardiography to rule out acute coronary syndromes or an arrhythmia. If indicated, a lumbar puncture to evaluate for infectious and neoplastic processes or an electroencephalogram looking for seizure activity should be performed [4, 10–12].

Most of all, it is important to prevent delirium, if possible. Research in the hospital setting has shown that up to one third of cases of delirium are either potentially preventable or iatrogenic [14]. Interventions used in the hospital that may also help prevent delirium in the LTC setting are listed in Table 11.3.

## DEPRESSION

Because estimates of the prevalence of major depressive disorder in the elderly range from 12 to 20% and estimates of some kind of depressive symptoms are as high as 70%, suspicion that a resident in LTC could have depression should be very high. Depression is also more likely to occur in patients with dementia or other chronic comorbidities that are frequently seen in the LTC population such

TABLE 11.3. Interventions that prevent or ameliorate delirium [20]

| Problem | Intervention |
| --- | --- |
| Cognitive impairment | Reorientation to time, location, care team |
|  | Provision of cognitively stimulating activities |
| Sleep deprivation | Caffeine-free warm beverages |
|  | Music |
|  | Back massage |
|  | Noise reduction measures in patient care areas |
|  | Minimization of sleep deprivation by care staff or medication aide |
| Immobility | Encourage early ambulation or active range of motion |
| Vision impairment | Use of glasses, magnifying lenses, and other adaptive equipment |
| Hearing impairment | Disimpaction of cerumen, use of hearing aids and portable amplifiers |
| Dehydration | Volume repletion (encouragement of oral intake) |

as stroke, cancer, coronary artery disease, or Parkinson's Disease. Although depression in the LTC population is very common, it can be easily missed when its symptoms are confused with those of other illnesses. When depression goes untreated, it can worsen any coexisting medical illness and may lead to poorer outcomes and increased risk of suicide [1, 4, 16].

**Differentiating Depression from Dementia**

The symptoms of depression and dementia frequently overlap, which can make it difficult for clinicians to differentiate between the two. The Cornell Scale for Depression in Dementia is a tool that uses interviews with the patient and the caregiver to elicit a possible diagnosis of depression (see Diagnosis/screening tools below). Any resident with newly recognized memory or cognitive impairment should also be evaluated for depression, as they may actually be suffering from pseudodementia rather than dementia. Pseudodementia has been described as cognitive impairment related to a depressive disorder [1]. Aggressive treatment of depression in the resident with suspected pseudodementia will lead to a gradual improvement or resolution of the cognitive impairment associated with their depression [17]. However, even those patients with complete resolution of pseudodementia are at high risk for the development of dementia within a few years [4].

Depression is frequently undiagnosed or underdiagnosed in the geriatric patient population. It is postulated that this occurs for many different reasons. The reasons include an overlap between symptoms of depression and those of dementia, a lack of a biologic gold standard test that would diagnose geriatric psychiatric disorders, and preconceptions that depression is a natural part of aging. There is also concern that clinicians have inadequate diagnostic skills and are unable to recognize the frequently subtle clinical features of depression in geriatric patients [4, 17].

**Diagnosis of Depression**
It is important to note that a resident may experience a depressed or sad mood and yet not meet the criteria for depression. The key to the diagnosis and treatment of depression is determining whether or not the mood makes a significant negative impact on the resident's quality of life. The diagnosis of depression may be guided by Diagnostic and Statistical Manual of Mental Disorders – version IV-TR (DSM IV-TR) [18]. If a resident has significant psychiatric disease, comorbid substance abuse, or depression with psychotic features, it may be helpful to consult a psychiatrist for help with a resident's diagnosis and treatment.

The specific diagnostic criteria by DSM IV-TR for a major depression disorder are:

Five or more symptoms present nearly every day during the same 2-week period, which represent a change from previous functioning

These five symptoms must include the presence of depressed mood most of the day or markedly diminished interest or pleasure in all or mostly all activities most of the day (anhedonia) as well as:

- Significant weight loss or gain, or significant change in appetite
- Insomnia or hypersomnia
- Psychomotor agitation or retardation
- Fatigue or loss of energy
- Feelings of worthlessness or excessive or inappropriate guilt
- Diminished ability to think or concentrate, or indecisiveness
- Recurrent thoughts of death, recurrent suicidal ideation without a specific plan, or suicide attempt or specific plan for committing suicide.
- The symptoms do not meet criteria for a mixed episode
- The symptoms cause clinically significant distress, or impairment in function

- The symptoms are not due to effects of substance (medication or substance of abuse) or a medical condition
- The symptoms are not better accounted for by bereavement.

A major depressive disorder can occur as either a single episode or two or more episodes separated by at least two consecutive months in which criteria are not met for a major depressive episode. DSM IV-TR lists many forms of depressive disorders that include mild, moderate, and severe episodes of major depression, severe episode of major depression with psychotic features, minor depression disorder, recurrent major depressive disorder with hypomanic features, dysthymic disorder, and adjustment disorder with depressed mood or with mixed anxiety and depressed mood [16].

The evaluation of depression, as with the evaluation of delirium and dementia, requires a thorough history and physical examination to determine any causative or contributing factors. The investigation should be guided by the goals of care and life expectancy of each patient. For example, in the case of a patient whose life expectancy can be measured in weeks, it may be less important to determine the cause of the depression than it is to treat the depression with therapy that will provide relief of symptoms quickly.

Many medications and some drug–drug interactions may cause or worsen depression. Medication changes and dose reductions should be made to lessen these affects. Commonly used medications that may cause symptoms of depression include:

- Cardiac medications such as antiarrhythmic or antihypertensive drugs.
- Psychotropic medications such as benzodiazepines or barbiturates.
- Antiseizure medications.
- Steroids.
- GI preparations such as H2 blockers and metoclopramide.
- Opioid analgesics.
- Carbidopa/levodopa [16].

Laboratory tests that should be considered include: electrolytes, a complete blood count, thyroid function studies, B12 and folate levels, as well as blood levels of antiseizure drugs, digoxin, theophylline, tricyclic antidepressants, and lithium. Other investigations may include evaluation for infection such as urinalysis with culture and an EKG to evaluate for a cardiac arrhythmia [4].

## Diagnostic Tools

A simple screening tool for evaluating depression includes: SIGECAPS, which is a mnemonic reminder with eight questions (a version of this tool shown in Table 11.4). Five or more positive answers (indicated in bold) on SIGECAPS may indicate depression. Other screening tools include the Geriatric Depression Scale (GDS) with either 15 or 30 questions (Table 11.5), and the Cornell Scale for Depression in Dementia [19]. SIGECAPS and the GDS include questions that are asked *only of the resident* as opposed to the Cornell Scale that is comprised of questions asked of *both*

TABLE 11.4. SIGECAPS Mnemonic

| | |
|---|---|
| S | Are you **S**ad? (**YES**/NO) |
| I | Do you suffer from **I**nsomnia (**YES**/NO) |
| G | Do you have feelings of **G**uilt (**YES**/NO) |
| E | Do you have a lack of **E**nergy (**YES**/NO) |
| C | Do you have difficulty **C**oncentrating (**YES**/NO) |
| A | Have you had changes in your **A**ppetite (**YES**/NO) |
| P | Do you receive **P**leasure from anything in your life (YES/**NO**) |
| S | Have you had thoughts of **S**uicide (**YES**/NO) |

TABLE 11.5. Geriatric depression scale – short form, a mood scale

Choose the best answer for how you have felt over the past week

Are you basically satisfied with your life? YES/**NO**
Have you dropped many of your activities and interests? **YES**/NO
Do you feel that your life is empty? **YES**/NO
Do you often get bored? **YES**/NO
Are you in good spirits most of the time? YES/**NO**
Are you afraid that something bad is going to happen to you? **YES**/NO
Do you feel happy most of the time? YES/**NO**
Do you often feel helpless? **YES**/NO
Do you prefer to stay at home, rather than going out and doing new things? **YES**/NO
Do you feel you have more problems with memory than most? **YES**/NO
Do you think it is wonderful to be alive now? YES/**NO**
Do you feel pretty worthless the way you are now? **YES**/NO
Do you feel full of energy? YES/**NO**
Do you feel that your situation is hopeless? **YES**/NO
Do you think that most people are better off than you are? **YES**/NO

*the caregiver and the resident.* SIGECAPS and the GDS are in the public domain and therefore available for use by anyone.

Answers in *bold* indicate depression. Although differing sensitivities and specificities have been obtained across studies, for clinical purposes a score >5 points on either scale is suggestive of depression and should warrant a follow-up interview. If the patient has a score >10, they almost always have a depression.

Every person with depression must be asked about suicidal ideation and if they have a suicide plan. Those who are at highest risk are white males older than 80 years of age, followed by white males 65–80 years of age. The most important risk factors for suicide are [4]:

- Severity of depression
- Psychotic depression
- Alcoholism
- Recent loss or bereavement
- Abuse of sedatives/hypnotics
- Development of disability
- Analgesic abuse

**Treatment of Depression**

Psychotherapy and medication are the mainstays for the treatment of depression. The benefit of psychotherapy may be limited by the cognitive abilities of the resident. In a resident who is more cognitively intact, cognitive-behavioral therapy and learning-based therapy have been shown to help with depression. These therapies may be provided by a primary care practitioner, social worker, or psychologist [16]. Other nonpharmacologic measures include lessening the institutional appearance of the facility, especially the resident's own space, and providing opportunities for meaningful interaction and social, physical, spiritual, and religious activities.

Classes of medication for the treatment of depression include serotonin-reuptake inhibitors (SSRIs), tricyclic antidepressants, monoamine oxidase inhibitors, serotonin/norepinephrine reuptake inhibitors (SNRIs), serotonergic agents such as trazodone, and medications chemically unrelated to the other antidepressants including mirtazepine and bupropion. An antidepressant should be chosen on the basis of the characteristics of the resident's depression. In the case of depression with a significant anxiety component, it may be more appropriate to choose an SSRI such as citalopram or sertraline. Mirtazepine may better treat depression associated with anxiety, insomnia, and anorexia. If a resident has profound vegetative features and requires quick relief of their symptoms, it may be appropriate to choose a stimulant, such as methylphenidate or modafinil, while awaiting for the eventual antidepressant effects of the concurrently prescribed antidepressant to occur.

Different antidepressants affect different brain neurotransmitter systems such as the dopaminergic (bupropion) and noradrenergic and serotonergic (tricyclics), rather than only the serotonergic system (SSRIs). The SNRIs are like the tricyclics because they affect both norepinephrine and serotonin. This class includes venlafaxine and duloxetine. Knowing in which neurotransmitter system an antidepressant acts can aid the clinician in choosing a second antidepressant when the first one chosen does not have an adequate therapeutic response.

Remember that medications for depression have only been extensively studied in younger patients, so care must be taken in the older patient whose drug metabolism is frequently different. Side effects are less common with the newer antidepressants.

Before the SSRIs were developed, tricyclic antidepressants were commonly used. They are as effective as SSRIs, but have more significant side effects and so are now used as a second (such as over the counter cough suppressants) or third line of treatment. Common side effects of tricyclics include dry mouth, constipation, bladder problems, sexual dysfunction, blurred vision, dizziness, drowsiness, and cardiac abnormalities.

Monoamine oxidase inhibitors are less commonly recommended because they cannot be taken with decongestants or food that contain high levels of the monoamine *tyramine*. The interaction of tyramine with MAOIs can precipitate a sharp increase in blood pressure.

Side effects of SSRIs include hyponatremia, sexual dysfunction, nausea, diarrhea, nervousness and insomnia, agitation, and decreased sweating with increased body temperature. These side effects may be amplified when combined with other medications (such as over-the-counter cough suppressants) or herbs (such as St. John's Wort) that affect serotonin and can result in a potentially serious or even fatal *serotonin syndrome*, characterized by fever, confusion, muscle rigidity, and cardiac, liver, or kidney problems.

Although the SNRIs affect the same neurotransmitters as the tricyclics and have similar types of side effects, the side effects seen are fewer. Mirtazepine and bupropion have similar side effects to the SSRIs. Bupropion should not be used in a resident with a history of a seizure disorder as it may lower the seizure threshold [17].

The expected response rate for any single optimally dosed antidepressant is approximately 60% in six to twelve weeks. Another antidepressant should be tried after four weeks if there are no signs of symptom improvement. Even when a person responds to an antidepressant, they may have residual symptoms and may need their antidepressant changed to another or augmented with a second antidepressant or adjuvant. The length of time that depression should be treated in the LTC population has not been fully determined, but a period of 6–12 months has been proposed [3].

If medication has not helped the depression, or if the resident's condition is rapidly deteriorating, electroconvulsive therapy should be considered. Electroconvulsive treatment has been shown to be effective in older adults [4].

## SUMMARY

Dementia, delirium, and depression in the LTC community have many commonalities in their presentation and clinical evaluation. Treatment should be tailored to the goals of care of each resident, guided by the resident's prognosis, level of functioning, comorbidities, and life expectancy. A careful evaluation and a good understanding of each of these three conditions will lead to appropriate intervention and treatment. It is important to remember that some residents may suffer from all three conditions concurrently.

## PEARLS FOR THE PRACTITIONER

### Dementia
- Dementia is a chronic, irreversible, progressive condition with insidious onset.
- There is a high prevalence of dementia as a primary diagnosis in the LTC setting.
- Residents with dementia can exhibit behaviors as a natural part of their disease process.

### Delirium
- Delirium is a potentially life-threatening condition.
- Hyperactive delirium is more easily recognizable than hypoactive delirium.
- Interventions to prevent delirium have been shown to be effective.

### Depression
- The prevalence of some kind of depressive disorder in the long-term care population has been estimated to be as high as 70%.
- Depression is not an inevitable consequence of aging.
- Depression frequently occurs in the setting of other medical conditions.

## WEBSITES

- Alzheimers Association. www.alz.org.
- American Geriatrics Society. www.americangeriatrics.org.
- American Medical Directors Association for their Clinical Practice Guidelines. www.amda.com.
- Hospitalized Elder Life Program for information on delirium. www.elderlife.med.yale.edu.
- Folstein Mini Mental Status Exam (MMSE), the official form has been copyrighted and must be purchased from www.minimental.com.
- St. Louis University Mental Status Exam (SLUMS) is available at: http://medschool.slu.edu/agingsuccessfully/pdfsurveys/slumsexam_05.pdf.
- St. Louis University Geriatrics www.aging/SLU.edu.

## REFERENCES

1. Gagliardi JP. Differentiating among depression, delirium, and dementia in elderly patients. Virtual Mentor 2008; 10, 6:383–388.
2. National Nursing Home Survey 2004. Centers for Disease Control. June 2009 http://www.cdc.gov/nchs/data/series/sr_13/sr13_167.pdf. Accessed January 9, 2010.
3. Rosenblatt A. The art of managing dementia in the elderly. Cleve Clinic J Med 2005; 72, (Suppl 3): S3–S13.
4. Hazzard WR, Blass JP, Halter JB, Ouslander JG, Tinetti ME. Principles of Geriatric Medicine & Gerontology, 5th Edition. McGraw-Hill: New York. 2003.
5. American Medical Directors Association. Dementia in the Long Term Care Setting Clinical Practice Guideline. Columbia, MD: AMDA 2009.
6. Turner M, Moran N, Kopelman M. Subcortical dementia. Br J Psychiatry 2002; 180: 148–151.
7. Doshi JA, ShafferT, Briesacher BA. National estimates of medication use in nursing homes: findings from the 1997 medicare beneficiary survey and the 1996 medical expenditure survey. J Am Geriatr Soc. 2005; 53: 438–443.
8. Fick DM, Cooper JW, Wade WE, Waller JL, Maclean JR, Beers MH. Updating the beers criteria for potentially inappropriate medication use in older adults. Arch Intern Med. 2003; 163: 2716–2724.
9. Buhr GW, White HK. Difficult behaviors in long-term care patients with dementia. J Am Med Dir Assoc 2007; 8: E.101–E.113.
10. American Medical Directors Association. Delirium and Acute Problematic Behavior in the Long-Term Care Setting Clinical Practice Guideline. Columbia, MD: AMDA 2008.
11. Inouye SK. Delirium in Older Persons. N Engl J Med 2006; 354: 1157–1165.
12. Fick DM, Agostini JV, Inouye SK. Delirium Superimposed on dementia: a systematic review. J Am Geriatr Soc 2002; 50: 1723–1732.

13. Ozbolt LB, Paniagua MA, Kaiser RM. Atypical antipsychotics for the treatment of delirious elders. J Am Med Dir Assoc 2008; 9: 18–28.
14. Elie M, Cole MG, Primeau FJ, Bellavance F. Delirium risk factors in elderly hospitalized patients. J Gen Intern Med 1998; 13: 204–212.
15. Cole MG, Primeau FJ, McCusker J. Effectiveness of Interventions to Prevent Delirium in Hospitalized Patients: A Systematic Review. Can Med Assoc J 1996; 155: 1263–1268
16. American Medical Directors Association. Depression Clinical Practice Guideline. Columbia, MD: AMDA 2003
17. Peskind ER. Management of Depression in Long-Term Care of Patients with Alzheimer's Disease. J Am Med Dir Assoc 2003; Supp Nov/Dec: S141–S145.
18. Handbook of Differential Diagnosis DSM-IV-TR, American Psychiatric Publishing, Inc, Washington, DC: 2002.
19. Alexopoulos GS, Abrams RC, Young RC, Shamoian CA. Cornell Scale for Depression in Dementia. Biol Psychiatry. 1988 Feb 1; 23(3): 271–84.
20. Aging in the Know. www.americangeriatrics.org Accessed January 9, 2010.

# Chapter 12
# Ethical and Legal Issues

David A. Smith and Randall D. Huss

**Keywords:** Ethical issues • Legal issues • Health care ethics • Resident rights • Elder abuse • Driving • Competency • End-of-life issues • Liability

## INTRODUCTION

Ethical and legal issues are common in long-term care and are separate, but integrally interrelated. Health care ethics is the application of *values* (patient, caregiver, and societal) to the process of clinical decision making. This process requires the intellectual and empathetic weighing of values, facts, and prognostications to produce a supportable decision. Clinicians often encounter competing values, e.g., the right of self-determination of an individual versus the interests of society as a whole, and must take into consideration the facts and the likelihood and consequences of various outcomes.

The *law* is a society's compilation of rules, which are intended to be uniformly applied (equal protection under the law), mandatory (ignorance of the law is no excuse), and modifiable only through the legislative process. Fortunately, the principles of health care ethics have not been ignored in the process of evolution of the law as it interfaces with clinical medicine.

There is no shortage of challenges for the long-term care practitioner in applying health care ethics within the tenets of existing state and federal law. It should be noted that all state and federal regulations related to the survey of long-term care facilities are dictated by law. Clinicians are admonished to know the laws of their jurisdiction and to seek legal counsel when needed. The contents of this chapter are educational only and not formal legal advice.

## PRINCIPLES OF HEALTH CARE ETHICS

The principles of health care ethics include *autonomy*, *beneficence*, *justice*, *nonmaleficence*, and *fidelity*. These principles do not stand alone or in a hierarchy, but must be considered in the context of each other. Frequently, different aspects of each ethical principle compete and an ethical judgment must be made by considering one or the other more strongly, yet made within the framework of the law.

*Autonomy* is the principle attesting to an individual's right to sovereignty over oneself. It encompasses the right to self-determination and to privacy. This right does not automatically "trump" other principles, but must be balanced with other rights. The *right to privacy* would be subordinate to the principles of beneficence and justice, for instance, in the case of an individual with chronic active hepatitis B who willingly refuses to follow guidelines to prevent the transmission of the disease to others. The law recognizes the right to privacy in statutes that codify the privacy of medical records such as the Health Insurance Portability and Accountability Act (HIPAA), informed consent, and the individual's right to decline life-sustaining treatments. Competency and mental capacity issues, discussed later, may alter the principle of autonomy.

*Beneficence* is the principle that holds that an individual has responsibility to do good for others. Good Samaritan laws are designed to protect individuals when they act by this principle. Similarly, laws that require health care professionals to report suspected elder abuse are another example of this principle. Also, laws related to guardianship and other forms of surrogate decision making for those adjudicated incompetent by a judge in a court of law or clinically determined to be mentally incapacitated derive from the principle of beneficence.

*Justice* is the principle espousing the responsibility of the medical professional to treat a patient fairly, to treat all patients equally, and to consider not only one's patient but also the good of society in medical decision making. A common example of applying this principle is the physician's role in terminating driving privileges for a person who can no longer safely operate a motor vehicle.

The principle of *nonmaleficence* is the responsibility of the medical professional to do no harm. Avoiding unnecessary surgery and optimizing patient safety are examples. Laws regarding medical malpractice are based on this principle and claims for punitive damages stem from what plaintiffs perceive as breaches of this principle.

Finally, the principle of *fidelity* involves the medical professional's responsibility to keep the terms of the "doctor/patient contract." Truthfulness and substantial compliance with informed consent are components of fidelity as is *nonabandonment*. A medical professional should not summarily cease to act for the benefit of one's patient even when that patient has not lived up to their side of the doctor/patient contract (e.g., noncompliance) or exerted their autonomy and chosen a course of medical action with which the physician disagrees. The physician should attempt to provide the best possible outcome in the context of the patient's noncompliance and their treatment choices. Alternatively, the medical professional may exit the doctor/patient contract by providing emergency care as needed while affording the patient sufficient time to establish themselves with another health care professional.

The vast majority of applications of these principles are played out not in the legal arena, but in everyday medical decision making. Every day, the practice of medicine within the long-term care continuum involves issues related to diminished mental capacity and mental illness, treatments with narrow risk/benefit ratios, end-of-life care, potential for elder abuse and exploitation, and high utilization of limited and expensive medical resources, all of which challenge every practitioner to hold dear these principles and to competently apply them with skill and confidence. The input from others on the interdisciplinary team and from the family is essential to apply these principles and to choose the most appropriate course of action. Finally, every practitioner must be able to communicate and balance these principles as they apply to the specifics of the clinical scenario and to succinctly record his/her reasoning in the medical record.

## COMMON AREAS OF CONCERN

### Resident Rights
A fundamental principle is that no individual loses his/her human rights upon entering into a nursing facility, other facility, or program within the long-term care continuum. Providers have an obligation to inform residents of their rights and to encourage and assist them in exercising those rights. It is illegal for a facility, program, or any employee to infringe upon an elder's human rights by threatening, coercing, intimidating, or retaliating against an elder who is exercising their rights. A facility or program should educate elders on the process of a human rights complaint. Specific responsibilities are outlined in the section on Abuse, Neglect and Exploitation.

A statement of nursing facility resident rights, as outlined in state and federal regulation, is detailed in Table 12.1 [1].

A resident's rights may only be restricted when it is necessary to protect them or another individual from potential harm or to protect the rights of another resident, e.g., infringements on another's privacy or confidentiality. Facility rules that have been fully disclosed before admission, such as scheduled smoking breaks or a nonsmoking policy, can only be enforced if the resident or their legally recognized surrogate has agreed to these as a condition of admission. Furthermore, problem behaviors may be addressed by providers through behavior modification programming or behavioral contracting with the resident, or even as a condition of continued residence in the facility if done as part of a therapeutic plan of care and in keeping with nursing facility regulations. A resident with mental incapacity still retains all of the human rights outlined in Table 12.1. However, these rights are both advocated and managed by the legally designated surrogate decision-maker. For instance, a mentally incapacitated resident with diabetes mellitus who wants to spend all of their money on candy and soda may be care planned to receive budgeted amounts of spending money from their facility account and be supervised in spending this on diabetic snacks and sugar-free soft drinks if the care plan is agreed upon by their surrogate decision-maker. Providers and practitioners should note that litigation alleging infringement on human rights may not be covered by medical malpractice insurance.

### Elder Abuse, Neglect, and Exploitation

Residents within the long-term care continuum represent a population vulnerable to abuse, neglect, and exploitation by a family member, another person, a member of the health care team, or even at an institutional level. Abuse, neglect, and exploitation may be purposeful or due to inadequate knowledge and training.

*Abuse* is an act of commission intended to do harm. Abuse can be physical, sexual, or emotional in nature. Many episodes of physical and emotional abuse are sporadic and occur as an unguarded response to an elderly, demented, or mentally ill person's behavior toward the caregiver. Resistive, combative, and assaultive behaviors by the resident may trigger retaliation if the caregiver fails to understand the behavior as part of the disease process. Caregivers are more likely to be abusive if they lack knowledge of alternative behavioral approaches, become overly obsessed with completion of caregiving tasks (feeding, bathing, etc.), have unresolved stress, are depressed, have a cultural acceptance of violence and punishment,

TABLE 12.1. Statement of resident rights

*You have a right to*

All care necessary for you to have the highest possible level of health

Safe, decent, and clean conditions

Be free of abuse and exploitation

Be treated with courtesy, consideration, and respect

Be free from discrimination based on age, race, religion, sex, nationality, or disability and to practice your own religious beliefs

Privacy, including privacy during visits and telephone calls

Complain about the facility and to organize or participate in any program that presents residents' concerns to the administrator of the facility

Have facility information about you maintained as confidential

Retain the services of a physician of your choice, at your own expense or through a health care plan, and to have a physician explain to you, in language you understand, your complete medical condition, the recommended treatment, and the expected results of the treatment, including reasonably expected effects, side effects, and risks associated with psychoactive medications

Participate in developing a plan of care, to refuse treatment, and to refuse to participate in experimental research

A written statement or admission agreement describing the services provided by the facility and the related charges

Manage your own finances or to delegate the responsibility to another person

Access money and property you have deposited with the facility and to an accounting of your money and property that are deposited with the facility and of all financial transactions made with or on behalf of you

Keep and use personal property, secure from theft or loss

Not be relocated within the facility, except in accordance with nursing facility regulations

Receive visitors

Receive unopened mail and to receive assistance in reading or writing correspondence

Participate in activities inside and outside the facility

Wear your own clothes

Discharge yourself from the facility unless you have been adjudicated mentally incompetent

Not be discharged from the facility, except as provided in the nursing facility regulations

Be free from any physical or chemical restraints imposed for the purposes of discipline or convenience and not required to treat your medical symptoms

(continued)

TABLE 12.1. (continued)

Receive information about prescribed psychoactive medication from the person who prescribed the medication or that person's designee, to have any psychoactive medications prescribed and administered in a responsible manner, as mandated by the Health and Safety Code, § 242.505, and to refuse to consent to the prescription of psychoactive medications

Place an electronic monitoring device in your room that is owned and operated by you or provided by your guardian or legal representative

---

or in the case of children, had been abused by their now elderly parent when they were children.

*Neglect* is an act of omission, i.e., the failure to meet one's obligation to anticipate and meet the needs of a vulnerable elderly person. Elders who have not yet been recognized as mentally incapacitated may be neglectful of themselves, refusing assistance, living in squalor, and not attending to health, hygiene, or safety (a common situation in Adult Protective Services). Neglect may be purposeful or retaliatory. This is more likely when the elder shows no gratitude or is critical of the care they receive. But more often, it is the result of inadequate understanding and anticipation of a vulnerable elder's needs. Poor knowledge and training on the specifics of caregiving for a vulnerable elder, inadequate care planning to delineate anticipated needs, lack of "job ownership," unprofessional attitudes, and low motivation are all potential risk factors for neglect. Elders with burdensome needs due to morbid obesity or slow assisted feeders are at increased risk as well. Neglect often occurs when caregivers fail to recognize progression of disability and its associated increased demands. Changes in the plan of care should not wait for a quarterly care plan update, but should occur when a change of resident condition is recognized.

Neglect may also occur at the institutional level due to understaffing, inadequately trained staff, or as a result of inadequate supervision, poor orientation or in-service training, inadequate equipment and resources, poor work group cohesion or excessive turnover of staff.

*Exploitation* refers to acts of misappropriation of a vulnerable elder's money or property. This is not necessarily for the purpose of enriching the perpetrator. For example, consider the scenario where two daughters hurriedly sell their mentally capacitated mother's house and furnishings while she was in a nursing facility recuperating from a surgery in order to prevent her returning to live unsafely at home alone since they thought that was in their mother's best interest. More often, however, exploitation is overt fraud or theft, for example, families misappropriating their elder's pension and Social Security checks for their own use, illegal transfers of property without proper consent or even the theft of the nursing home resident's property, or medications by staff. Occasionally, guardians and those designated as Power of Attorney may perpetrate exploitation. Courts require yearly reports from guardians as a method to discourage exploitation, but no such oversight is required for persons with other forms of surrogate decision making. The practitioner in long-term care should be alert to evidence of exploitation and report concerns to the appropriate authority. Consider the situation of an aged and nonambulatory resident with schizophrenia who wanted to buy a thermos to keep coffee in his room. This was conveyed to the facility's social worker who indicated the resident should have a small amount of spending money after nursing home payment from his Social Security check. When, 1 month later, the resident did not have a thermos, the physician discovered the resident's family routinely pocketed all his spending money. While the state government agency for nursing home surveys is typically the authority to investigate abuse of a nursing home resident by the facility or its staff, Adult Protective Services is the appropriate authority to investigate abuse, neglect, or exploitation of or by an individual who lives in the community.

Abuse, neglect, and exploitation perpetrated by a family member, unpaid caregiver, or other private individual are usually resolved without bringing criminal charges. In contrast, abuse, neglect, and exploitation at an institutional level, or by a certified or licensed caregiver within the long-term care continuum, are handled by the formal survey process and increasingly by licensure procedures and even criminalization. *Where tort reform has placed a cap on noneconomic damages, occasionally events alleged to be medical malpractice have been determined to be criminal abuse, thereby, arguably, making caps on noneconomic damages for medical malpractice irrelevant.*

The Centers for Medicare and Medicaid Services State Operations Manual requires nursing facilities to make efforts at abuse prevention by:

- Having abuse prevention policies and procedures
- Screening potential employees to be hired
- Providing initial and ongoing in-service training on elder abuse
- Making an effort to identify potential abuse events including setting expectations among staff for reporting

- Doing investigations of alleged abuse events and incidents that might constitute abuse
- Protecting residents from retaliation or distress during investigations
- Reporting incidents, alleged abuse events, investigations, and facility actions in response to investigations as required by state and federal authority

## Driving

Rarely will nursing facility providers need to address issues of the older driver, but other facilities within the long-term care continuum are likely to be challenged by this. Families will often raise this concern to the clinician and occasionally law enforcement or the Division of Motor Vehicles (DMV) will request the clinician's determination of an elder's fitness to drive. Best practices would include a clinician periodically considering fitness to drive as a part of geriatric health maintenance.

For the older drivers, a challenge to their fitness to drive will usually be perceived as a threat to their independence. At a practical level, inability to drive any longer would also restrict their ability to transport themselves to social and community activities and to meet basic needs such as shopping for food and accessing health care.

There is a perception that older drivers are more likely to be unsafe. In contrast, some maintain that experience, caution, and fewer miles driven make older drivers relatively safer than younger cohorts. Nevertheless, the rate of fatal motor vehicle accidents per mile driven is nine times greater for those 85 years of age or older than for drivers of 25 through 69 years of age [2].

From a public health perspective, driving carries some degree of risk for every person who goes behind the wheel and the diagnostic task for the clinician involves weighing this risk as increased by the elder's deficits in function or cognition with their need for independence and the circumstances under which they typically use a motor vehicle. The opinion of the clinician would likely differ for an urban elder with an available and supportive family and more options to meet transportation needs in contrast to the elder living in a rural setting with no support from family, despite an equal status of impairment in function and/or cognition.

Only a few states require a health care provider to report concern for an elder's fitness to drive and, as such, should be aware of their obligation to do so in their jurisdiction. Nevertheless, a majority of physicians hold the opinion that they should report concerns to authorities [3]. Addressing the issue of fitness to drive challenges the clinician to balance their ethical obligation with regard to an elder's autonomy and the clinician's fidelity to the elder with the principles of beneficence, to do what is best for the elder, and justice, to do what is best for the general public.

Elders need not lose their privilege to drive as clinicians may discover and correct remedial problems that are the cause of inadequate driving skills and prescribe adaptive equipment. Authorities may issue a limited license, e.g., daytime driving only. "Refresher" driver courses may help. These may be particularly useful if an elder who participates in such a course cannot redevelop adequate skills. Then the clinician can make a recommendation to the DMV based on more solid and objective evidence. A negative report to the DMV has significant potential to damage the doctor–patient relationship, but if framed in an empathetic manner, can focus on the elder's driving performance as the determinant and not have the elder blame the clinician for an arbitrary negative decision.

A thorough treatment of the assessment of elders' fitness to drive is beyond the scope of this chapter. A comprehensive review has been published by Marottoli [3]. Additionally, there are useful resources available at the American Medical Association website [4].

## Mental Capacity, Competence, and Options for Surrogate Decision Making

By law, all adult persons are considered mentally competent unless adjudicated otherwise. Thus, a designation of competency or incompetency is made by a court. Physicians and other providers as recognized by individual state law may make a determination of an individual's mental capacity or incapacity. This may be partial or complete and it may be specific to a particular circumstance. Capacity, then, is somewhat decision-related. Similarly, incapacity may be permanent as in dementia or temporary as in delirium or intoxication. While often used interchangeably, competency is a legal determination and mental capacity is a clinical one.

*There are several distinct types of competency under the law.* A person is competent to stand trial for crime if they know the difference between right and wrong and are able to participate in their own defense. Different criteria exist for making or changing a will, e.g., *testamentary capacity*. In this circumstance a person is considered competent if they know who are their heirs and understand the extent and the value of their assets. A person making or changing a will must be free of undue influence or coercion.

Practitioners are rarely asked to determine mental capacity as it relates to competence to stand trial, though in cases of resident-to-resident physical or sexual assault, this may occur. More often, practitioners are asked to evaluate mental capacity as it relates to making or changing a will. When this is likely to be contested, the practitioner may wish to obtain appropriate consents and then do the capacity evaluation on videotape or in a lawyer's office with full transcription. Asking questions that relate to the aforementioned scenario as well as performing a standard test of cognition would seem prudent.

Assessing mental capacity is often needed in long-term care practice to determine an elder's ability to make decisions in their own best interest of a personal, medical, and financial nature. Often an adult child listed as the *"Responsible Party"* on the nursing facility demographic face sheet with no formal legal authority is relegated to make decisions without any attempt to determine whether the resident is partially or fully mentally capacitated. This practice runs contrary to the ethical principle of autonomy and exemplifies ageism. Indeed, cases have occurred where a mentally capacitated individual has been kept in nursing home care against their will through the combined efforts of the facility, attending physician, and family.

Conversely, there are nursing or assisted living facilities which list the resident as the "Responsible Party," even though they are moderately or severely demented, psychotic, or neuropsychologically impaired, and thus clearly do not have decisional capacity. This usually occurs when the resident has no close family or proxy legal representative.

When an elder is found mentally incapacitated, the law can provide for several options of surrogate decision making. In many states, statutes exist listing a *hierarchy of family decision making* usually beginning with the spouse, then the oldest adult child, and so forth, who assume the decision-making role without need for a more involved legal process. Clinicians simply make a determination of *temporary* or *permanent* mental incapacity in the medical record, and then contact the family member highest on the list who is both capable and willing to undertake surrogate decision making. Should a clinician initially or subsequently believe that this individual is not acting in the best interest of the patient, the clinician should challenge their surrogate decision making status by submitting a report to Adult Protective Services or perhaps to the court as appropriate to that jurisdiction and circumstance.

Other forms of surrogate decision making include *Power of Attorney* and *conservatorships*. The latter typically deals only with financial matters, while Powers of Attorney may be designated as to decision making related to "person" or "estate" or both.

A *general power of attorney* is a legal instrument by which a mentally capacitated (presumed competent) person chooses another to make decisions on his or her behalf commencing from the time the instrument is executed and *endures until either death or a future time of mental incapacity*. These instruments may convey broad powers or may be very specific, e.g., to complete a real estate transaction.

A *springing power of attorney* may be made by a mentally capacitated person to give their chosen surrogate decision-making powers at some future time when the person may become mentally incapacitated.

A *durable power of attorney* goes into effect at execution (if agreed to by the capacitated person) and continues to grant surrogate decision-making power to the chosen person beyond the occurrence of mental incapacity of the person who established the power of attorney.

Long-term care providers should remain alert to the circumstance under which a family and lawyer draw up a Power of Attorney and encourage a mentally incapacitated person to sign it. These instruments can only be executed by a person who remains mentally capacitated. Once a person is mentally incapacitated, another form of surrogate decision making other than a Power of Attorney must be established such as a *guardianship*.

*Guardianship.* This may be temporary or permanent. A physician will often be asked to provide an opinion on an elder's mental incapacity (in part or total) stating the reason for incapacity and elaborating on any medical condition and medications that might affect the elder's mental status. This is typically done on a standardized legal form and submitted to the court. Upon making a ruling of incompetence, the court will name a guardian for surrogate decision making. These powers are not total. For example, a guardian may not sign consent for admission to inpatient psychiatric care, sign a Do Not Resuscitate (DNR), or authorize withdrawal of life-sustaining treatment. Such medical decisions require separate court action and can differ from state to state. In most states, a surrogate decision-maker cannot give permission for the nursing facility to hide antipsychotic medication in food, or give it by force or by injection on a routine basis, even to a severely demented or mentally ill person who has objected to taking the medication. This usually does not apply to the treatment of a psychiatric emergency in which the behavior puts the patient at imminent danger to self or others. In some states, the need for psychiatric treatment is sufficient to seek a forced medication order, but in most the standard of imminent danger to self or others must be met.

In decision making, the guardian should attempt to represent resident/patient choices that follow existing advanced directives. If no such directives exist, the guardian should make a best effort to make choices on behalf of their ward that are consistent with the historical value system, culture, and life history of the ward. When partial capacity exists, the wishes of the ward should be respected for those decisions for which they remain capacitated. When totally incapacitated, the guardian and caregivers should still attempt to ascertain the resident/patient opinions on different choices, more so when the probable outcomes of various choices are likely inconsequential. Wherever possible, *assent* should be solicited even when *consent* cannot.

### *Evaluation of Capacity*

When undertaking a capacity evaluation, the practitioner must maintain a high level of intellectual honesty. An elder's capacity is challenged when they make a decision with which others disagree. Obviously, this cannot be a stand-alone criterion. Neither can the level of cognitive impairment, similarly, be a sole criterion. Capacity is less an issue when various choices differ little in their risk and benefit. Of note, poor judgment that is lifelong does not necessarily indicate mental incapacity. People have a right to make mistakes, and some exercise this right again and again. However, poor judgment resulting from disease of the central nervous system and representing a decline from prior intellectual functioning is noteworthy evidence of mental incapacity.

A capacity evaluation should include a formal mental status examination, which includes:

- Mental status testing
- Judgment
- Orientation (time, person, place)
- Memory (recent, remote)
- Ability to think in the abstract
- Ability to calculate
- Ability to explain the nature of the needed decision at hand
- Ability to explain personal implications of choices, understand risks/benefits
- Ability to explain the rationale for choices
- How their decision best matches their personal goals
- Ability to persist in a decision unless new facts or circumstances arise
- Ability to negotiate (unless the issue at hand is a core value)
- Evaluation for undue influence or coercion
- Consideration for the effect of mental illness on decision making

Formal mental status testing such as with the Mini Mental Status Examination (MMSE) or the Saint Louis University Mental Status Exam (SLUMS) evaluates memory and orientation as well as other domains of cognition.

Judgment can be tested with hypothetical scenarios such as requesting a solution to the problem, "What would you do if you were the first person in a crowded movie theater to discover that it was on fire?" Answers not recognizing the need to avoid causing a panic would indicate faulty judgment. If the need for a specific and important decision has induced the evaluation, the clinician may specifically explore the individual's ability to explain the nature of the decision at hand, the individual's thoughts on the personal ramifications of various choices, and their assessment of the risks and benefits. An individual with capacity should also be able to articulate how they have come to a decision, what factors were important to them, and what values or principles they applied to come to the decision. The clinician must make allowances if hearing or eyesight interfere with the individual's grasp of the issues at hand.

Adequate *judgment* also involves the *ability to negotiate*. A capacitated individual should be able to negotiate in their best interest unless the issue at hand is related to one of their fundamental human and religious values. Thus, an individual who declines a blood transfusion, because they are a Jehovah's Witness, can be capacitated, though unwilling to negotiate on this issue in any way. But, an elder with a compelling need to be admitted to long-term care, yet who absolutely refuses to discuss the matter, insisting that her daughter will meet her needs for housekeeping, medical care, and personal assistance even though the daughter has categorically stated she will not be able to do, would fail to meet this test of mental capacity. Sometimes, if the potential medical consequences are not too high, a dilemma may best be handled by allowing the elder to experience the consequences of their decision. *Self-neglect* by the elder should be recognized and would support a determination of mental incapacity.

The *ability to think in the abstract* can be evaluated by asking the individual to explain the "underlying or poetic" meaning of a familiar proverb. The proverb should be one with which the individual is likely familiar. A concrete (nonabstract) answer may indicate low IQ, low educational level, or an organic impairment of the brain.

*Ability to calculate* can be tested by requesting the individual to subtract seven serially from 100. When specific to decisions at hand, a value comparison of certain assets may be helpful, e.g., "Which is worth more-your farm or your antique car?"

*A dysfunctional or "enmeshed" family* is at increased risk for placing undue influence or coercion on an elder family member. However, practitioners should also be aware that in certain cultures the opinion of a family leader or a family consensus is the accepted norm for decision making and would not be considered undue influence or coercion.

*Mental illness*, e.g., depression and psychosis, often is the basis of a finding of mental incapacity. However, decisions that conform to the individual's historical value system, culture, and life history prior to the onset of mental illness may well be capacitated decisions. Additionally, the reasoning underlying a decision should be examined such that choices made as a result of the individual's mental illness may be incapacitated, while others may be capacitated. For instance, a patient with paranoid schizophrenia who is refusing evaluation and treatment of a breast mass "because it's probably nothing" while scowling at the examiner probably lacks capacity. Or a patient with suicidal depression who declines electroconvulsive therapy because "it won't do any good" or because "I don't deserve to feel better" is likely incapacitated, while a similar patient who declines because "I'm scared I'll have memory loss, you told me ECT can cause that" is likely capacitated.

*Dementia does not automatically imply mental incapacity.* Determination of mental capacity depends on the severity of cognitive loss, the domains affected by cognitive loss, the kind and complexity of the issues at hand, and the potential consequences of the decision. Having said this, level of cognition is important to the determination of capacity. In a study by Marson et al. most participants with Alzheimer's disease showed capacity to make and communicate choices, consequences of choices, and their rationale for choices if they had a MMSE score of 19 or greater [5]. The clinician should not use this as a sole criterion when determining capacity. Standardized, structured capacity evaluations do exist such as the MacArthur Capacity Assessment Test [6], but these are not designed to determine if an elder is capacitated at a certain score.

**End-of-Life Issues**
Residents of long-term care facilities often have a limited life expectancy. Thus, end-of-life issues are common for clinicians. It has become a federal mandate upon admission to hospital or a long-term care facility to inquire whether a patient has made an *advance directive*, though it is not law that the patient must have one. Persons without a known advance directive are, in emergencies, presumed to have elected to pursue lifesaving and

life-sustaining treatment. In some states, persons with an advance directive that includes a decision of "Do Not Resuscitate" (DNR) are presumed to have verbally withdrawn their DNR if they call for an ambulance. Should a person wish to have such an advance directive for DNR continue to be respected, he or she may need to exercise a second advance directive that may be called an *Out-of-Hospital DNR*.

Any advance directives should be routinely and compassionately reviewed on admission to hospital or long-term care. Crisis-driven prerogatives by caregivers for a patient to create an advance directive should be viewed with apprehension that there may be other motives than the desire of the caregiver to follow the wishes of the patient.

An Advance Directive for health care may take the form of a *Living Will*. The Springing and Durable Powers of Attorney are also forms of advance directives, but these involve use of a proxy decision-maker. The Living Will is a document outlining the general and/or specific wishes of a capacitated individual (or previously capacitated person) for various health care procedures and strategies to be (or not be) carried out irrespective of his or her future mental capacity. If a capacitated person has a known, potentially fatal medical condition, it is wise to construct the Living Will within one's wishes in the event of clinical circumstances that are possible or likely given the natural history of that terminal disease. As most lack sufficient detail to speak directly about a specific disease or an actual clinical circumstance, Living Wills often leave room for doubt and controversy. However, they can provide a general framework that is useful to family as a guideline for that person's substituted judgment in the specific situation. This may lessen discord among family members and relieve potential guilt.

Note that a Living Will may state a person's wishes to receive aggressive treatment such as cardiopulmonary resuscitation (CPR), use of a respirator or feeding tube, etc., though this is seldom seen.

Areas of concern not usually addressed by Living Wills but that should be considered by the individual completing a Living Will include:

- Whether the individual wishes or declines to give a Power of Attorney the prerogative to consent to enter the person into research
- Whether they wish to be an organ donor
- Whether they wish to accept or decline psychotropic drug treatments by class and accept/decline electroconvulsive treatment

- Whether they wish to be allowed to enter into an emotional, physical, or sexual relationship with another person when they demonstrate assent
- Whether they wish to continue to have a physical relationship with their spouse when they demonstrate assent. Practitioner should be aware that some state surveyors and caregivers (both formal and informal) believe that once mentally incapacitated, an individual can no longer consent to be intimate with their spouse

The wishes expressed by an individual in their Living Will or by their surrogate, however, do not oblige the practitioner to perform *futile care*. The American Medical Association defines futile care as medical treatment that has very little or no potential for benefit. Practitioners may not recognize this obligation to avoid futile medical care. In some cases offering this (e.g., CPR in an unwitnessed cardiopulmonary arrest in the nursing home or feeding tube placement in a patient with end stage dementia), as if it were a reasonable treatment option, breaches the medical ethics of nonmaleficence and fidelity and may cause guilt in a family that declines such care. It may be prudent to educate families about futile medical treatments and discuss them as such. *There is no ethical difference between withholding a treatment and withdrawing it at such time as it becomes apparent that it is futile.* For instance, placing a person on a respirator when in acute respiratory failure does not oblige one to continue artificial ventilation when it is evident that the patient has intractable adult respiratory distress syndrome.

End-of-life issues, of course, include controversial issues such as of *active euthanasia* and *physician-assisted suicide*. The AMA and American Medical Directors Association (AMDA) have both spoken about these and other end-of-life issues. The reader is referred to policy statements and white papers stating the collective wisdom of these professional organizations. Table 12.2 lists these resources [7, 8].

### Ethical and Legal Aspects of Research in Long-Term Care

Given the unresolved care issues in long-term care, the value of research cannot be understated. Studies rarely focus on the long-term care population as those potential research subjects have many confounding diseases and conditions and are at risk to drop out of a study due to unexpected death or intervening comorbidity. They are also considered a "vulnerable population" with a higher than usual ethical and legal standard for informed consent to participate in research.

TABLE 12.2. American Medical Association and American Medical Directors Association Policy Statements, white papers and resolutions regarding end-of-life issues

### *AMA*

Policies on provision of life-sustaining medical treatment:
Optimal use of orders-not-to-intervened and advance directives
Sedation to unconsciousness in end-of-life
Advanced care directives
Medical futility in end-of-life care
Futile care
Quality of life
Withholding and withdrawing life-sustaining medical treatment
Euthanasia
Physician-assisted suicide
Do-not-necessitate orders
Surrogate decision making

### *AMDA*

White paper on the role of a facility ethics committee in decision making at the end of life (2008)
White paper on palliative care and hospice in long-term care (2007)
Surrogate decision making and advance care planning in long-term care (2003)
Hospice in long-term care (2000)
Access to high quality end-of-life care in nursing homes (March 2006)
Position statement on video surveillance in the long-term care Continuum (March 2005)
Ethical and professional responsibilities of long-term care physicians Providing expert witness (January 2004)
Ethics of long-term care research (March 2003)
Video surveillance cameras in nursing homes (March 2002)
Quality indicators for end-of-life care (March 2001)
Euthanasia of infants and children (March 2000)
End-of-life care planning in nursing facilities (March 1999)
Cardiopulmonary resuscitation in long-term care facilities (March 1999)

The high prevalence of cognitive impairment makes the long-term care population vulnerable to abuse in recruitment for research. The protections and processes required for the ethical and legal recruitment of incapacitated persons do allow for a legally recognized surrogate decision-maker to consent to research on behalf of the incapacitated person. However, an elder who in any way demonstrates lack of assent to the research should be either not enrolled or withdrawn. Further information on the ethical and legal aspects of research in vulnerable populations is reviewed in Reference [9].

### Liability in Long-Term Care

A discussion of medical malpractice and liability issues is crucial to practitioners and also germane to patient access, delivery of care, and care transitions. An AMDA survey in 2005 on attitudes and responses to the risk of litigation indicated that more than half had in some way limited their work as a medical director to avoid risk. Some 38% had limited their long-term care patient numbers as an attending physician. Almost the same number increased their use of consultations. Seven percent of respondents reported they had left long-term care practice due to risks of liability [10].

Most practitioners agree that when medical errors occur as a result of either negligence or purposeful misdeeds, the injured party should be reasonably compensated. Common liability issues in long-term care include:

- Dehydration
- Elopement
- Emotional distress
- Falls/fractures
- Improper use of restraints
- Medication errors
- Pressure ulcers
- Sexual assault
- Single event injuries
- Weight loss

Many long-term care providers feel that inevitable bad medical outcomes, inevitable decline in function or cognition, and unavoidable accidents are frequently litigated irrationally or unfairly. A negatively held view of long-term care by the public, frequently validated by the press, predisposes the facility and practitioners to criticism and liability.

In order for a *medical malpractice* action to have merit, plaintiffs must show:

- The defendant(s) had a *duty* to the patient
- Made a breach of an existing standard of care
- The breach was a *proximate cause* of harm suffered by the plaintiff
- Define the harm, injuries (e.g., *damages*), and what is their value

Given that most nursing facility residents have a limited remaining life expectancy and are not employable, actual damages in these cases are often not of great magnitude. But, *noneconomic damages*, e.g., pain and suffering or family/spouse loss of counsel and consortium, may increase damage claims. Additionally, *punitive damages* designed as a financial punishment for outrageously bad practices by the defendant(s) may be sought.

*Duty* exists when a long-term care practitioner or facility has an existing relationship with the patient, e.g., the patient is a resident of the nursing facility or is attended by a certain physician. Practitioners are duty bound to act in accordance with their *professional standards*. Facilities, likewise, are duty bound and also must act within existing state and federal regulations. Institutional policies and procedures that exceed professional standards or regulations can appear to raise the standard. *A practitioner is expected to exercise the degree of care and skill that would be expected of a reasonably prudent practitioner of that same kind under the same or similar circumstances.*

*Standards of care* once thought to be unique to a local geographic area are now viewed as national. *Regulations, clinical practice guidelines,* and *evidence-based practice* are often used to establish standard of care as well as the testimony of expert witnesses. *A breach of a standard of care may be either a matter of omission or commission.* While State and federal regulations are often claimed as creating the standard of care, the standard of care is created by medical professionals.

Not all breaches of a standard of care will connect to causation of harm. For example, failing to chart one meal intake as ordered by the physician is a breach of a nursing standard of care, but could not reasonably be the cause of weight loss. A *proximate cause* is an event or act that results in an injury that would not have occurred were it not for that event or act. It should be recognized that there could be more than one proximate cause for an injury. Breaches of standard of care (that do not connect to causation) are of great interest and concern to quality improvement processes, but may only be relevant to medical malpractice as supplemental evidence of a defendant's inadequate training, experience, or professional conduct.

Practitioners should be aware of several pitfalls in nursing facility litigation. Creating risk are inadequate documentation, criticisms or bickering between practitioners in the medical record, failure to follow policies and procedures without documentation of a clinically supportable reason to do so, doing routine documentation of care in a manner not concurrent with that care (end-of-shift rote charting that can foster documentation of care not delivered such as turning and repositioning charted at a time when the resident was out of the facility), and failure to notify the physician and family of changes in condition (sometimes facilitated or motivated by the excessive use of PRN orders for problems such as pain, nausea and vomiting, fever, etc.). Outdated and unnecessary policies and procedures create risk. Care plans not updated to reflect the current condition of the resident and the care being delivered, failure to follow the care plan, and unrealistic goals documented in the care plan all predispose the facility, staff, and physician to litigation. Once a malpractice action is initiated, failure to protect the integrity of the medical record and alterations of the medical record (whether these relate to the cause of action or not) can be severely damaging to the defense.

When *medical errors* do occur, there is an evolving literature on disclosure and apology. Proponents believe that residents and families who have suffered harm from a medical error will appreciate honest disclosure of fault, heartfelt apologies, and providers' and practitioners' thoughts on how changes in policies and care practices will prevent future mishaps. Practitioners should become familiar with these issues, risk management, loss control (i.e., prevention), expectations at their facility, medical group, etc., before undertaking this course of action. At the present time, early and honest disclosure of fault with or without an offer to remedy the matter offers no protection from the plaintiff's constitutional right to litigate. In the future, a system of recognizing errors through the quality improvement process, incident reports and complaints followed by disclosure, and apology may be possible. Caregivers could then make legitimate and fair offers for compensation for injuries and assure an injured party of changes in policies and care process to prevent future error. Such a system would do much to incentivize quality of care and allow caregivers to adhere to the principles of medical ethics as we all aspire to do.

## SUMMARY
Ethical and legal issues abound in the everyday practice of long-term care medicine. The clinician must have a thorough understanding of medical ethics and the law in one's jurisdiction and be able to communicate these issues to other members of the interdisciplinary team, the family, and patients in a way that will foster collaboration and consensus within an ethical and legal framework. A clinician skilled and confident in these areas can do much to guide patients, families, and other caregivers through the process of medical decision making that will provide clarity, comfort, and consistency to the plan of care within the goals and personal

values of the person receiving that care. Our adherence to the principles of medical ethics defines our professionalism and creates the matrix within which all clinical care must be delivered.

## PEARLS FOR THE PRACTITIONER

- Clinicians making ethical medical decisions often encounter competing values and must weigh these in view of the facts and circumstances, and within the framework of the law, to come to a supportable decision.
- The basic principles of medical ethics include autonomy, beneficence, justice, nonmaleficence, and fidelity.
- Providers have an obligation to inform long-term care residents of their rights and to encourage and facilitate them in exercising those rights.
- Elders who have been found inadequate in driving skills need not lose their privilege to drive if the clinician can discover and correct remedial problems that are the cause or if a limited license can be issued making the inadequacy moot.
- Mental capacity to make decisions for oneself may be partial or complete and may be specific to a particular circumstance or decision.
- A capacity evaluation should include assessment of judgment, orientation, memory, ability to think in the abstract, to do calculations, and freedom from undue coercion.
- Wishes for medical care expressed by a patient or surrogate do not obligate the practitioner to perform futile care.
- There is no ethical obligation to even offer any proposed intervention incapable of providing a benefit to the patient, or one whose burdens outweigh its benefits, in fact it is ethically unjustifiable to provide such an intervention to a patient.
- The act of withholding a proposed medical intervention and that of later withdrawing the same intervention once begun is the same ethical decision.
- Withdrawing life-sustaining therapy such as artificial hydration, feeding or ventilation when it is deemed to be incapable of providing further benefit to the patient, or when its continued application provides greater burden than benefit, is not an affirmative act causing the death of the patient. It is the underlying medical condition that is being allowed to go to its conclusion that is the cause of death of the patient.
- Medical malpractice action is meritorious if (a) the defendant(s) had a duty to the patient, (b) there was a breach of an existing standard of care, (c) that breach was a proximate cause of harm, and d) there are quantifiable damages.

- Any proposed medical intervention must first be capable of providing a benefit to the patient, and further that the benefits must outweigh any burdens to the patient from its application.
- Artificial feeding and hydration are medical interventions, not basic care, and as such, are subject to the same benefits/burdens analysis as for any other proposed medical intervention.

## WEBSITES
- Texas Department of Aging & Disability Services www.dads.state.tx.us
- AMA Physician's Guide to Assessing and Counseling Older Drivers www.ama-assn.org/ama/pub/category/10791.html
- American Medical Directors Association (AMDA) White Papers www.amda.com/governance/papers.cfm
- AMDA Ethics of Long-Term Care Research www.amda.com/governance/resolutions/m03.cfm
- Physician's Guide to Assessing and Counseling Older Drivers http://www.nhtsa.dot.gov/people/injury/olddrive/OlderDriversBook

## REFERENCES
1. www.dads.state.tx.us
2. AMA Physician's Guide to Assessing and Counseling Older Drivers. http://ama-assn.org/ama/pub/category/10791.html
3. Marottoli R (2000). Older driver assessment. In: Osterweil D, Brummel-Smith K, Beck JC, Eds. Comprehensive Geriatric Assessment. New York: Mc-Graw-Hill, 443–464.
4. http://ama-assn.org/ama/pub/category/10791.html and www.nhtsa.dot.gov/people/injury/olddrive/physician
5. Marson DC, Ingram KK, Cody HA, et al. (1995). Assessing the competency of patient's with Alzheimer's disease under different legal standards. Archives of Neurology, 52, 949–954.
6. Grisso T, Applebaum PS, Hill-Fotouhi C., (1997) The MacCat-T: clinical tool to assess patient's capacity to make treatment decisions. Psychiatric Services, 48, 1415–1419.
7. www.ama-assn.org/ama/pub/physician-resources/medical-ethics
8. www.amda.com/governance/papers.cfm
9. www.amda.com/governance/resolutions/m03.cfm
10. AMDA liability survey shows more than half limit work as medical director. AMDA Health Policy Advisor 9(2), 2005.
11. Huss R, Smith DA (2009). Nursing facility litigation and liability: a case-based tutorial. In: Presented 32d Annual Symposium of American Medical Directors Association, Charlotte, NC.

# Chapter 13
# Caring for Families

David Brechtelsbauer

**Keywords:** Family • Skills in dealing with families • Family spokesperson • Family meeting • Cultural barriers

## INTRODUCTION

Too often physicians and other members of the interdisciplinary team (IDT) shudder when the note, "Please call Mrs. Jones' daughter" appears on the chart. The goal of this chapter is to examine attitudes, review and apply knowledge, and illustrate skills that will improve the performance of all practitioners who must work with families in the LTC setting.

Family caregivers, usually adult children, face many challenges. Family members vary widely in their level of knowledge of their loved ones condition and of how to work effectively with the health care system. Poorly implemented hospital-nursing facility patient transfers can leave family caregivers frustrated and confused [1]. Adult children are often uncomfortable with the role-reversal experienced when caring and advocating for an elderly parent. The realities of being separated by long distances and having employment and nuclear family obligations can limit an adult child's opportunities to assess the situation firsthand, or to actively participate in care giving. Family members are often unprepared when thrust into the new role of caring for a parent, and need education and support [2].

The 2008 Institute of Medicine report, *Retooling for An Aging America* [3], recommends an even greater role for family and other informal caregivers as part of the response to workforce challenges created by the baby boomer generation's entry into old age and the resulting stresses on the health care system, especially long-term care. This demographic reality will require LTC professionals to become even more efficient and effective when working with families.

This chapter will provide guidance and a concise reference for physicians and other LTC professionals who wish to improve their performance when working with families.

## ATTITUDES

It is useful to examine one's attitudes towards families and the issues that commonly arise when working with families. Prejudicial assessments, blind spots in problem solving, and ineffective interventions can result when the professional is unaware of his or her own beliefs and values relative to how families are defined and how they (should) function.

Some of the discomfort in dealing with family issues probably relates to the lack of attention to communication, particularly communication with persons other than the patient, in many professional training programs. The emphasis placed on the doctor-patient relationship and confidentiality is often the first attitudinal barrier that must be negotiated before one can work effectively with families. Practitioners who feel they are exclusively responsible to the designated patient may respond by trying to avoid dealing with families, a response that only worsens most issues.

*Overcoming an exclusive focus on the patient will allow the professional to consider the family system, as well as the patient, to be a focus of care.* Many times this can result in a collaborative relationship between the IDT and the family, to the benefit of the resident and the facility. Other families, due to personal preferences or the barriers created by living far away or holding down two jobs, will want to be kept informed, but will not be able to share in the care of the resident. Finally, a few families (the vast majority in the experience of the author) have no desire to be involved. It is useful to determine the level of involvement desired by each family, and periodically check to determine if the desired level of involvement has changed.

*It is important to recognize the influence of one's family of origin on attitudes toward family issues.* While professionals are encouraged to set aside personal biases when engaged in a professional relationship, *feelings* about traditional verses nontraditional family structures, gender roles, locus of decision-making, and filial obligation all can impact a professional's attitudes, and therefore effectiveness, when dealing with families.

A major attitudinal issue is reflected in the use of the word "*dysfunctional*" when describing families. Too often the word signals a professional caregiver's feeling hopeless or powerless to intervene in a difficult family situation. Whenever a care team member utters this word, that person needs to be encouraged to examine exactly what he/she understands the word to mean and why use of "dysfunctional" seems necessary or appropriate in the situation at hand. At times dysfunctional may be an accurate description, but dwelling on that aspect of the problem will interfere with problem solving.

*Cross-cultural issues* can also raise attitudinal issues and create blind spots in one's thinking. Increasing diversity in the population is a second demographic trend that requires reexamination of systems of care and communication skills. Cultural issues will be discussed later in this chapter.

## KNOWLEDGE

The physician's knowledge of the resident and of the *health care system* are important prerequisites to success when working with families. It is important for the LTC professional to remember that families are generally not expert in how the health care system works, and much of the knowledge families do have was gained through experience obtained in the acute care setting. For example, it is useful to discuss restraints preemptively as the family has probably seen their loved one "protected" by side rails in the hospital and will be at best confused, and at worst angry, that such a simple and common sense safety device is not available in the nursing home.

Displaying and sharing knowledge of the health care system in a noncondescending manner is an important first step in building credibility and rapport with the resident and family. Studies have shown that the move to a long-term care setting, which for many LTC professionals is routine and straightforward, is a major stressor for residents and families [4]. Compassionately and effectively guiding the family through the initial transition from acute care to long-term care will get the physician-patient and physician-family relationship off to a positive start, and in turn help create a collaborative and positive tone for the ongoing relationship between the *professional (formal)* and *family (informal) caregivers*.

Subsequent situations that are likely to be new to the family and that will benefit from proactive efforts by the physician and IDT to meaningfully engage the family include: the response to the first incident, the first acute illness or exacerbation of a chronic illness, the need to explicitly address goals of care and possible limitation of treatment options, formal code status discussions, and end of life care issues [4].

Beyond knowledge of the resident's medical condition and the functioning of the medical system, some knowledge of *clinical psychology* and *family systems* medicine is useful to provide a foundation for effective work with families. Full discussion of this knowledge base is beyond the scope of this chapter. Excellent texts [5] and review articles [6, 7] discussing this aspect of care with particular reference to long-term care are available.

*Chronic illness* in general, and particularly moving from the family home, creates stress for residents and their families. Most families cope well most of the time. Explicitly asking, "What stressful events have you (your family) dealt with in the past? and How did you cope?" is helpful. The best predictor of future behavior is past behavior. Knowledge of past coping skills can inform plans being made to deal with a new crisis. Responses to the above questions can raise "red flags" for ineffective coping and dissatisfaction with care. Communication difficulty is more likely to occur if family members bring with them a pattern of chronic financial stress, active substance abuse, chronic psychiatric problems, or criminal behavior [8].

Prudence requires that the physician and other members of the care team proactively engage family members when red flags are noted. Make extra and persistent efforts to communicate. Seek agreement or at least acknowledgement of realistic goals of care, and monitor the resident's progress and the family's progress in managing their stress. Give family members permission to take time for themselves as a way to manage stress and preserve caregiver health. If things are not going well, consider referral to a family therapist, religious counselor, or a community resource (Alzheimers Association, Adult Day Care Program, etc.).

## SKILLS

*Skills in dealing with families are learned and improve with practice.* If one finds him/herself struggling when returning phone calls from family members, avoiding family contact, or, unable to participate in family meetings, it is helpful to find someone who is skilled and effective in this area. Practicing these skills under the watchful eye of a mentor, and being open to feedback and the use of new or refined approaches will lead to improvement.

In an encounter likely to be emotionally charged it is important to choose one's words very carefully [9]. The phrase "there is nothing more to do" often is spoken when dealing with fail elderly residents and their families. A more complete, accurate, and less provocative phrase would be, "There is nothing more to do *to cure the illness*." This statement opens the door to discussion of symptom management, psychosocial and spiritual support, and other measures that promote comfort and dignity for the resident and caring and support for the family.

A similar problematic question posed to residents or their families is, "Would you like us to do everything?" Clinicians often equate this with the use of high tech interventions and need for acute hospital level of care. For families, it is a question that often precipitates a "yes" answer when they are thinking about everything to relieve pain and suffering, not about transferring their loved one back to the hospital. A better phrase is, "I recognize your mother is in distress, and that in turn is distressing to you. I don't think sending her to the hospital for more tests would help her distress, but let me explain what we can do here in the nursing home to get her pain (or any distressing symptom) under better control."

There are times a resident may need to be admitted for symptom control, but many symptoms can be managed by a skilled nursing facility IDT without hospitalization. The physician's awareness of the nursing facility team's level of skill and confidence will also influence the recommendation to treat in the nursing facility or in the hospital [10].

### Selection of a Family Spokesperson

In most circumstances communication efficiency is enhanced when the physician and other IDT members communicate with the family through a family spokesperson. This person's contact information needs to be conveniently available. While the physician or IDT may have a preference as to which family member should be the spokesperson, the choice rests with the family. The family's choice is often revealing as it typically reflects how the family has functioned in the past.

The team needs to inquire as to the spokesperson's preferred method of communication – telephone (home, work, cell), email, face-to-face, and the alternative plan if the designated spokesperson is not available. It is also useful to let the spokesperson know the best times and locations for contacting team members, generally which team members are most knowledgeable in which areas, and who to contact when it is not obvious to the spokesperson. Typically, the administrator is ultimately the point person for facility issues, and the attending physician or medical director for medical issues.

### Responding to a Phone Call from an Unhappy Family Member

A useful phrase to use when returning phone calls is, "Hello Mrs. Jones. This is Dr. Smith. *I understand you are concerned about your mother.*" Use of this phrase communicates to the family member that you have some level of awareness about the concern. If you don't have an idea about what is going on, call the nurse, social worker, or other staff member to get basic information about what might be going on before returning the call. If it's a particularly dicey situation, making a face-to-face visit to the resident and more thorough data collection is important if it can be accomplished without causing too much delay in returning the call. The need for prompt communication needs to be balanced with the need for preparation.

Mrs. Jones is likely to have to agree with your opening statement, which gets the conversation off on the right foot. Next, *very briefly* state your understanding of the issue – "I think at least some of your concerns relates to your mother's bruises, but please explain to me what you are noticing." Then, with the chart available in order to record what you are about to hear, do what too many professionals find difficult: listen to the whole story before attempting to explain. On one level, families often are as concerned that they are not being heard as they are about the problem itself. Important things to listen for are family perceptions and interpretations that you did not expect, and if the caller is an eager or reluctant family spokesperson. Sometimes the caller has been put up to calling by another family member and the caller's own feelings and perceptions are not congruent with the feelings and perceptions of the family member with the concern. While working through a family spokesperson is generally recommended, in this case the professional might want to ask the spokesperson if it would be better to speak directly to the person with the concern.

After listening, and with review of your notes, reflect back what you heard with enough detail for the family member to be convinced that you have heard and understood what was said. Depending on the issues involved, you may be able to provide education, reassurance, or an action plan that will satisfy the caller. If you are not able to do so, in the absence of a true emergency, the best response is, "I'm going to have to look into your concerns in order to better understand what is going on. I will visit the nursing facility tomorrow and get back to you later in the day. What is the best way to reach you tomorrow afternoon after three?"

Effective communication by phone, including keeping a succinct record of what was said, is an extremely important skill.

Consider the following example of a phone call from a family member whose loved one had been transferred from the nursing facility to the hospital the day earlier. The phone call was transcribed verbatim (names have been changed) in order to enter it into the medical record.

> This is Donna Smith. I am Richard Jones' daughter. Richard was taken yesterday from Sunset Manor to the hospital, at first with thoughts of a stroke or whatever. I guess we are just really, really frustrated. Nobody, Dr. B or I know he has students or whatever that come in and are under him [the caller is referring to resident physicians], my mom has not heard anything from him as far as treatment, what is the plan, what are they going to do? If it was a stroke, what the blood test results were? We need to know. He has been laying up there for a full day with nothing to eat, we don't know if he can eat. He can't speak. It is pretty frustrating and I believe probably somebody needs to get on the ball and find out what is going on and let the family know. My number is xxx-xxxx, and my mother's number is xxx-xxxx. Her name is Darla Jones and she is retired. She is on her way up to the hospital right now. Again, we do want some answers and we want to know what is going on. Thank you.

Obviously the ball was dropped in this situation. When this call is returned, an apology needs to be promptly stated. What is really informative however, in this example is the concerned tone of the message when it was reviewed by *listening to the voice mail*, in contrast to the hostile character one quickly picks up when reading the transcription. A major lesson here is not to read too much into a transcribed message. In situations where there seems to be hostility (and, in contrast to the example, there may be hostility), it's best to respond by phone in order to hear the tone of voice and inflection, or even face-to-face so the clinician can observe and respond to nonverbal cues.

It is becoming more common for families to communicate by email. Email allows the convenience of asynchronous communication and convenient record keeping. Like the above example however, email messages generally cannot accurately convey the emotional state of the family member sending the message or the empathy of the responding professional. When the content of the email message is not routine it is generally better to pick up the phone than to hit the reply button. It is also very important to carefully proofread your email before sending it, and be extremely careful if you are sending it to the correct person; inadvertently striking the "reply all" key can create problems.

Emerging technology may allow virtual face-to-face encounters. These hold promise to overcome some of the disadvantages of current technology, but their use and role are still in evolution [11].

### Convening and Conducting a Family Meeting

Effective phone communication and face-to-face meetings with the family spokesperson can sometimes resolve family concerns. Other situations, either because of complex family dynamics, or because of the complex medical or ethical issues that are causing the concern, require a much more formal process to achieve resolution. The "rules" for family meetings are a product of the "Family Systems" literature and are summarized here. A more detailed description is referenced at the end of this chapter [12].

*Preparation for a family meeting* needs to be even more thorough and thoughtful than preparation for a phone call. The practitioner needs to learn as much as possible about the resident, be as familiar as possible with the facility environment and culture, and understand the medical issues as completely as possible. This often involves an examination of the resident and review of the chart for the purpose of clarifying the current status of the medical issue(s), obtaining as much knowledge as possible about the family, and discussing the concern with relevant staff members including the floor nurse and certified nursing assistant, the social worker, and chaplain. If the issue involves a conflict about nursing facility regulations or internal polices, the administrator should also be consulted. Once the above preparation is complete, set a date, time, and place for the meeting. Professionals need to, as much as possible, clear schedules to allow for uninterrupted participation. All *relevant* professionals should attend, but avoid having too many staff members attend in order not to appear to be ganging up on the family. By the same token, all family members should attend. Out of town family members should be encouraged to participate via conference call or speakerphone.

*The person moderating the meeting should begin with introductions and state the "rules" for the meeting.* Many physicians, with training and experience, are comfortable in the moderator role, but the moderator can be anyone on the professional team. Many social workers have formal training and are skilled moderators of family meetings.

*The first rule is that everyone will be invited to state his or her perception of the problems.* This is to be done without interruption, if another person at the table wants to make a comment the comment should be written down and reported during that person's time to speak. Generally speaking, the resident, if present, or the least empowered person should speak first. The person who is least empowered may be the person who is present only by speakerphone, or the person with the least familiarity with the problem or the least formal education. In an effort to put family members at ease, assure everyone that all comments are useful to help understand the concerns that precipitated the need for the meeting. If you are aware that a particular family member might be intimidating to other family members, or has very strong feelings about the issue at hand, call on that person last.

This may seem like a time consuming process, especially with large families. Often however, family members begin to report that they agree with a previous speaker and have nothing to add.

*After the family has spoken, the moderator should summarize what has been said and secure assent that the summary is basically correct.* Then each professional is called upon to state his/her perception of the issue. Avoid offering solutions at this point. Once again, after the professional team has spoken, the moderator should offer a brief summary of what was said.

*Next the person with the most credibility (this is often, but not always, the physician) can provide education and suggest realistic goals and expectations.* Discussion, problem solving, and hopefully agreement on next steps follow. It is useful to explicitly define what will be measured to monitor the results of the intervention(s). Ask, "If this plan works, how will we know?" Also, agree on how the results of the monitoring will be communicated to both the family and the IDT, particularly the front line caregivers.

Most of the time this will lead to a plan that is acceptable to the family and the IDT. If things go poorly it may be possible only to state that the outcome, for now at least is "we can only agree we disagree."

The team and family at this point can be *assigned tasks* (obtaining a second opinion, obtaining a copy of the advance directive, searching the internet for references) that may impact the situation and provide useful information for a future meeting. It is sometimes helpful to have the next meeting moderated by a skilled and disinterested family therapist. Other options are to refer the situation to an ethics committee or formal arbitration.

While in the long run formal family meetings often save time (and improve outcomes and satisfaction) and can sometimes be quite efficient, there are barriers to equitable reimbursement for the time involved in preparation and participation in a family-IDT meeting. If the resident is present the physician can bill and be reimbursed for education, counseling, and coordination of care using appropriate nursing facility subsequent visit codes. Some facilities will recognize the value of family meetings, both in terms of resident/family satisfaction and risk management, and be willing to pay the moderator a reasonable consultation fee.

## Writing a Progress Note for Families

The *degree of involvement families desire* in the care of their loved ones varies dramatically. For the family who has frequent questions it can be useful to, with the consent of the resident, send a copy of the physician's progress note after each routine nursing facility visit. It is of course necessary to write a less technical note, or provide a brief cover letter, to make this a useful intervention. Sending a copy of progress notes routinely can sometimes dramatically decrease the number of phone calls to the physician or facility.

Families quickly learn that, generally speaking, no news from the nursing facility is good news. Ongoing communication about routine and nonurgent matters can build rapport and a common understanding of the resident's situation. This in turn can make communication at critical times more efficient and productive. An example of a cover letter to the family spokesperson is as follows:

Dear Mrs. White,

A copy of my note from your sister's most recent nursing home check-up is enclosed. Tilly was pleasant and cooperative during my visit. I did not find any major changes.

If you have any questions or comments please feel free to call the office (XXX–XXXX) and leave a message with my office nurse, Sandy H.

Sincerely,
Dr. Good Apple

## Creating and Using a Genogram

Creation of genograms, a diagrammatic representation of a family, is taught in many social work and nursing training programs, but is less familiar to most medical professionals. The ability to create *a genogram is a useful skill, providing an efficient way to document and recall the "anatomy" of the family*.

By convention, male family members are represented as squares and females as circles. An arrow indicates the resident. A horizontal line connecting the two individuals involved indicates a marriage, a slash though the line indicates a divorce. Each generation occupies a separate "layer" on the genogram. Notations can be added indicating supportive or problematic relationships [13]. An example of the Brown family, whose matriarch is unhappy with being placed in a nursing facility, is as follows:

A review of the genogram illustrates Grandma Ethel's likely belief that "in our family we take care of people at home" and the likely pressure this family story creates for daughter Beth and daughter-in-law Heidi. The genogram also provides a "snapshot" of potential family resources and likely sources of conflict.

Families change over time and the genogram needs to periodically be updated. Reference to the genogram before returning a phone call or participating a family meeting can quickly refresh one's memory of family structure and dynamics, making the call or meeting more productive and efficient.

## WHEN THERE ARE CULTURAL BARRIERS

Like unexamined attitudinal issues, *cultural barriers can also create blind spots and interfere with success when working with families.* In an age where political correctness sometimes trumps confronting a problem directly, examining possible cultural issues can be intimidating.

*Begin by examining your personal and professional cultures.* What assumptions might others make based on knowing you are an African-American physician, or a Pilipino nurse? If things often thought about a cultural or professional group were true, how much would they apply to you?

*Next, consider the cultural background of the resident and his/her family.* What do you know, or think you know, about the culture in question? No one expects a healthcare professional to have an intimate knowledge of each resident's culture, but some basic knowledge is useful. Professional colleagues from the culture of the resident may be helpful. Other resources are your local librarian, Brigham Young University's "CultureGrams" (www.culturegrams.com) [14] ,and the US Department of State (www.state.gov) [15].

Just as you may recognize yourself as being an American physician, but meet none of the stereotypes, you cannot assume the resident and the resident's family will be well characterized by generalizations made about their culture. A useful way to begin to address this is to ask; "I have heard that it is common in Bulgaria for adult children to care for their elderly parents. How true is that for your family?"

Sometimes, despite being knowledgeable and respectful of the family and the family's cultural background, communication still seems ineffective. In this case it is *usually helpful to find a mutually acceptable mediator.* This person selected is often a community or religious leader from the cultural group involved. This person can often "bridge the gap" between the prevailing and/or professional culture and the minority and/or lay culture.

Effective communication when a translator is necessary requires behaviors that may not be intuitive. When a translator is being used it is important to talk directly to the resident and not to the translator. "How are you feeling today?" is more likely to engender engagement and a meaningful response than "Ask her how she is feeling today." Talking directly to the resident also makes the translator's job easier.

Professional translators are preferred over use of family members, although financial and logistical barriers often force the use of untrained family members. Companies offering telephone-based translators can be found by searching "language line" on the Internet. Prices and available languages vary.

## SUMMARY

A practitioner seeking to achieve excellence in working with families in the long-term care setting needs to critically examine his or her attitudes towards families, and display detailed knowledge of the resident, facility, IDT function, and the family system. Excellence can only be achieved through the development of communication skills, including communication in the setting of a family meeting. The ability to create and utilize a genogram is a powerful asset that will enhance communication with families.

Cultural issues can make communication more difficult. Successful communication can be assured by a obtaining a basic knowledge of the culture, and when necessary the skilled use of a translator.

## PEARLS FOR THE PRACTITIONER

- Recognize and acknowledge that chronic illness and LTC placement are major stressors for residents and their families.
- In almost every situation it is important to listen before offering solutions.
- Determine the level of involvement the family desires, whenever possible support that involvement.
- Practice until you can comfortably and skillfully
- Return a phone call from a family member
- Respond to an email communication from a family member
- Participate effectively in a family meeting
- Create and utilize a genogram
- Communicate with a resident/family when using a translator
- Develop resources that can efficiently provide background information when dealing with residents/families from cultures different from the dominant culture

## WEBSITES

- Culture Grams: http://www.culturegrams.com
- AMDA: http://www.amda.com

- End of Life/Palliative Education Resource Center: http://www.eperc.mcw.edu
- EPERC has valuable, practical and succinct information in "Fast Facts" – select "Communication" for information most relevant to this chapter, including particularly Fast Fact 222 Preparing for the Family Meeting, and Fast Fact 223 The Family Meeting: Starting the Conversation.
- U.S. Department of State: http://www.state.gov

## REFERENCES

1. Marziali E, Shulman K, Damianakis T. Persistent family concerns in long-term care settings: meaning and management. J Am Med Dir Assoc. 2006;7:154–162.
2. Henry SM. The Eldercare Handbook: Difficult Choices, Compassionates Solutions. New York: Harper-Collins; 2006.
3. Institute of Medicine. Retooling for an Aging America: Building the Health Care Workforce. Washington: National Academies Press; 2008.
4. Bern-Klug M. The emotional context facing nursing home residents' families: a call for role reinforcement strategies from nursing homes and the community. J Am Med Dir Assoc. 2008;9:36–44.
5. Conn DK, Herrmann N, Kaye A, et al., eds. Practical Psychiatry in the Long-Term Care Home: A Handbook for Staff. 3rd ed. Cambridge: Hogrefe & Huber; 2007.
6. Winn P, Cook JB, Bonnel W. Improving communication among attending physicians, long-term care facilities, residents, and residents' families. J Am Med Dir Assoc. 2004;5:114–122.
7. Bluestein D, Bach PL. Working with families in long-term care. J Am Med Dir Assoc. 2007;8:265–270.
8. Kidder SW, Smith DA. Is there a conflicted surrogate syndrome affecting quality of care in nursing homes? J Am Med Dir Assoc. 2006;7:168–172.
9. Pantilat SZ. Communicating with seriously ill patients: better words to say. JAMA. 2009;301:1279–1281.
10. Cheng HY, Tonorezos E, Zorowitz R, et al. Inpatient care for nursing home patients: an opportunity to improve transitional care. J Am Med Dir Assoc. 2006;7:383–387.
11. Hensel BK, Parker-Oliver D, Demiris G, Rantz M. A comparison of video-based resident-family communication in a nursing home and a congregate living facility. J Am Med Dir Assoc. 2009;10:342–347.
12. Bloom MV, Smith DA. Brief mental health interventions for the family physician. New York: Springer; 2001:262–263.
13. McGoldrick M, Greson R, Shellenberger S. Genograms: Assessment and Intervention. 2nd ed. New York: W. W. Norton & Co.; 1999.
14. CultureGrams. www.culturegrams.com. Accessed October 3, 2101.
15. U. S. Department of State. www.state.gov. Accessed October 3, 2101.

# Part 4
Special Issues in Long-Term Care

# Chapter 14
# Documentation and Coding

Alva Baker and Leonard Gelman

**Keywords:** Documentation • Medical decision-making • CPT codes • Coding • Billing

## INTRODUCTION

The provision of care to residents of long-term care facilities presents different complexities in documentation and coding for both physician and practitioner services than those provided in the office or hospital setting. Proper documentation of the care provided and use of the appropriate billing code is essential to receiving appropriate reimbursement for rendered services. Practitioner familiarity with a glossary of common terms (see Figure 14.1) is critical to ensure accurate documentation, coding, and billing.

## DOCUMENTING THE VISIT

The AMA is responsible for establishing and maintaining the CPT codes. The AMA defined documentation guidelines for Evaluation and Management (E/M) codes in 1995 and these were revised in 1997. These are available on the CMS website. Either set can be used but one cannot mix the guidelines for any one encounter. AMDA has issued a Guide to Long Term Care Coding, Reimbursement and Documentation based upon the AMA's CPT guide (available for ordering at www.amda.com).

There are seven components that define provider encounters. In most cases the first three are called the *key components* and are used to define the level of E/M service.

> *Admission* – when a patient enters a NF or SNF and there are no open clinical or financial records pertaining to the current stay
> *Re-Admission* – there is no clarity from CMS concerning the definition of this term, and it may be used in two ways, the more logical of which, based on the CMS wording in the Medicare Carrier Manual, is number two below
> 1. When a patient returns to a NF or SNF after leaving with a bed hold status; the clinical and financial records have remained open and the patient is considered to be continuing the current stay that began prior to leaving with the bed hold status; all services are billed using the subsequent care codes (99307-99310)
> 2. When a patient returns to a NF or SNF after leaving with a discharged status; the clinical and financial records from the prior stay have been closed and the patient is considered to be starting a new stay; an initial visit is again required and this is billed using the initial care codes (99304-99306)
>
> *Discharge* – when a patient leaves a NF or SNF to go to another venue of care (home, hospital, assisted living, group home, etc.) and the clinical and financial records pertaining to the current stay are closed, even if there is a possibility or probability that the patient will return to the same NF or SNF
> *Bed Hold* – when a patient leaves a NF or SNF to go to another venue of care (usually, hospital) and the clinical and financial records pertaining to the current stay remain open in expectation of the patient's return
> *MDS* – acronym for Minimum Data Set, the comprehensive multidisciplinary evaluation performed for a patient on admission and periodically thereafter as long as the patient remains a resident in the NF or SNF; the MDS is electronically to State and Federal agencies
> *Initial Visit* – "the initial comprehensive assessment visit during which the physician completes a thorough assessment, develops a plan of care and writes or verifies admitting orders for the nursing facility resident."
> *CMS* – acronym for The Centers for Medicare and Medicaid Services
> *Nursing Facility (NF)* – an institution (or a distinct part of an institution) which is primarily engaged in providing skilled nursing care and related services for residents who require medical or nursing care, or rehabilitation services for the rehabilitation of injured, disabled, or sick persons. *Patients (residents) in a NF do not receive Medicare Part A benefits.*
> *Skilled Nursing Facility (SNF)* – an institution (or a distinct part of an institution) which is primarily engaged in providing skilled nursing care and related services for residents who require medical or nursing care, or rehabilitation services for the rehabilitation of injured, disabled, or sick persons. *Patients (residents) in a SNF are receiving skilled services that are being paid for by the resident's Medicare Part A benefits.*

FIGURE 14.1. Glossary of common terms.

- History
- Physical examination
- Medical decision making
- Patient counseling
- Coordination of care
- Severity of the presenting problem
- Time or duration needed to render the service

The three key components each have four levels of extensiveness or complexity.

### History

The four types of history and their definitions are as follows:

- Problem focused: *brief* history of present illness or problem.
- Expanded problem focused: *brief* history of present illness: *problem pertinent* system review.

- Detailed: *extended* history of present illness; *problem pertinent* review of systems; pertinent past, family and/or social history directly related to patient's problems.
- Comprehensive: *extended* history of present illness; review of systems that is directly related to the problem(s) identified in the history of the present illness plus a review of all additional body systems; *complete* past, family and social history.

A Chief complaint is needed for each encounter.

### Examination

The four types of physical examination are defined as follows:

- Problem focused: A *limited* examination of the affected body area or organ system.
- Expanded problem focused: A *limited* examination of the affected body area or organ system and other symptomatic or related body area(s) or organ system(s).
- Detailed: An *extended* examination of the affected body area(s) and other symptomatic or related body area(s) or organ system(s).
- Comprehensive: A general multisystem examination or a complete examination of a single organ system and other symptomatic or related body area(s) or organ system(s).

### Medical Decision Making

The four types of medical decision-making are based on:

- The number of possible diagnoses
- The number of management options that are considered
- The amount and complexity of medical records and other information that must be reviewed
- The risk of significant complications, i.e., morbidity and/or mortality, in addition to comorbidities and their respective severity and how all these can impact management options

The four levels of complexity of medical decision-making are as follows:

- Straightforward: *minimal* number of diagnoses or management options; *minimal* or no data to be reviewed; *minimal* risk of complications, morbidity, and mortality.
- Low complexity: *limited* number of diagnoses or management options; *limited* amount or complexity of data to be reviewed: *low* risk of complications, morbidity, and mortality.

- Moderate complexity: *multiple* diagnoses or management options: *moderate* amount of complexity of data to be reviewed: *moderate* risk of complication, morbidity, and mortality.
- High complexity: *extensive* diagnoses or management options; *extensive* amount or complexity of data to be reviewed; *high* risk of complication, morbidity, and mortality.

### Time

Time can be used to define a level of E/M service if counseling and coordination of care predominates the encounter (>50% of time spent). Time is also used for prolonged service codes (see below). Otherwise the times associated with the E/M codes (Tables 1–4, 8 and 9) are *not* used to define the level of service provided and are to be only used as estimates. Document time spent with the patient in conjunction with the medical decision-making involved and a description of the coordination of care or counseling provided. Documentation must be in sufficient detail to support the claim.

### CODING AND BILLING FOR NURSING FACILITIES

The E/M service code selection is based upon fulfilling the requirements of the individual CPT codes as well as fulfilling medical necessity requirements. Having provided the service and properly documented the care, the selection of the most accurate CPT code is relatively straightforward.

### Skilled Nursing and Nursing Facility Visits

For attending physician services, there are four groups of service codes:

- *Initial Nursing Facility Care* (services provided on admission to the SNF or NF for the initial comprehensive assessment): 99304, 99305, 99306. The patient's attending physician of record must append the modifier "AI" to the bill when performing initial visits
- *Subsequent Nursing Facility Care* (services provided subsequent to or prior to the initial comprehensive assessment): 99307, 99308, 99309, 99310
- Services provided for discharge: 99315 or 99316
- Services provided for annual health evaluation: 99318

Note that all codes apply to either new or established patients.

The appropriate *Initial Nursing Facility Care* code is determined by the extensiveness and complexity of the components of the E/M service provided: with the most comprehensive service being billed at level 99306 (see Table 14.1). All the initial codes require that all

TABLE 14.1. Initial SNF or NF visit codes: 99304–99306

99304
- Requires three of three E/M components
  - Detailed or comprehensive HX
  - Detailed or comprehensive exam
  - Medical decision making:
    - Straight forward, low complexity
  - 25 min
- Used for
  - Initial admission/readmission
  - Usually, the problem(s) requiring admission are of low severity

99305
- Requires three of three E/M components
  - Comprehensive HX
  - Comprehensive exam
  - Medical decision making:
    - Moderate complexity
  - 35 min
- Used for
  - Initial admission/readmission
  - Usually, the problem(s) requiring admission are of moderate severity

99306
- Requires three of three E/M components
  - Comprehensive HX
  - Comprehensive exam
  - Medical decision making:
    - High complexity
  - 45 min
- Used for
  - Initial admission/readmission
  - Usually, the problem(s) requiring admission are of high severity

three E/M components be performed (history, physical, medical decision making). These codes are used for the initial admission (or readmission, if the patient has previously resided in the nursing facility and had been discharged, i.e., no bed hold). The *Subsequent Nursing Facility* care codes are reviewed in Table 14.2. Again, the appropriate subsequent care code is determined by the complexity of the components of the E/M service provided, with the most complex and comprehensive services being coded at the 99310 level.

Note that when billing for subsequent care, only two of the three E/M components need to be performed, though optimal medical care is likely best provided if all three components are performed.

The codes for services provided upon discharge from a SNF or NF include 99315 and 99316 (see Table 14.3). For these discharge

Table 14.2. Subsequent SNF or NF visit codes: 99307–99310

99307
- Requires two of three E/M components
  - Problem focused HX
  - Problem focused exam
  - Medical decision making:
    - Straightforward
  - 10 min
- Used for
  - Patient stable, recovering, or improving
  - "Routine/regulatory" visit

99308
- Requires two of three E/M components
  - Expanded problem focused HX
  - Expanded problem focused exam
  - Medical decision making:
    - Low
  - 15 min
- Used for
  - Patient responding inadequately to RX or developed minor complication
  - "Routine/regulatory" visit

99309
- Requires two of three E/M components
  - Detailed HX
  - Detailed exam
  - Medical decision making:
    - Moderate
  - 25 min
- Used for
  - Patient developed significant complication or significant new problem
  - "Routine/regulatory" visit

99310
- Requires two of three E/M components
  - Comprehensive HX
  - Comprehensive exam
  - Medical decision making:
    - High
  - 35 min
- Used for
  - The patient may be unstable or may have developed a significant new problem requiring immediate physician attention

TABLE 14.3. SNF or NF discharge visit codes: 99315 or 99316

99315 – 30 min or less duration of time
99316 – More than 30 min duration of time
- Used for
  - Final exam
  - Instructions for continuing care
  - Preparation of discharge records
  - Prescriptions
  - Referral forms
  - Communications with after-discharge providers

TABLE 14.4. Annual (periodic) nursing facility health evaluation code: 99318

99318
- Requires three of three E/M components
  - Detailed interval HX
  - Comprehensive exam
  - Medical decision making:
    - Low to moderate
  - 30 min
- Used for
  - Annual exam
  - Usually, the patient is stable, recovering, or improving

services, the differentiation of the appropriate code is determined by the time spent performing all of the tasks and services required for the patient's discharge (final exam, instructions for continuing care, preparation of discharge records, prescriptions, referral forms and communications with providers of care for the patient following discharge). It is important to remember that these discharge visit codes, as do all the other visit codes, require a face-to-face visit, and that if the visit is performed on a day different than the actual day of discharge, the date of service for the billing should be the actual date of the visit. These same codes can be used for a visit when a patient has died, but are only billable if the physician fulfills the requirement of a face-to-face visit and actually pronounces the death.

The code for services provided for the annual (or periodic) health evaluation is 99318 (see Table 14.4). The visit for this health evaluation and the billing with this code are to be used in place of, not in addition to, a routine or regulatory visit code.

CMS requires that any E/M code for a SNF visit be noted with the Place of Service Code "31" and that for a NF visit with the Place of Service Code "32."

## Other Coding Issues in Nursing Facilities

### Consultations

A specialist consultant or a primary care physician may perform consultations in the nursing or skilled nursing facility. A billable consultation requires the request from the physician caring for the patient. As of January 1, 2010 (see below for CMS informational website) the initial consultation evaluation is billed using the nursing facility initial assessment E/M codes (99304–99306). The patient's principal physician of record must append the modifier "AI" to the bill when performing initial visits to differentiate the attending initial visit from a consultant performing an initial visit as a consultation at which time no modifier is needed. The principal physician of record is identified in Medicare as the physician who oversees the patient's care from other physicians who may be furnishing specialty care.

Any follow-up visits for consultation are billed using the subsequent nursing facility visit codes (99307–99310).

### Hospice Care

If the patient is receiving care under the Medicare hospice benefit, there are additional guidelines for billing for provided services that depend on the relationship that the provider may have with the hospice and whether care is related to the terminal illness or not (see Table 14.5). However, physicians should ask their Medicare Administrative Contractor (formerly called Medicare Fiscal Intermediary or Carrier) to verify whom to bill for physician services related to the terminal diagnosis (i.e., whether the hospice or Medicare Part B).

TABLE 14.5. Billing for patients receiving the Medicare hospice benefit

For care *not* related to terminal illness:
  Bill Medicare Part B – modifier GW
For care *related* to terminal illness:
  Check with your Medicare administrative contractor
  - If the physician is not associated with the hospice:
    - Bill Medicare Part B – modifier GV
  - If the physician is associated with/employed by the hospice:
    - Bill Hospice unless services are covered by the contract or agreement with hospice

TABLE 14.6. Group practice

Same group – same specialty
- Bill and be paid as though they were single physician
- One E/M code per day per problem
- Can combine same day visits and submit appropriate code
- Unrelated problems: can submit different bills; documentation critical

Same group – different specialty
- Bill and be paid without regard to membership in group

## *Physicians in Group Practice*

In certain circumstances, provider members of a group practice of the same specialty may bill for services provided to a patient on the same day as indicated in Table 14.6.

## *Multisite Same Day Visits*

The only case in which Medicare will pay for two different services provided by the same physician to the same patient on the same day at different sites of service is for hospital discharge management (99328, 99329) and the nursing facility admission (99304, 99305, 33906). Documentation must be adequate at each site of service to demonstrate that each service with all the appropriate E/M components was actually provided.

## *Split or Shared Visits*

Medicare does not recognize split or shared E/M visits in the nursing facility and thus these may not be billed.

## *"Incident To" Services*

"Incident To" services provided in the nursing facility are not recognized by Medicare and will not be reimbursed. However, if the physician establishes an office in the nursing facility (a discrete space that the physician rents and controls the use of for patient care visits), "incident to" services provided in that discrete office space are billable to and reimbursable. In this case, the "incident to" services are billed utilizing the office service codes.

## *Visits by Qualified Nonphysician Practitioners*

Nonphysician practitioners (NPP) include Nurse Practitioners (NP), Physician Assistants (PA) and Clinical Nurse Specialists (CNS). All E/M visits must be within their State scope of practice and licensure requirements where the visit is performed. All the federal and state requirements for physician collaboration and physician supervision must also be met. Refer to Table 14.7 for the

TABLE 14.7. Nonphysician practitioner services

| | Order to admit | Admission treatment orders | Initial comprehensive visit | Other required visits | Other medically necessary visits | Other medically necessary orders | Certification recertification |
|---|---|---|---|---|---|---|---|
| SNF | | | | | | | |
| NP & CNS employed by facility | N | N | N | Y | Y | Y | N |
| NP & CNS not a facility employee | N | N | N | Y | Y | Y | Y |
| PA regardless of employer | N | N | N | Y | Y | Y | N |
| NF | | | | | | | |
| NP, CNS & PA employed by facility | N | N | N | N | Y | Y | Y |
| NP, CNS & PA not a facility employee | Y | Y | Y | Y | Y | Y | Y |

TABLE 14.8. Prolonged care services: 99356–99357

99356 – First hour of prolonged service
99357 – Each additional 30 min beyond the first hour
- Including both SNF or NF
- Time of prolonged service included in these codes is face to face, continuous or not, beyond the typical time for the E/M visit code plus 30 min
- Documentation not required to be sent with the bill, but is required in record as to duration and content of the service provided

Federal regulations related to which services may be provided by the various NPPs in differing employment and care settings.

### *Prolonged Services*
Medicare does pay for prolonged care services in the nursing facility. These are billed in association with and in addition to the visit charge for a standard E/M visit. The prolonged care timing starts at the completion of the typical time for the E/M visit being billed plus additional time as summarized in Table 14.8. The service must be face-to-face. For further guidance on this complex issue go to http://www.cms.hhs.gov/transmittals/downloads/R1490CP.pdf.

### *Services Provided in the NF or SNF That Are Not Reimbursable by Medicare*
Care plan oversight, telephone calls, medical team conferences (interdisciplinary team meetings), and prolonged services without face-to-face service are *not* reimbursable.

## Coding and Billing for Assisted Living Facilities
Levels of E/M services are defined by the same components. See Table 14.9 for the billing codes used for assisted living facilities, group homes, custodial care facilities and residential substance abuse facilities. It is important to use the correct place of service code for each of these venues (13, 14, 33, and 55, respectively).

## Coding and Billing for Home Visits
Visit services provided in the patient's home are billed using still a different set of codes. These nevertheless follow the same pattern of E/M service intensity and also linked to typical duration of service. These codes are used for services provided in the patient's private residence (place of service code 12) and may not be used for services provided to persons residing in any type of congregate/

TABLE 14.9. Assisted living visit codes

| Initial | | Subsequent | |
|---|---|---|---|
| Code | Time (min) | Code | Time (min) |
| 99324 | 20 | 99334 | 15 |
| 99325 | 30 | 99335 | 25 |
| 99326 | 45 | 99336 | 40 |
| 99327 | 60 | 99337 | 60 |
| 99328 | 75 | | |

Note: These visit codes with typical service duration are for assisted living facilities, Group Homes, custodial care facilities, and residential substance abuse facilities

TABLE 14.10. Home visit codes

| Initial | | Subsequent | |
|---|---|---|---|
| Code | Time (min) | Code | Time (min) |
| 99341 | 20 | 99347 | 15 |
| 99342 | 30 | 99348 | 25 |
| 99343 | 45 | 99349 | 40 |
| 99344 | 60 | 99350 | 60 |
| 99345 | 75 | | |

Note: Visit codes with typical service duration for E/M services provided in the patient's home

shared facility living arrangement, including assisted living facilities and group homes. See Table 14.10 for a listing of these codes.

## PEARLS FOR THE PRACTITIONER

- Appropriate medical necessities along with fulfilling the requirements of the individual CPT codes are necessary for choosing the level of E/M code.
- Appropriate and thorough documentation in the medical record must support the level of service E/M code chosen.
- The extensiveness of the history and physical examination and the complexity of medical decision-making must be appropriate to the presenting complaint(s) or clinical situation.
- The three Key components of any E/M code are history, physical examination, and medical decision-making.
- For billing purposes, it is essential to use the appropriate place of service and modifier codes.

- Contact your Medicare Administrative Contractor for information on billing and coding in your locale.
- The home visit codes are not to be used for practitioner visits performed at assisted living facilities, residential care facilities, group homes, custodial care facilities, and residential substance abuse facilities.
- Be cognizant that the E/M code numbers and documentation requirements do change over time and the responsibility rests with practitioners to keep informed of these changes.

## WEBSITES
- AMA Website CPT Code/Relative Value Search Engine based on Current CPT codes and Medicare payment information https://catalog.ama-assn.org/Catalog/cpt/cpt_search.jsp
- Find-A-Code, a commercially available website that helps find ICD and CPT codes http://www.findacode.com
- Centers for Medicare & Medicaid Services Manual Update on Prolonged Service Codes from April 2008 http://www.cms.hhs.gov/transmittals/downloads/R1490CP.pdf
- CMS Revisions to Consultation Services Payment Policy, information for physicians http://www.cms.hhs.gov/MLNMattersArticles/downloads/MM6740.pdf
- AMDA's Website where a Guide to Long Term Care Coding, Reimbursement and Documentation http://www.amda.com/resources/print.cfm

## REFERENCES
1. Current Procedural Terminology CPT, Professional Edition, 2009, American Medical Association. All rights reserved.
2. Guide to Long Term Care Coding, Reimbursement and Documentation, AMDA, 2009.

# Chapter 15
# Medication Management in Long-Term Care

Susan T. Marcolina and Keith Swanson

**Keywords:** Adverse drug event • Anticoagulants • Antipsychotic medications • Beta-blockers • Hypertension • Pharmacokinetics • Polypharmacy • Subclinical hypothyroidism

## INTRODUCTION

Most clinicians recognize that the elderly take a disproportionately large number of medications compared to younger people and, as a result, they are two to three times more likely to experience adverse drug events (ADEs) [1]. Since pharmacologic therapy for chronic disease treatment is an essential component of the care of geriatric patients, optimization of their drug regimen is an important public health issue in the United States. The geriatric population is the fastest growing segment in the United States in that by 2030, 20% of the US population will be 65 or older. Appropriate prescribing, especially for frail residents of long-term care facilities (LTCF), is challenging due to multiple chronic diseases, limited physiologic reserves, changes in pharmacokinetics and pharmocodynamics, and impaired immune and inflammatory mechanisms. The physical disabilities of these frail elders can be significant. According to the Agency for Healthcare Research and Quality, 83% of nursing home residents receive assistance with three or more activities of daily living (ADL) that include bathing, dressing, toileting, transferring from bed or chair, feeding, and walking. Therefore, these frail elders with their disabilities are highly susceptible to the serious consequences of ADEs, such as hip fractures, weight loss, cognitive, and functional decline. As 27% of LTCF patients take 9 or more prescription medications daily, it should not be surprising that over 65% have ADEs over a 4-year period, while 1 in 7 of these ADEs results in a hospital transfer [2]. Therefore, the prevention and recognition of medication-related problems in patients is a principal healthcare quality and safety issue for LTC facilities, hospitals, and the ambulatory care settings.

**Polypharmacy**
The risk of suffering an ADE is directly related to the number of medications taken by the elderly individual. In contrast to the typical elderly person living in a LTCF, elders living in assisted living facilities and the community take approximately 7 and 5 medications, respectively [3]. The occurrence of polypharmacy is a predictable situation and can be simply defined as the use of multiple medications to treat multiple medical and psychiatric conditions, whether appropriate or not. This may include either an excessive or unnecessary drug regimen than clinically indicated (i.e., the wrong drug, for the wrong patient's clinical condition, given at the wrong time, at the wrong dose, or for the wrong length of time). It is important for practitioners to understand the benefit/risk for each drug within the context of geriatric physiology and pharmacology.

**Pharmacokinetics**
The physiologic changes that occur with aging can have important influences on the pharmacokinetics or disposition of a specific drug within the body that includes each day's absorption, distribution, metabolism, and clearance. Significant changes in these four parameters are summarized as follows:

Absorption

- Passive diffusion and bioavailability unchanged for most drugs.
- Reduced active transport and decreased bioavailability for some vitamins/drugs (example: vitamin B12).
- Reduced GI motility and absorptive surface area: decreases drug absorption.
- Reduced first-pass extraction and increased bioavailability for some drugs (examples: oral nitrates, beta-blockers, estrogens, and calcium channel blockers).
- Concomitant administration of medications decreases absorption of certain drugs (example: thyroid medication with iron supplements).

Distribution

- Reduced volume of distribution (Vd) for water-soluble drugs (examples: digoxin, lithium, theophylline, morphine).
- Increased Vd and increased disposition half-life for fat-soluble drugs (example: benzodiazepines such as diazepam).
- Altered (increased or decreased) free fraction (unbound) drug due to changes in serum proteins and/or binding characteristics (examples: warfarin, phenytoin).
- Increased body adipose stores, which increases the volume of distribution of fat-soluble drugs (examples: benzodiazepines, hormones, amiodarone). Such drugs take longer to reach steady-state levels and exhibit longer elimination times.
- Diminished concentrations of plasma proteins, especially albumin. This results in higher levels of free drug and therefore increased effects of such highly protein-bound drugs as warfarin and phenytoin.

Metabolism (hepatic)

- Reduced clearance for drugs dependent upon hepatic blood flow (examples: morphine, propanolol, verapamil, impramine).
- Reduced clearance for drugs cleared through oxidative (Phase I) metabolism (example: valium).

Clearance (renal)

- Reduced clearance/increased half-life for renally eliminated drugs and active metabolites (examples: many antibiotics (penicillins, cephalosporins, vancomycin, aminoglycosides, floroquinolones, sulfonamides, metformin, $H_2$ antagonists, lithium, digoxin).
(Adapted from reference [4].)

**Absorption**
Medications enter the systemic circulation via oral, rectal, inhalation, percutaneous, subcutaneous, and intramuscular routes. Absorption from these sites can be affected by aging. The effect of aging on gastric and intestinal motility and permeability has not shown consistent effects on drug absorption. The hypochlorhydria seen with normal aging affects the absorption of some oral medications such as ketoconazole. The widespread use of acid suppression therapies with proton pump inhibitors (PPIs) and H2 antagonists has made this issue more evident [5]. Long-term use

of PPIs has been associated with eventual development of vitamin $B_{12}$ deficiency.

Comorbid medical conditions can further alter oral absorption of medications. Congestive heart failure with bowel wall edema interferes with absorption of diuretic medications such as furosemide, thus diminishing its clinical efficacy. With regard to the transdermal or intramuscular absorption of medications, several changes occur in the geriatric integumentary system that can result in significant decreases in absorption:

- Diminished peripheral blood flow with impaired microcirculation (especially in patients with cardiovascular and peripheral vascular disease).
- Increased keratinization.
- Decreased hydration and surface lipid content which affect both water- and fat-soluble topical medications.
- Decreased permeability with increased percentage of intramuscular connective tissue [6].

### Distribution

After absorption, how a drug is distributed within the body compartments depends upon its lipid and water solubility and the extent to which it is bound to plasma proteins. The volume of distribution (Vd) is the pharmacokinetic variable that relates the drug dose administered to its concentration in body fluids. Aging decreases the body's lean-to-fat ratio and total body water 10–15% by age 80 [7]. Cumulatively, this results in a reduced Vd for water-soluble drugs and those drugs distributed to lean body tissues. Therefore, a reduced loading dose is necessary for these medications. Conversely, the age-related increase in body fat content increases the Vd for lipid-soluble compounds, thereby resulting in reduced clearance or elimination time from the body.

Although the concentrations of albumin and alpha 1-acid glycoprotein, the common plasma proteins to which drugs are bound, do not normally decline significantly with aging, reduced nutritional status or catabolic states may lead to clinically important declines. Medications that are highly protein-bound such as the anticoagulant warfarin and the anticonvulsant phenytoin will have higher free serum concentrations in those with reduced plasma proteins [8].

### Metabolism

Liver mass and blood flow decrease significantly with aging, reducing clearance and increasing the half-life and bioavailability for medications that undergo extensive first-pass metabolism such as propanolol and labetolol [5]. On the other hand, several ACE inhibitors such as enalapril and perindopril, which require hepatic activation, have reduced bioavailability with advancing age [9]. Some hepatic metabolic pathways performed through the cytochrome P450 mixed function oxidase systems diminish predictably with age, including many Phase I reactions (reduction, oxidation, hydroxylation, and demethylation). Several cytochrome P450 isoenzyme pathways are significantly reduced in geriatric patients. One example is the CYP3A isoenzyme system, which catalyzes the metabolism of many drugs such as cyclosporine, lovastatin, warfarin, nifedipine, erthyromycin, methylprednisolone, carbamazepine, and midazolam. Blockage of the metabolism of these drugs can decrease clearance, increase half-life, and thus increase the risk of toxicity. Therefore, coadministration of drugs that are known inhibitors of the CYP3A enzyme system such as erythromycin, ketoconazole, itraconazole, ritonavir, the calcium channel blockers (CCBs) diltiazem, nicardipine, and verapamil and grapefruit juice should be avoided [4].

**Elimination**

Renal elimination is the most significant pharmacokinetic change seen in the geriatric population. Renal mass decreases an average of 20% from the fourth to the eighth decades of life with concomitant age-associated reductions in glomerular filtration rate, renal blood flow, and tubular secretion. Thus, drugs that depend upon renal excretion require a dosage reduction [10].

Due to decreased muscle mass in the geriatric population, serum creatinine by itself is not an accurate measure of renal function. Calculators based on equations such as the Cockcroft–Gault Equation, which take into account a patient's measured serum creatinine, sex, age, and estimated lean body weight, give a more accurate approximation of creatinine clearance [11]. Another method to estimate creatinine clearance, the modification of diet in renal disease (MDRD) equation, is being used in clinical practice, but is neither yet recommended for adjustment of medication doses in the elderly nor routinely utilized in drug information sources and labeling for dosage recommendations [12]. In one study of 10,000 long-term care residents, 40% had significant renal insufficiency [13].

**Pharmacodynamic Changes**

Pharmacodynamics is the interaction between a drug and its effector organ(s) that results in either a therapeutic or adverse response or both. The elderly can exhibit increased sensitivity to the therapeutic as well as the toxic effects of many medications due to comorbid illness such as Alzheimer's disease, Parkinson's disease, strokes, congestive heart failure, and other disorders that increase frailty and reduce the ability of the body to maintain homeostatic balance. The following are some age-related pharmacodynamic changes commonly seen in the elderly:

**Increased response:**

- Increased sensitivity to CNS effects of benzodiazepines and alcohol.
- Greater analgesic response to opioids.
- Increased sensitivity to anticoagulants (warfarin, heparin).
- Increased risk of delirium from anticholinergic medications.
- Increased risk of bladder outlet obstruction from anticholinergics.
- Increased risk of extrapyramidal side effects and tardive dyskinesia from antipsychotics.

**Decreased response:**

- Reduced sensitivity to beta-adrenergic agonists and antagonists [4, 5].

### Preventing Adverse Drug Events in Long-Term Care

A consensus panel of experts established the Beers' criteria. This is a list of medications best avoided in the elderly due to the high likelihood of *potential* adverse effects and has been included in State surveys of LTCFs. The Beers'criteria include medications with anticholinergic effects such as antihistamines (diphenhydramine) and antiemetics (promethazine) and other medications with a propensity to cause worsening mental status, falls, urinary retention, orthostatic hypotension, dehydration, and movement disorders including extrapyramidal signs and tardive dyskinesia. Long-acting benzodiazepines are also included because they increase the risk of mental status changes, sedation, and falls (see Table 15.1) [14].

A more recent screening tool, the STOPP (Screening Tool of Older Person's Prescriptions), has been increasingly implemented for the evaluation of potential problematic prescription medication and may be more user friendly than the Beers' list. The STOPP tool was created because many clinicians considered that certain drugs designated as inappropriate by the Beers' criteria were debatable, e.g., avoidance of amiodarone and doxazosin in older people regardless of the diagnosis. Amiodarone may be the only agent for effective control of an arrhythymia, and although not often a first-choice agent, may be entirely appropriate in

TABLE 15.1. Potentially inappropriate drugs to use in the elderly

| Considering the diagnosis | Drug Class | Drug (or anything containing this drug) |
|---|---|---|
| | Antibiotics | Nitrofurantoin (Macrodantin) |
| | Antidepressants | Amitriptyline (Elavil) |
| | | Fluoxetine (Prozac) |
| | | Doxepin (Sinequan) |
| | Antihistamines and anticholinergics | Chlorpheniramine (Chlor-Trimeton) |
| | | Cyproheptadine (Periactin) |
| | | Dexchlorpheniramine (Polaramine) |
| | | Diphenhydramine (Benadryl) |
| | | Hydroxyzine (Vistaril, Atarax) |
| | | Oxybutynin (Ditropan) |
| | | Promethazine (Phenergan) |
| | | Tripelennamine guanadrel (Hylorel) |
| | Antipsychotics | Mesoridazine (Serintil) |
| | | Thioridazine (Mellaril) |
| | Anorexic agents | All |
| | Amphetamines | All |
| | Barbiturates | All |
| | Cardiovascular agents | Amiodarone (Cordarone) |
| | | Digoxin >125 µg/day (Lanoxin) |
| | | Disopyramide (Persantine) |
| | | Doxazosin (Cardura) |
| | | Ethacrynic acid (Edecrin) |
| | | Guanethidine (Ismelin) |
| | | Methyldopa (Aldomet) |
| | | Nifedipine (Procardia – short acting) |
| | | Ticlopidine (Ticlid) |
| | | Isoxsuprine (Vasodilan) |
| | Diabetic agents | Chlorpropamide (Diabinese) |
| | Gastrointestinal antispasmodic agents | Clidinium-chlordiazepoxide (Librax) |
| | | Dicyclomine (Bentyl) |
| | | Hydroxyzine |
| | | Hyoscyamine |
| | | Propantheline |
| | | Trimethobenzamide |

(continued)

TABLE 15.1. (continued)

| Considering the diagnosis | Drug Class | Drug (or anything containing this drug) |
|---|---|---|
| | High-dose short–intermediate acting benzodiazepines | Alprazolam (Xanax) |
| | | Diazepam (Valium) |
| | | Lorazepam (Ativan) |
| | | Oxazepam (Serax) |
| | | Temazepam (Restoril) |
| | | Triazolam (Halcion) |
| | Hormones | Dessicated thyroid |
| | | Methyltestosterone (Android, Virilon, Testrad) |
| | Long-acting benzodiazepines | Chlordiazepoxide (Librium, Mitran) |
| | | Clorazepate (Tranxene) |
| | | Flurazepam (Dalmane) |
| | | Halazepam (Paxipam) |
| | | Meprobamate (Miltown, Equanil) |
| | | Quazepam (Doral) |
| | Non-COX selective NSAID | Indomethacin (Indocin, Indocin SR) |
| | | Naproxen (Naprosyn) |
| | | Oxaprozin (Daypro) |
| | | Piroxicam (Feldene) |
| | Muscle relaxants | Carisoprodol (Soma) |
| | | Chlorzoxazone (Paraflex) |
| | | Cyclobenzaprine (Flexeril) |
| | | Hyoscyamine (Levsin) |
| | | Metaxalone (Skelaxin) |
| | | Orphenadrine (Norflex) |
| | | Methocarbamol (Robaxin) |
| | Miscellaneous | Bisacodyl (Dulcolax) |
| | | Cascara sagrada |
| | | Ergot mesyloid (Hydergine) |
| | | Cyclandelate (Cyclospamol) |
| | | Mineral oil or castor oil (Neoloid) |
| | | Ketorolac (Toradol) |
| | | Meperidine (Demerol) |
| | | Propoxyphene (Darvon) |
| | Supplements | Ferrous sulfate >325 mg/day |

(continued)

TABLE 15.1. (continued)

| Considering the diagnosis | Drug Class | Drug (or anything containing this drug) |
|---|---|---|
| Bladder outflow obstruction | Antidepressant Anticholinergic | More anticholinergic |
| Cognitive impairment | Anticholinergic Antispasmodic | Any<br>Belladonna alkaloids |
| Syncope/falls | Cardiac | Clonidine (Catapress)<br>Digoxin <125 µg/day<br>Reserpine >0.25mg (Serpalan, Serpasil) |
| | Short–intermediate acting benzodiazepines | Alprazolam (Xanax)<br>Diazepam (Valium)<br>Lorazepam (Ativan)<br>Oxazepam (Serax)<br>Temazepam (Restoril)<br>Triazolam (Halcion) |
| | Tricyclic antidepressants | Amitriptyline (Elavil)<br>Doxepin (Sinequan)<br>Imipramine (Tofranil) |
| Chronic constipation | Tricyclic antidepressant | As above |
| | Calcium channel blocker | Any in class |
| COPD | Long-acting benzodiazepines | As above |
| Gastric or duodenal ulcers | NSAID and aspirin | Any in class |
| Miscellaneous | Hormones<br>$H_2$-blocker | Estrogen<br>Cimetidine (Tagamet) |

Adapted from reference [15]

particular cases. Doxazosin in turn may be appropriate in patients with resistant hypertension. Similarly, nitrofurantoin may be the only antimicrobial to which an infecting pathogen is sensitive and thus would be appropriate. The STOPP criteria were designed to incorporate commonly encountered prescribing pitfalls that practitioners encounter. Drug–drug and drug–disease interactions, drugs that adversely affect older patients at risk of falls, as well as duplicate drug class prescriptions all were included in the STOPP criteria.

The STOPP and Beers' criteria's ability to identify patients taking inappropriate medications have been compared. The Beers' criteria identified 44 patients as "inappropriately" receiving drugs that were felt justified by the STOPP criteria. Whereas when the STOPP criteria were used, they were able to find 33 instances of potentially inappropriate prescriptions not found with the Beers' criteria. Examples include excessive duration and dose of PPI therapy, and duplicate drug class prescriptions. Not only does the STOPP criteria help the clinician look for specific clinical situations where a class of drugs has the potential to cause harm and thus is inappropriate to prescribe, but also for circumstances where drugs add unnecessarily to the cost and to the complexity of the drug regimen without providing any additional therapeutic benefit. Because the STOPP criteria are applied to specific clinical situations, it acknowledges the rationale to prescribe some medications where they may be clinically indicated, despite being potentially inappropriate by the Beers' criteria, e.g., use of low-dose amitriptyline in chronic pain syndromes or neuropathic pain. This approach is more flexible than that of the Beers' criteria. In order to be more clinically useful, the STOPP criteria are not only accompanied by an explanation as to why a medication is potentially inappropriate, but also classified according to each medication's relevant physiological system.

Both the Beers' and STOPP criteria do not substitute for thorough clinical assessment and good judgment, as clinicians must always consider whether medications are the possible cause of any symptoms seen in older people. By optimizing and minimizing medication in the elderly, unnecessary and potentially harmful adverse side effects and prescribing cascades can be lessened or avoided. A prescribing cascade occurs when one medication is used to treat the side effects of another, e.g., using a neuroleptic to treat the adverse CNS effects caused by an anticholinergic drug. The STOPP criteria are summarized in Table 15.2 together with some potential adverse outcomes of inappropriate prescribing [16].

### Use of Antipsychotic Medications

Geriatric patients are especially vulnerable to adverse effects from antipsychotic medication including delirium, extrapyramidal symptoms, postural hypotension, falls, and cardiac arrhythmias. If used, it is important to consider the risk to benefit ratio for each newly prescribed medication [17]. For example, the Food and Drug Administration (FDA) recently issued an advisory warning of fatal cardiovascular adverse events in patients with dementia who are treated with either atypical or conventional antipsychotics [18].

TABLE 15.2. STOPP Criteria for potentially inappropriate prescriptions

| Medication by physiological system | Prescribing pitfall | Potential adverse outcome |
|---|---|---|
| **Cardiovascular system** | | |
| Digoxin | >125 μg per day with impaired renal function | Digoxin toxicity from decreased renal clearance |
| Thiazide diuretics | With history of gout | Gout attack, nephropathy |
| β-blockers | With COPD | COPD exacerbation |
| Diltiazem or verapamil | Class III or IV heart failure | CHF exacerbation |
| Calcium channel blockers | Chronic constipation | Worsening constipation, Impaction |
| Dipyridamole | As monotherapy for cardiovascular secondary prevention | Orthostatic hypotension |
| Aspirin | With history of PUD without histamine H2 antagonist or PPI<br>≥150 mg/day<br>With no history of coronary, cerebral, or peripheral vascular symptoms or occlusive event | Gastrointestinal bleeding |
| **Central nervous system** | | |
| TCAs | With dementia<br>With cardiac conductive abnormalities<br>With constipation<br>With prostatism or history of urinary retention | CNS adverse effects<br>Cardiac arrhythmia<br>Impaction, worsening constipation<br>Urinary retention |

(continued)

TABLE 15.2. (continued)

| Medication by physiological system | Prescribing pitfall | Potential adverse outcome |
|---|---|---|
| Long-term, long-acting benzodiazepines | Any use | Falls, confusion, lethargy, overdose |
| Long-term neuroleptics | In those with Parkinsonism or dementia | CNS and extrapyramidal adverse effects, cardiovascular events |
| First-generation antihistamines | Prolonged use | Falls, CNS adverse effects |
| Gastrointestinal system | | |
| Diphenoxylate, loperamide, or codeine phosphate | For treatment of diarrhea of unknown cause | Delay in treatment of bacterial causes of diarrhea |
| | For severe infective gastroenteritis, i.e., bloody diarrhea, high fever, or severe systemic toxicity | Bacteremia, sepsis, death |
| Proton pump inhibitors | For peptic ulcer disease at full therapeutic dosage for >8 weeks | Aspiration pneumonia, B12 deficiency |
| Respiratory system | | |
| Theophylline | As monotherapy for COPD | Poorly controlled COPD, theophylline toxicity |
| Systemic corticosteroids | Instead of inhaled corticosteroids for maintenance therapy in moderate–severe COPD | Any corticosteroid side effect, especially hyperglycemia, osteoporosis, cataracts, confusion |

| | | |
|---|---|---|
| Musculoskeletal system | | |
| NSAIDs | With history of PUD or gastrointestinal bleeding, unless with concurrent histamine H2 receptor antagonist, PPI, or misoprostol (Cytotec) | Gastrointestinal bleeding |
| | With moderate to severe HTN | Poorly controlled HTN |
| | With heart failure | Exacerbation of HF |
| | With warfarin (Coumadin) | Bleeding |
| | With chronic renal failure | Worsening renal function |
| | For relief of mild–moderate joint pain in osteoarthritis | All of the above |
| Long-term corticosteroid | As monotherapy for rheumatoid or osteoarthritis | Corticosteroid adverse effects (see above) |
| Long-term NSAID or colchicine | For chronic treatment of gout where there is no contraindication to allopurinol | NSAID or colchicine adverse effects |
| Urogenital system | | |
| Bladder antimuscarinic drugs | With dementia | CNS adverse effects |
| Antimuscarinic drugs | With chronic prostatism | Urinary retention |
| Endocrine system | | |
| β-blockers | In those with DM | Unrecognized hypoglycemia |

(continued)

TABLE 15.2. (continued)

| Medication by physiological system | Prescribing pitfall | Potential adverse outcome |
|---|---|---|
| Drugs that adversely affect persons who are at risk to fall | | |
| Benzodiazepines | | Fall with or without injury |
| Neuroleptic drugs | | |
| Vasodilator drugs | With postural hypotension | |
| Long-acting benzodiazepine | | |
| Long-term opiates | In those with recurrent falls | |
| Analgesic drugs | | |
| Long-term potent opioids | Use as first-line therapy for mild–moderate pain, e.g., morphine or fentanyl patch | CNS adverse effects, Falls with or without injury, hypotension |
| Long-term opioids | In those with dementia unless used for palliative care | |
| Regular scheduled opioids | For more than 2 weeks in those with chronic constipation without concurrent use of laxatives | Impaction, worsening constipation, bowel perforation, and ischemia |
| Duplicate drug class prescription | | |

Adapted from reference [16]

## Diabetic Medications

Several recent studies have suggested that older persons with diabetes and high levels of comorbidity receive diminished cardiovascular benefit from intensive blood glucose control (Hgb A1C less than 6.5–7%), due to an increased risk for hypoglycemia, and would benefit more from better control of other risk factors including serum lipids, dietary fats and sodium, and blood pressure [19, 20]. Certain diabetic medications such as metformin are contraindicated in older patients with renal disease, ischemic heart disease, and heart failure (HF) because of the increased risk for lactic acidosis. Thiazolidinediones can exacerbate bone loss and can cause fluid retention, which in turn can exacerbate HF. Rosiglitazone may increase risk for myocardial infarction [21] (see Chap. 5 on Common Medical Conditions for further discussion of the treatment of DM).

## Analgesics

The most recent pain treatment guidelines published by the American Geriatric Society (AGS) in 2009 discourage both the use of nonselective NSAIDs (especially those with a long half-life such as naproxen and piroxicam) and COX-2 selective inhibitors due to their potential cardiac (fluid and sodium retention), gastrointestinal (inflammation, bleeding), CNS (altered mental status, psychosis), and renal effects (altered blood flow) [22]. Both these classes of medication have significant drug interactions with ACE inhibitors (potential for hyperkalemia), diuretics (diminished diuresis due to changes in renal blood flow), methotrexate (decreased clearance), anticoagulants (potentiated effects), and lithium (decreased renal clearance and potentiated lithium toxicity). Additionally, there is concern that concomitant use of a NSAID (especially ibuprofen) or a COX-2 inhibitor with a once-daily cardiovascular dose of aspirin will negate aspirin's cardioprotective effect [23].

In 2009, a FDA Advisory Panel recommended sweeping safety restrictions on the use of acetaminophen alone and in combination with opioids such as hydrocodone/acetaminophen and oxycodone/acetaminophen due to increasing reported cases of liver damage and acute liver failure associated with acetaminophen overuse. The panel ruled that because combination prescription opioid/acetaminophen analgesics increase the possibility of accidental overdose and acute liver failure, they either should not be used or their drug labeling should contain a black box warning in order to increase consumer awareness regarding the amount and content of acetaminophen in over-the-counter preparations. The panel also recommended that the maximal amount per unit dose of acetaminophen be lowered to 325 mg in lieu of the current 500 and 650 mg tablets currently available on the market and that the maximum daily dosage for osteoarthritis be *less* than the current recommended maximal dose of 4 g per day recommendation, possibly 3,250 mg [24].

Useful medication guidelines for many drugs can be downloaded from the FDA website. These guidelines provide specific information for patients and caregivers and may help prevent ADEs [25].

*Transition in Care and Medication Errors*
Transitions between care settings are a common scenario for potential medication errors as the patient commonly changes care providers. Comprehensive and up-to-date records that accompany the patient through each care transition can help alleviate medication errors.

## MEDICATION SELECTION IN THE ELDERLY

In LTCFs, the primary responsibility for prescribing, ordering and procuring, initiating, dosing, monitoring, and when appropriate, altering or discontinuing therapy involves the triad of prescriber, nursing personnel, and pharmacy provider/consultant. Each holds specific responsibilities to assure that the patient receives the most appropriate medical therapy. Although studies assessing suboptimal prescribing often focus on identification of overuse and misuse of medications, it is equally important to ensure against the underuse of medication or the omission of a medically indicated drug for the treatment or prevention of disease. Such occurrences are reported in up to 50% of community-dwelling elders [26]. Examples of possible therapy omissions in LTCFs include the lack of GI protection with PPIs for those taking prednisone, no ACE inhibitor therapy for diabetics, no calcium and vitamin D supplementation for individuals at risk for osteoporosis, and lack of venous thromboembolism (VTE) prophylaxis.

The START (Screening Tool to Alert Doctors to Right Treatment) is a new tool to help identify potentially beneficial medications that may have been omitted from a LTCF resident's treatment regimen. START is similar to STOPP because they were both validated in the elderly, derived from evidence-based prescribing indicators and arranged according to physiological systems; but unlike the STOPP, the START identifies possible prescribing omissions in older adults, not medication overuse. Such tools can enable practitioners to better evaluate an older person's prescription drug regimen in the context of their current clinical diagnoses [15].

## Special Considerations

*Hypertension*

The elderly are a subgroup of hypertensive patients at high risk for cardiovascular events and thus should be monitored and treated for hypertension, especially isolated systolic hypertension. Large, placebo-controlled randomized trials have shown that blood pressure reduction decreases both death from strokes and any cardiovascular event. Increasing age is a major predictor of death from stroke with mortality rates of 52% in persons 80 years of age and older [27]. The Hypertension in the Very Elderly Trial (HyVET) established a target BP goal of 150/80 [28]. Oates et al, in a retrospective cohort analysis of patients older than 80 years of age, reported *decreased* survival for those receiving antihypertensive medications with systolic blood pressures below 140 mmHg after adjustment for known predictors of death [29].

If clinically appropriate, it is particularly important in geriatric patients to optimize therapy with lifestyle modifications, including the implementation of the Dietary Approaches to Stop Hypertension (DASH) diet with sodium restriction of 1,500 mg/day (4 g or two thirds of a teaspoon of table salt) [30]. Restrictive diets are not recommended in the frail elderly because of their potential to cause weight loss. The National Institutes of Health has an informative educational brochure for implementation of the DASH diet [31]. If, however, dietary intervention is insufficient to control the blood pressure, low-dose thiazide diuretics and long-acting dihydropyridine CCBs can be prescribed, unless there are comorbidities that merit specific antihypertensive therapy, as follows:

Clinical Situations Meriting Specific Antihypertensive Therapy

- *Angina* – Beta-blockers decrease myocardial oxygen consumption and long-acting dihydropyridine CCBs improve diastolic dysfunction.
- *Postmyocardial infarction* – Beta-blockers decrease risk of recurrent myocardial infarction (MI); angiotensin converting enzyme inhibitors (ACEIs) and angiotensin receptor blockers (ARBs) mitigate congestive heart failure and ventricular remodeling.
- *Diabetes* – ACEIs and ARBs can help preserve normal renal blood flow and function early in the course of kidney disease.
- *Heart failure* – ACEIs, ARBs, and diuretics improve afterload reduction and beta-blockers improve survival.
- *Gout* – Avoid thiazide diuretics if possible due to elevation in uric acid level.

- *Chronic obstructive lung disease* – Avoid beta-blockers which may exacerbate bronchospasm. (Adapted from [32]).

See Chap. 5 on common clinical conditions for further discussion of the treatment of HTN.

*Beta-Blockers Postmyocardial Infarction*
Beta-blockers are important medications for patients in the early course of acute MI and as secondary prevention to reduce cardiac morbidity, mortality, and MI recurrence. However, age greater than 75 is associated with the underuse of beta-blockers. This is concerning given that mortality rate has been reported to be 43% less among beta-blocker recipients than nonrecipients [33].

*Anticoagulants in Nonvalvular Atrial Fibrillation*
Warfarin is recommended as a first-line agent in patients older than 75 years of age with atrial fibrillation due to the increased rate of stroke. Warfarin is also recommended for patients with atrial fibrillation between the ages of 65 and 75 if other risk factors for stroke are present (i.e., hypertension, diabetes mellitus, CHF, previous stroke, or transient ischemic attack). The Congestive Failure, Hypertension, Age, Diabetes, Previous Stroke (CHADS2) calculator can be used to predict the yearly stroke risk in patients with chronic atrial fibrillation [34]. Patients with a CHADS2 score greater than 2 are at high risk for embolic stroke with a greater than 8.5% risk of an event per year without warfarin. As in the general population, the INR should be in the recommended range of 2–3 in order to provide the maximal benefit. Although the risk of bleeding during warfarin therapy is of concern, careful patient selection and frequent, regular monitoring of therapy minimizes the risk, particularly with use of specialty coagulation clinics [35].

*Subclinical Hypothyroidism*
Identified in up to 18% of elderly persons, progression from subclinical to overt hypothyroidism occurs at a rate of 5–18% per year [36]. Use of medications such as lithium, alpha interferon, and amiodarone increases the risk for hypothyroidism. Lithium, amiodarone, propanolol, and glucocorticoids inhibit peripheral conversion of T4 to T3, whereas alpha interferon and amiodarone can cause thyroiditis. Subclinical hypothyroidism has been associated with subtle cardiac function abnormalities, atherogenic serum lipid profiles, blood pressure dysregulation, impaired endothelial function as well as alterations in cerebral blood flow and impairment of memory [37]. Bedtime dosing of thyroid replacement normalizes serum TSH levels more optimally than daily dosing in the morning [38]. Replacement dosing should be advanced gradually in geriat-

ric patients as they may have undiagnosed heart disease and can develop dysrhythmias, angina, or myocardial infarctions if started on full replacement dosages or if their dose is increased too rapidly. Treatment of subclinical hypothyroidism, even at TSH levels of 5–10 mU/L, produces beneficial effects on lipoprotein profiles. However, in elderly patients this must be balanced with a decreased initial levothyroxine dose of 25–50 µg/day, with subsequent dose increments of 25 µg every 4–6 weeks until target TSH goals are reached. This slow titration is necessary to avoid increased myocardial oxygen consumption and subsequent cardiovascular complications. Additionally, serum TSH levels can occasionally rise to levels consistent with primary hypothyroidism during the recovery phase of acute illnesses. In such situations, it is prudent to repeat the TSH measurement after recovery is complete prior to initiation or adjustment of thyroid medications. The Clinical Practice Guidelines of the American Association of Clinical Endocrinologists for the management of patients with hypothyroidism are posted on their website [39]. (See Chap. 5 on Common Medical Conditions for further discussion of the treatment of Thyroid Disease.)

*Gradual Dose Reduction in SNFs/NFs*
Federal nursing facility regulations require that *gradual dose reductions* (GDR) of patients' medication be attempted at least quarterly for all sedative/hypnotics that are used routinely and taken beyond the manufacture's recommendations for duration of use.

However, GDR can be declined on clinical grounds if (1) continued use of the medication is in accordance with the current standard of practice and a GDR would likely impair the patient's function or cause psychiatric instability by either exacerbating an underlying medical condition or psychiatric disorder *or* (2) the patient's target symptoms for which the medication had been prescribed either returned or worsened after the most recent GDR and further GDR attempts would likely impair the patient's function or psychiatric stability.

Practitioners should note that current State Operations Manual (SOM) guidelines to surveyors state that medications should be prescribed *only* when necessary and in the lowest effective dose. Once symptoms have resolved or stabilized, these guidelines also suggest that attempts be made to either discontinue the medication or reduce the dose through GDR.

Previously, efforts to reduce unnecessary medication use focused solely on antipsychotics, benzodiazepines and other centrally acting drugs. The current guidelines encourage GDR be attempted for *all medications* unless the patient's current condition would be adversely effected.

## SUMMARY

Early and aggressive pharmacologic treatment for new or worsening medical conditions is still recommended in the elderly who are relatively healthy and who have a favorable life expectancy, but the expected positive outcomes of any medication must be balanced against the real risk of an adverse drug effect, a subtherapeutic response, or other medication-related event.

Efforts to optimize appropriate, effective, and safe medication use in the elderly has become a priority goal for healthcare systems, clinicians, and the state and federal governments. Screening tools such as the Beers', STOPP, and START criteria can remind practitioners of potentially inappropriate medication use as well as alert them to possible omissions of therapeutic drugs for particular disease conditions which, if prescribed, could have the potential for primary and secondary prevention and improved quality of life. Keeping in mind that the addition of each new medication increases the risk of an adverse event, it is incumbent upon practitioners to collaborate with pharmacists, nursing personnel and caregivers to regularly assess for both negative and positive outcomes and to decide whether to continue pharmacologic treatments based upon patient goals and preferences for care, prognosis, and time needed to treat to obtain the desired therapeutic benefits. (See Chap. 8 for a further discussion of medication management at the end of life.)

## PEARLS FOR THE PRACTITIONER

- Polypharmacy is characterized by excessive or unnecessary use of medications (often at doses higher than necessary for the clinical situation) or drug combinations that put the elderly at excessive risk due to drug–drug, drug–disease, or drug–nutrient interactions.
- Regularly request elderly individuals and their caregivers to bring in all medications, including over-the-counter and herbal medications to each office visit.
- Regularly review LTCF resident medication lists, looking for unnecessary medications that have no apparent indication, subtherapeutic or excessive doses, prolonged duration of action, drug interactions, inappropriate dosage forms and excessive cost.
- Consider a potential ADE in the differential diagnosis of any change in the clinical status of an elderly individual.
- The old axiom, "start low and go slow" is always appropriate when starting a new medication in the elderly, particularly when prescribing thyroid hormone replacement in a patient who may have underlying ischemic cardiovascular disease.

- The Beers' and STOPP criteria can be used to help clinicians avoid prescribing potentially inappropriate medication in older adults, especially those with anticholinergic properties or hypotensive effects.
- Anticipate decreased renal and hepatic oxidative clearance and individualize doses when initiating or modifying drug therapy in the elderly.

**WEBSITES**

- National Kidney Foundation. Calculators for Health Care Professionals-GFR by MDRD Study Equation and Cockcroft-Gault equations. http://www.kidney.org/professionals/kdoqi/gfr_calculator.cfm. Accessed on October 1, 2010.
- Warning of Fatal Reactions in Geriatrics Patients of Typical and Atypical Antipsychotics. http://www.fda.gov/NewsEvents/Newsroom/PressAnnouncements/2008/ucm116912.htm. Accessed on November 1, 2009.
- Pharmacological Management of Persistent Pain in Older Persons: American Geriatrics Society Panel on the Pharmacological Management of Persistent Pain in Older Persons. http://www.americangeriatrics.org/files/documents/2009_Guideline.pdf. Accessed on October 2, 2010.
- US Food and Drug Administration Medication Guides. http://www.fda.gov/Drugs/DrugSafety/ucm085729.htm. Accessed on December 10, 2009.
- AAFP News Now. FDA Panel Recommends Acetaminophen Restrictions Available at: http://www.aafp.org/online/en/home/publications/news/news-now/clinical-care-research/20090702acetamin.html. Accessed December 10, 2009.
- Your Guide to Lowering Your Blood Pressure with DASH. The DASH Eating Plan. Available on http://www.nhlbi.nih.gov/health/public/heart/hbp/dash/new_dash.pdf. Accessed on December 11.
- MD + CALC. CHADS2 Score for Atrial Fibrillation Stroke Risk. http://www.mdcalc.com/chads2-score-for-atrial-fibrillation-stroke-risk. Accessed December 3, 2009.
- Clinical Practice Guidelines of the American Association of Clinical Endocrinologists for management of patients with hypothyroidism and suspected hypothyroidism. 2006 Updates www.aace.com/pub/pdf/guidelines/hypo_hyper.pdf. Accessed December 11, 2009.

## REFERENCES

1. Nolan L, O'Malley K. Prescribing for the elderly. Part I: Sensitivity of the elderly to adverse drug reactions. J Am Geriatr Soc 1988;36:142.
2. Cooper JW. Probable adverse drug reactions in a rural geriatric nursing home population: a four-year study. J Am Geriatr Soc 1996;44: 194–197.
3. Briesacher B, Limcangco R, Simoni-Wastila L, et al. Evaluation of nationally mandated drug use reviews to improve patient safety in nursing homes: a natural experiment. J Am Geriatr Soc 2005;53: 991–996.
4. Oates JA, Wilkinson GR. Chapter 68: Principles of Drug Therapy. In: Fauci AS, Braunwald E, Isselbacher, KJ, et al (eds). Harrison's Principles of Internal Medicine 14th Ed. volume 1 New York: McGraw-Hill, 1998;411–424.
5. McLean AJ, Le Conteur DG. Aging biology and geriatric clinical pharmacology. Pharmacol Rev 2004;56:163–184.
6. Roskos KV, Maibach HI, Guy RH. The effect of aging on percutaneous absorption in man. J Pharmacokinet Biopharm 1989;17:617–630.
7. Parker BM, Cusack BJ, Vestal RE. Pharmacokinetic optimization of drug therapy in elderly patients. Drugs Aging 1995;7:10–18.
8. Greenblatt DJ, Sellers EM, Shader RI. Drug disposition in old age. NEJM 1982; 306: 1081–1087.
9. Todd PA, Fitton A. Perindopril. A review of its pharmacological properties and therapeutic use. Drugs 1991;42:90–114.
10. Bennett WM. Geriatric pharmacokinetics and the kidney. Am J Kidney Dis 1990;16:283.
11. Cockcroft DW, Gault MH. Prediction of creatinine clearance from serum creatinine. Nephron 1976;16:31–41.
12. GFR Calculator Using Cockcroft-Gault, MDRD equations. http://nephron.org/cgi_bln/MDRD_GFR/cgi. Accessed on November 9, 2009.
13. Garg AX, Papaioannou A, Ferko N, et al. Estimating the prevalence of renal insufficiency in long-term care. Kidney Int 2004;65(2):649–653.
14. Beers MH. Explicit criteria for determining potentially inappropriate medication use by the elderly. Arch Intern Med 2001;135:703.
15. Fick DM, Cooper JW, Wade WE, Waller JL, MacLean JR, Beers MH. Updating the Beers criteria for potentially inappropriate medication use in older adults: Results of a US consensus panel of experts. Arch Intern Med 2003;163:2716–2724.
16. Gallagher P, Ryan C, Byrne S. STOPP(Screening Tool of Older Person's Prescriptions) and START (Screening Tool to Alert Doctors to Right Treatment). Consensus Validation. Int J Clin Pharmacol Ther 2008; 46(2):72–83.
17. Maixner SM, Mellow AM, Tandon R. The efficacy, safety, and tolerability of antipsychotics in the elderly. J Clin Psychiatry 1999; 60(Suppl 8):29–41.
18. Warning of Fatal Reactions in Geriatrics Patients of Typical and Atypical Antipsychotics. http://www.fda.gov/NewsEvents/Newsroom/PressAnnouncements/2008/ucm116912.htm. Accessed on November 1, 2009.

19. Gerstein HC, Miller ME, Byington RP, et al. Action to Control Cardiovascular Risk in Diabetes Study Group. Effects of intensive glucose lowering in type 2 diabetes. N Engl J Med 2008;358:2560–2572.
20. Duckworth W, Abraira C, Moritz T, et al. VADT Investigators. Glucose control and vascular complications n veterans with type 2 diabetes. N Engl J Med 2009;360:129–139.
21. Home PD, Pocock SJ, Beck-Nielsen H, et al. Rosiglitazone Evaluated for Cardiac Outcomes in oral agent combinations therapy for type 2 diabetes mellitus (RECORD): a multicenter, randomized, open-label trial. Lancet 2009; 373(9681): 2125–2135.
22. AGS Clinical Practice Guidelines for Pharmacological Management of Persistent Pain in Older Persons. http://www.americangeriatrics.org/education/pharm_management.shtml. Accessed on November 5, 2009.
23. McGettigan P, Henry D. Cardiovascular risk and inhibitors of cycloxogenase: a systemic review of observational studies of selective and non-selective inhibitors of cyclooxygenase-2. JAMA 2006;296(13): 1633–1644.
24. Kuehn J. FDA Focuses on drugs and liver damage: labeling and other changes for acetaminophen. JAMA 2009;302:369–371.
25. US Food and Drug Administration Medication Guides. http://www.fda.gov/Drugs/DrugSafety/ucm085729.htm. Accessed on December 10, 2009.
26. Higashi T, Shekelle PG, Adams JL, et al. The quality of pharmacologic care for vulnerable older patients. Ann Intern Med 2004;140:714–720.
27. Hollander M, Koudstaal PJ, Bots ML, etal. Incidence, risk and case fatality of first ever stroke in the elderly population: the Rotterdam Study. J Neurol Neurosurg Psychiatry 2003;74:317–321.
28. Bulpitt C, Fletcher A, Beckett N. Hypertension in the very elderly trial (HyVET). Drugs Aging 2001;18(3):151–164.
29. Oates DJ, Berlowitz DR, Glickman ME, et al. Blood pressure and survival in the oldest old. J Am Geriatr Soc 2007;55:383–388.
30. Sacks FM, Svetkey LP, Vollmer WM, et al. Effects on blood pressure of reduced dietary sodium and the dietary approaches to stop hypertension (DASH)diet. N Engl J Med 2001;344:3–10.
31. Your Guide to Lowering Your Blood Pressure with DASH. The DASH Eating Plan. Available on http://www.nhlbi.nih.gov/health/public/heart/hbp/dash/new_dash.pdf. Accessed on December 11.
32. Chobanian AV, Bakris GL, Black HR. Seventh report of the Joint National Committee(JNC) on the prevention, detection, evaluation and therapy of high blood pressure. Hypertension 2003;42:1206–1252.
33. Soumerai SB, McLaughlin TJ, Spiegelman D, et al. Adverse outcomes of underuse of beta-blockers in elderly survivors of acute myocardial infarction. JAMA 1997;277(2):115–121.
34. MD + CALC. CHADS2 Score for Atrial Fibrillation Stroke Risk. http://www.mdcalc.com/chads2-score-for-atrial-fibrillation-stroke-risk. Accessed December 3, 2009.
35. Dhond AJ, Michaelena HI, Ezekowitz MD. Anticoagulation in the elderly. Am J Geriatr Cardiol 2003;12(4):243–250.

36. Hollowell JG; Staehling NW, Flanders WD, et al. Serum TSH T4 and thyroid antibodies in the United States population (1988-94): National Health and Nutrition Examination Survey (NHANES III). *J Clin Endocrinol Metab* 2002;87:489–499.
37. Samuels MH, Schuff KG, Carlson NE, et al. Health status, mood and cognition in experimentally induced subclinical hypothyroidism. J Clin Endocrinol Metab 2007;92:2545–2551.
38. Bolk N, Visser TJ, Kalsbeek A, et al. Effects of evening vs morning thyroxine ingestion on serum thyroid hormone profiles in hypothyroid patients. Clin Endocrinol (Oxf) 2007;66:43–48.
39. Clinical Practice Guidelines of the American Association of Clinical Endocrinologists for management of patients with hypothyroidism and suspected hypothyroidism. 2006 Updates www.aace.com/pub/pdf/guidelines/hypo_hyper.pdf Accessed on December 15, 2009.

# Chapter 16
# Rehabilitation and Maximizing Function

Thomas Lawrence

**Keywords:** Rehabilitation • Medical comorbidities • Rehabilitation approaches • Pain management • Deconditioning

## INTRODUCTION

Federal nursing facility regulations require that care be provided for residents to "attain or maintain" the highest possible level of physical, mental, and psychosocial function and well-being [1, 2]. Rehabilitation services and care to promote maximum function are a fundamental component of nursing facility care.

Providing recuperative and rehabilitation services to patients following acute-care hospitalization is among the fastest growing segment of health care spending in the United States. A growing number of elders being discharged from hospitals will spend some time convalescing in the long-term care setting especially in nursing facilities. About 1.5 million American elders receive rehabilitation in nursing facilities each year [3]. This subset of nursing facility residents represents the largest percentage of short-stay nursing facility admissions.

The decision of *where* to provide rehabilitation therapy following an acute illness is dependent on several factors:

- How many therapy modalities are to be utilized
- The number and complexity of concurrent medical problems and their management

- The individual's physical ability to participate in therapy
  - Acute rehabilitation admission – if a patient is able to participate in at least 2–3 h of combined therapies per day
  - Nursing facility admission– if a patient is able to participate with less than 2–3 h of combined therapies per day

- Sites of care
  - Acute rehabilitation hospital
  - Nursing facility
  - Assisted living facility
  - Home care

- Rehabilitation services are also provided to long-stay residents of nursing homes at any time during their care at the facility if physical function is impaired by acute and/or chronic illness

In all settings, successful rehabilitation requires that a variety of therapeutic interventions be delivered in a coordinated and timely fashion in order to restore and maximize function [2, 4].

- Goals for rehabilitation in the nursing facility must be established by a multidisciplinary team including therapists, nurses, and the attending physician and must be aligned with the preferences of the resident.
- Goals should be realistic and attainable and should be aimed at improving function and independence, while respecting the individual's quality of life.
- Overall prognosis of elderly nursing facility residents is often a shifting target and can result in the therapy plan being suspended due to acute changes in status and changing and competing goals of care. For example, an acute illness can result in the decision to forego rehabilitation goals of care for palliative or hospice care.

## TYPES OF THERAPY SERVICES

Therapy services have evolved into three traditional rehabilitation disciples: *physical therapy, occupational therapy*, and *speech therapy*. Other therapy modalities that are growing in both importance and availability include *respiratory therapy*, *psychotherapy*, *cognitive therapy*, and *recreational therapy* (which includes music and pet therapy). Although some of these modalities (e.g., psychotherapy) are covered separately under Medicare and other insurance plans, most of these supportive therapy services are not reimbursed separately but are provided as an integral part of nursing facility care. All rehabilitation professionals coordinate their services with the comprehensive assessments conducted as part of the federally mandated nursing facility resident assessment protocol.

*Physical therapy* is the discipline that focuses on the restoration of maximum movement and functional ability involving the extremities with particular attention to the lower extremity functions of ambulation and transfer skills.

*Occupational therapy* as a discipline in the long-term care setting focuses on promoting the residents' ability to participate in activities of daily living including dressing, grooming, and bathing. It is often stated that physical therapy focuses on the function of the lower extremities while occupational therapy focuses on upper extremity function.

*Speech and language therapy* is a discipline that deals with disorders of speech, language, voice, communication, cognition, and swallowing. Speech therapists often work on developing plans for altered consistency diets in residents with swallowing dysfunction.

### Payment for Rehabilitation Therapy

Under Medicare, rehabilitation therapy is covered as part of the (PPS) prospective payment system out of the daily rate paid to nursing facilities for short-term rehabilitation following an acute-care hospitalization (following at least 3-day hospitalization). The complex Medicare payment system pays a daily rate that is calculated in part according to the variety and intensity of rehabilitation services that are needed and provided. For residents whose nursing facility stay is no longer covered by the Medicare Part A benefit or other private insurance, rehabilitation therapies are usually paid separately by the Medicare Part B benefit or other private insurance. This coverage is contingent upon the service meeting medical necessity requirements as being reasonable and necessary for the resident's care.

### Medical Comorbidities and Frailty

In many cases there is a rather small window of opportunity to initiate rehabilitation therapy services. Elders have an increasing number and complexity of both acute and chronic medical problems – medical comorbidities – that can hinder this process. Common conditions in this setting include cardiac, pulmonary, gastrointestinal, and renal disease, malnutrition, depression, as well as musculoskeletal and neurological problems (including dementia) that cause functional decline as well as muscle deconditioning and weakness. These conditions can interact in dynamic and complex ways to both trigger an episode of functional decline and limit the individual's response to a coordinated program of therapy. Rehabilitation outcomes are directly impacted by these associated medical conditions.

## PREVENTION

### Pressure Ulcer Prevention
Residents who are undergoing rehabilitation are often at high risk for pressure ulcer development due to the risk factors of immobility, urinary incontinence, and multiple comorbid medical conditions (including diabetes). Aggressive prevention strategies should be implemented as part of routine rehabilitation care. Principles of pressure ulcer prevention that are particularly appropriate for this population include: a frequent turning and positioning schedule, managing urinary and fecal incontinence, management of contractures, frequent skin inspection, maintenance of adequate nutrition and hydration, use of off-loading or pressure-redistribution devices, and proper transfer and lift techniques [5]. Complicated and poorly healing pressure ulcers can derail a planned course of therapy; however, optimal prevention and management of pressure ulcers can help promote best outcomes in rehabilitation (see Chapter 10 for further detail).

### Prevention of Venous Thromboembolism
Deep vein thrombosis and pulmonary embolism are common complications of residents receiving rehabilitation services. Nursing home residents are considered a frequently overlooked risk group for venous thromboembolism (VTE) [6]. Although widespread application of VTE prophylaxis to all nursing facility rehabilitation patients is an unproven treatment, there are several populations of residents for whom prophylaxis is essential. The proven application of VTE prophylaxis includes patients who have had hip fracture surgery and those who have had hip or knee arthroplasty. Various agents are approved for use and the duration of treatment for extended prophylaxis is variable, but usually continues for a minimum of 4 weeks. Ongoing research will help define other high-risk residents of long-term care facilities who may benefit from prophylactic treatment to prevent this serious complication of nursing home elderly. One clinical dichotomy that needs to be balanced in all cases is the fact that the elderly generally and nursing facility residents specifically are at very high risk for VTE

events; however, they are also at higher risk for bleeding when treated with anticoagulants [7]. Individual patient clinical factors and preferences for treatment need to be considered in deciding whom to give prophylactic treatment.

## REHABILITATION APPROACHES

### Stroke
The goals of rehabilitation for stroke patients include:

- Establishing medical stability and implementing stroke prevention interventions
- Preventing and managing short-term complications
- Promoting neurological and physical functional recovery

The rehabilitation phase is critical as up to 20% of first-ever stroke patients die within the first 30 days. Pneumonia, pulmonary embolism, and cardiac complications are the most common causes of death.

*Stroke* rehabilitation begins immediately *upon medical stabilization*. The approach should be to prevent recurrent stroke, avoid medical complications, mobilize the patient, and encourage self-care activities. Medical complications that require active prevention and management strategies include pressure ulcers, spasticity and contracture, bowel and bladder issues, and prevention of respiratory complications.

*Spasticity* occurs in over 60% of patients following stroke [8]. This involves an increase in muscle tone with exaggerated tendon jerks due to increased excitability of the stretch reflex. Although spasticity can sometimes help ambulation, it is more often painful and can be debilitating. Management involves daily stretching exercises and avoidance of stimuli that trigger spasticity. In the elderly oral antispasmodic drugs are poorly tolerated due to the common side effects of sedation and confusion. Focal injections of phenol or botulinum toxin are often effective as is serial casting for more severe cases. Muscle contracture occurs when there is permanent shortening of a muscle or tendon due to continued increased muscle tone such as with continuous spasticity. Contractures are very difficult to reduce and often require surgical intervention to correct, therefore prevention through managing spasticity and promoting stretching and maintaining range of motion is critical.

*Bowel and bladder dysfunction* following stroke occurs in 50–70% of patients, but can be a relatively short-term complication resolving in many patients within 3–6 months [8]. Most cases of stroke cause a hyperreflexic bladder and uninhibited bladder contractions can occur causing the symptom of urinary urgency. This is best managed with a timed voiding schedule. Monitoring urine output and postvoid residual bladder volume tracking is helpful. Urinary retention and overflow incontinence are less common complications following stroke. Prostate enlargement in men, medication effects on bladder function, and preexisting urinary incontinence can complicate bladder management following stroke. Bladder incontinence is also one of the major risk factors for pressure ulcer development and skin breakdown, so skin protective interventions are often utilized. Bowel incontinence following stroke is less common and less chronic, but is often complicated by fecal impaction. This is often precipitated by inactivity, poor nutrition, and inadequate fluid intake. As nutrition improves with higher fiber content and adequate fluid intake, bowel incontinence can usually be successfully managed.

*Respiratory complications are often precipitated by stroke-related dysphagia.* Aspiration usually occurs during the pharyngeal phase of swallowing and significant dysphagia can often occur without discrete clinical evidence of aspiration. Up to one third of patients with stroke-related dysphagia have episodes of aspiration [8]. Formal evaluation of swallowing function by a speech therapist is often needed and video fluoroscopic swallowing studies can be both diagnostic and helpful with selecting the most appropriate altered diet for the patient.

The incidence of pulmonary embolism after stroke is 10–15%, and VTE prophylaxis in this clinical setting may be warranted. Attaining ambulation of at least 50 ft per day reduces the risk of deep venous thrombosis and pulmonary embolism [8].

*Therapy interventions* can begin once neurological deficits are no longer progressing, often within 48 h. Initially when the affected extremities are more flaccid, interventions involve passive range of motion and bed positioning exercises with progressively increasing intensity. In the past the approach to the older stroke patient was mostly supportive and focused on preventing complications while allowing spontaneous recovery to occur. Modern approaches involve the application of a number of more aggressive strategies which include compensatory strategies, neurophysiologic techniques, task-oriented retraining, as well as strengthening exercises [8].

*Compensation* refers to using alternate approaches to task completion such as using the unaffected extremity to perform a specific task or using wheelchair to assist mobility. Certain elements of compensation are necessary for functional recovery. Neurophysiologic training involves using the affected side to perform tasks and relearn normal movement. This also minimizes spasticity. Task-oriented exercise utilizes the more affected limb and involves intensive practice with the affected extremity that can be carried out for relatively long time periods. This technique sometimes includes restraining the unaffected extremity in order to force greater use of the affected extremity. Strengthening exercises target both general fitness and extremity strengthening utilizing progressive resistance. Aerobic exercises targeted at general fitness and extremity muscle strengthening have been shown to influence outcomes such as gait speed and fall risk.

### Fracture Care

*Hip fracture* is both a common reason for admission to a nursing facility and a common consequence of a nursing home fall. The mortality rate in the elderly following hip fracture is extremely high (up to 36%) and optimal outcomes require successful management of the complex medical comorbidities that exist. Up to 50% of patients who suffer a fractured hip do not regain their previous ambulatory function and up to 20% may become nonambulatory [9]. Rehabilitation should start as soon as possible after surgery. The most important issue following hip fracture repair is early mobilization, and this is considered essential in order to prevent such complications as pneumonia, deep venous thrombosis, pulmonary embolism, and urinary tract infection. Other common complications that can occur during the rehabilitation of hip fractures are delirium, depression, anorexia and weight loss, and unsuccessful healing (nonunion, instability, and dislocation).

Early goals of therapy following hip fracture surgery are increasing strength and preventing muscle atrophy on the unaffected side. The initial approach is isometric exercise of the limb while fully extended. The speed of rehabilitation usually depends on the type of surgery performed, with prosthetic joint replacement progressing more quickly than after pinning. Full weight bearing begins as soon as day 2 after surgery if the joint is replaced, followed by balance retraining and ambulation exercises beginning within 4–8 days. Stair-climbing exercises are the final stage of rehabilitation beginning usually after 10 days or so. Strengthening of the trunk and quadriceps muscles is performed daily and taught to patients.

Occasionally, in cases of high surgical risk, rehabilitation without surgery is the selected treatment approach. Secondary disabilities such as pressure ulcers, muscle atrophy, joint contractures and general deconditioning are, however, quite common and usually limit the functional outcome with this approach.

*Pelvic fractures* involving the pubic and ischial rami are less common than hip fractures, but also result from falls. These are the most common sites of fracture in the pelvis, not the bony arches of the ilium. Because the ilium provides most of the weight bearing strength of the pelvis, patients with pelvic fractures that do not involve the ilium can usually begin to bear weight on their lower extremities as soon as the pain eases. Isolated pubic ramus fractures often heal without causing significant long-term functional decline. Many patients can walk short distances with a walker within a week and early mobilization similarly reduces major complications such as have been previously discussed with hip fractures.

*Thoracic and lumbar vertebral compression fractures* are often not traumatic, but occur spontaneously during ordinary activity in the setting of preexisting osteoporosis. In thoracic fractures the vertebrae are frequently deformed into a wedge shape causing kyphosis and subsequent impairment in respiratory function. In lumbar fractures the deformity is usually flattened. With accumulation of fractures, spinal deformity can result in chronic pain and permanent gait dysfunction. The goals of therapy are to control pain and restore function. Use of a brace may help in pain management, but will not prevent deformity. Newer techniques at vertebral fracture repair, including *kyphoplasty*, may help to relieve pain and prevent deformity in selected patients who can tolerate the procedure.

## Joint Replacement

Although joint replacement surgery can be performed on any joint in the body, rehabilitation following total hip and knee joint replacement surgery is increasingly being carried out in the nursing facility setting. This is especially true in recent years since Medicare has limited coverage for total joint replacement care in acute rehabilitation hospitals. In contrast to fracture surgery, rehabilitation from total joint replacement must carefully balance therapy aimed at preventing deconditioning while avoiding the overuse of the new joints. Typically patients with cemented joints can weight bear as tolerated immediately after surgery, whereas patients with cementless joints are put on partial weight bearing initially to allow bony in-growth to occur. Due to the relative uniformity of joint replacement procedures, rehabilitation can often take place according to a highly structured therapy protocol. Pain management in joint replacement is usually a much greater challenge with elderly patients.

## Amputation and Orthotics

The higher incidence of amputation, especially of the lower extremity, among the elderly relates to the higher prevalence of peripheral arterial disease and diabetes in this population. In this age group trauma and tumor are less common causes for amputation. These patients present additional challenges to therapists due to presence of medical comorbidities that include decreased cardiopulmonary capacity, neuromuscular disease, muscle weakness, poor nutrition, and visual impairment. In addition, coexisting functional decline makes high intensity prosthetic training more difficult.

Common amputation sites in the lower limb include below the knee (*transtibial*) and above the knee (*transfemoral*) [10]. The time immediately following an amputation is referred to as the pre-prosthetic period. During this time the rehabilitation focus is on good wound healing and initiation of the therapy process. Specific clinical issues include: wound management, pain control, edema control, strengthening, functional training, and maintenance of range of motion to prevent contracture.

Pain management should address both surgical procedure-related pain and phantom limb pain. Phantom limb sensation is a perception that all or part of the amputated limb is still present. Although this sensation is usually not painful, it can be quite disturbing, but often improves over time and can be responsive to desensitization treatments. Edema of the residual limb is a common complication, and reducing edema also helps to promote healing and control pain. Management of edema includes elastic wraps and elastic shrinker socks.

Once good healing is achieved, which can take weeks, the prosthesis can be fabricated. The components of the prosthesis include: the *socket* (interface between the residual limb and the prosthesis), the *suspension* (secures the prosthesis to the body), *joints* (such as a knee in a transtibial amputation), and *terminal devices* (such as a foot) [11]. Collaboration between the patient, therapist, prosthetist, and prescribing physician is critical to successful fabrication. Fit and comfort of the socket is a special challenge. Fit is accommodated by residual limb socks that can be used in several layers (rated in ply) to achieve optimal fit. Weight shifts and edema can lead to changes in fit and may necessitate refitting the socket.

Prosthetic training often involves significant cardiopulmonary stress; oxygen consumption increases by about a third in a transtibial amputee and nearly doubles for a transfemoral amputee [10]. Cardiac or respiratory disease can limit an individual's prognosis for independent function with the prosthesis. Psychological issues often surface during this phase of the rehabilitation process and the services of a psychologist or counselor can be an asset.

### Deconditioned State

It is very common that nursing facility residents are admitted from a hospital following an acute illness with generalized weakness. This condition is often referred to as *deconditioning*, and it is also an extremely common complication in long-stay nursing home residents when either acute problems or exacerbations of chronic conditions result in weakness and functional decline. Rehabilitation interventions, often with combined therapy modalities, can be implemented in these residents to restore strength and function. As mentioned previously, for long-stay Medicare residents, whose stay is not currently covered under the Medicare part A benefit, this therapy treatment is covered under the Medicare part B benefit. Most assisted living facilities can also arrange for therapy services covered under the Medicare part B benefit or other private insurance either on-site with a contracted therapy provider or at an outpatient therapy center.

## OTHER GUIDING PRINCIPLES

### Maximizing Function

As stated previously, federal nursing facility regulations require facilities to provide services to support and maintain a resident functioning at the highest possible level achievable by them. For residents with acute weakness, neurological deficits, or who are convalescing from an acute illness or surgery, therapy services are provided in a highly coordinated manner to achieve individual treatment goals. For residents with subacute or chronic decline, the variety of services may be less complex and intense, and the frequency of treatments may be less often, but the goals of rehabilitation still apply. There is another arm of long-term rehabilitation that focuses on maintaining functional improvement gained by acute rehabilitation; this intervention is often referred to as *restorative care*. Restorative care is a program of ongoing exercise and activities of daily living training that is individually developed for each resident by the therapy team and is usually carried out by the nursing staff of the facility, including the nursing assistants who provide most of the daily care in the nursing home, or by a specially designated restorative therapy aid. Maintaining the improvement in physical function gained by acute rehabilitation is an important goal in the overall care of the long-term care resident.

### Pain Management

Adequate analgesia for patients is a key priority in rehabilitation. Many elders receiving therapy have underlying conditions that cause pain, such as hip fracture or spasticity related to stroke, and experience pain during the therapy exercises. The administration of analgesics should be provided around the clock (not only as needed) for patients with continuous pain and additional medication (as needed) should be given for breakthrough pain. Because of the intensity of therapy treatments, it has become common practice for patients to receive pain medications close to the start of a therapy session to prevent excessive pain that may limit their performance in therapy. As physical function improves, or surgical sites heal, pain frequently lessens so that reevaluation of the medication regimen should take place routinely.

### Depression

Depression is an extremely common condition among residents of long-term care facilities with prevalence in excess of 50% among nursing home residents. Similar high rates of depression occur among long-term care residents who are undergoing rehabilitation for conditions such as stroke and hip fracture. Depression among rehabilitation patients may involve several mechanisms including multiple contributing medications, medical comorbidities, neuroendocrine imbalance related to the primary illness, or may have reactive features related to psychological stress or disability. Depressed patients are at risk for slower rehabilitation progress, longer length of stay, achieving worse outcomes, and not completing the therapy program designed for them. Practitioners should be vigilant in diagnosing depression, and treatment in this setting should be timely and comprehensive including both psychotherapy and pharmacologic agents. (For a more comprehensive discussion of depression please see chapter 11).

## SUMMARY

Rehabilitation is a critically important part of health care delivery to long-term care residents and serves essentially all residents at some time in their nursing home stay. Attention to preserving and restoring function is an essential element of quality long-term care. Two additional caveats apply to this population of frail elders:

- Firstly, impairment in cognition and comprehension, common among elderly nursing home residents, often makes reaching optimal rehabilitation goals very difficult.
- Secondly, resident treatment goals and their prognosis for achieving them is often a constantly shifting scenario and changes in the approach to care must be made frequently.

For long-stay nursing home residents, who all too frequently progress toward functional decline at the end of life, greater treatment priorities centered around maintaining the quality of life often supercede traditional rehabilitation goals. A plan of care centered on the individual's specific immediate and long-term needs is always most appropriate.

## PEARLS FOR THE PRACTITIONER
- Nursing facility as a site of care for rehabilitation is appropriate for patients who are unable to perform or tolerate the 2–3 h of daily combined therapy required in acute rehabilitation hospitals.
- It is helpful to remember physical therapy as the discipline that focuses on lower extremity function and ambulation and occupational therapy as the discipline that works with upper extremity performed tasks.
- Concomitant medical conditions, referred to as medical comorbidities, can interact in dynamic and complex ways to impact both outcomes and complications of rehabilitation.
- Pressure ulcers or poorly healing wounds can derail a planned course of therapy.
- Stroke rehabilitation begins immediately upon medical stabilization of the patient – often within 48 hours.
- Up to 50% of hip fracture patients do not regain their previous level of ambulation and up to 20% become nonambulatory.
- Generalized weakness following acute illness in the elderly, referred to as deconditioning, is an extremely common complication of both hospitalization and long-term nursing home stay.
- Restorative care is the provision of exercises and activities of daily living training in a nursing facility that continues long-term following an episode of acute rehabilitation.
- Depression among rehabilitation patients is extremely common and may involve several mechanisms including: medication effects, medical comorbidities, and neuroendocrine imbalance, as well as a psychological reaction to disability.
- Resident treatment goals and short-term prognosis are constantly changing and must be frequently reevaluated.

## WEBSITES

- American Geriatrics Society http://www.americangeriatrics.org
- American Academy of Physical Medicine and Rehabilitation http://www.aapmr.org
- Centers for Medicare and Medicaid Services http://www.cms.hhs.gov
- Cochrane Collaboration, Cochrane Reviews http://www.cochrane.org/reviews/
- National Institute of Neurological Disorders and Stroke, Post-Stroke Rehabilitation Fact Sheet http://www.ninds.nih.gov/disorders/stroke/poststrokerehab.htm

## REFERENCES

1. Centers for Medicare & Medicaid. State Operations Manual, Appendix PP – Guidance to Surveyors for Long Term Care Facilities, Rev. 55 12-2-2009. http://www.cms.hhs.gov/manuals/downloads/som107ap_pp_guidelines_ltcf.pdf.
2. Kochersberger G, Hielema F, Westlund R. Rehabilitation in the nursing home: how much, why, and with what results. Public Health Rep 1994;109:372–376.
3. Quinn CQ, Port CL, Zimmerman S, Gurber-Baldini AL, Kasper JD, Fleshner I, Yody B, Loome J, Magaziner J. Short-stay nursing home rehabilitation patients: transitional care problems pose research challenges. J Am Geriatr Soc 2008;56:1940–1945.
4. Cruise CM, Sasson N, Lee MH. Rehabilitation outcomes in the older adult. Clin Geriatr Med 2006;22:257–267.
5. American Medical Directors Association. Pressure Ulcers in the Long-Term Care Setting Clinical Practice Guideline. Columbia, MD: AMDA; 2008.
6. The Surgeon General's Call to Action to Prevent Deep Vein Thrombosis and Pulmonary Embolism. 2008. http://www.surgeongeneral.gov/topics/deepvein/.
7. Jaffer AK, Brotman DJ. Prevention of venous thromboembolism in the geriatric patient. Clin Geriatr Med 2006;22:93–111.
8. Shah MV. Rehabilitation of the older adult with stroke. Clin Geriatr Med 2006;22:469–489.
9. Zuckerman JD. Hip fracture. N Engl J Med 1996;334:1519–1525.
10. Pomeranz B, Adler U, Shenoy N, Macaluso C, Parikh S. Prosthetics and orthotics for the older adult with a physical disability. Clin Geriatr Med 2006;22:377–394.
11. Cristian A. The assessment of the older adult with a physical disability: a guide for clinicians. Clin Geriatr Med 2006;22:221–238.

**ERRATUM TO:**

## Chapter 9
# Weight and Nutrition

Todd H. Goldberg and Joel A. Levine

In Chapter 9 (Weight and Nutrition) the spelling of the second author's name was incorrect. His name is Joel A. Levien

# Index

**A**

Activities of daily living (ADLs)
   assisted living (AL), 19
   home care, 3, 4
   medication management, 285–286
   nursing facilities, 48
Acute care interface
   assisted living (AL), 140
   effective transitions barriers, 140
   improvement opportunities, 140–141
   Masonic Village (MV), 138, 139
   nursing home readmissions, 138
   rehospitalization, 138
   transition of care, 141, 142
Acute change
   acute care interface (*see* Acute care interface)
   Infection Disease Society of America (IDSA), 127
   long-term care (LTC), 125–126
   pneumonia
      diagnosing, 133–134
      lower respiratory infections, 132–133
      nursing home-acquired pneumonia treatment, 136–138
      pneumonia *vs.* pneumonitis, 135
      treatment, 134–135
   residents, 142–143
   standing orders, 144
   urinary tract infections (UTI)
      diagnosing guidelines, 126–130
      treatment, 131–132
Acute illness, 323–324
Acute or chronic immune activation (ACI), 86
AD. *See* Alzheimer's disease
ADLs. *See* Activities of daily living
Adverse drug events (ADEs)
   absorption, 287–288
   analgesics, 299–300
   antipsychotic medications use, 294, 299–300
   diabetic medications, 299
   distribution, 288
   elimination, 289
   medication errors, 300
   metabolism, 288–289
   pharmacodynamics, 289–298
   pharmacokinetics, 286–287
   polypharmacy, 286
   potentially inappropriate drugs, 290–293
   Screening Tool of Older Person's Prescriptions (STOPP) criteria, 294–298
   transition of Care, 300
Agency home health care
   future of, 10
   homebound status definition, 5, 6
   members of, 5
   physician reimbursement, 9
   requirements, 5–7

Alzheimer's association, 19
Alzheimer's disease (AD), 227–228
American Medical Directors Association (AMDA)
  assisted living (AL), 27–28
  end-of-life issues, 262–263
  medical director, 67–68
  wound care, 215–216, 220
Amputation, 331
Analog insulin therapy, 103, 104
Anemia
  acute or chronic immune activation (ACI), 86
  blood transfusions, 86
  causes of, 84–86
  CKD, 86
  complications, 82–83
  definition, 83
  diagnosis algorithm, 85
  erythropoietin secretion (EPO), 82
  impairments, 82–83
  iron-deficiency vs. chronic disease, 85, 86
  noninvasive diagnostic tests, 84–85
  outcomes, 83
  red cell morphology, 85
  signs and symptoms, 83–84
  treatment, 86, 87
Angina, 301
Anorexia, 166–167
Anticholinergic drugs, 192–193
Assisted living (AL)
  acute care interface, 140
  ADL dependence, 19
  advantages, 15
  Alzheimer's association, 19
  American Medical Directors Association (AMDA), 27–28
  assisted living communities (ALC), 16
  assisted living workgroup (ALW), 17

base rate costs
  variations, 21
care
  barriers, 24, 26–27
  direct care services, 22
  facility operations, 24
  medication management, 22–24
  provider responsibilities, 24, 26
  resident rights, 24–26
  staff training, 24
Center for Excellence in Assisted Living (CEAL), 17
community-dwelling resident, 23–24
definition of, 17–18
effective communication, 27
facility characteristics, 18–19
financing, 20–22
growth and structure factors, 34
history of, 16–17
medical director, roles and responsibilities, 32, 33
optimal medical care
  physician practice, 27–28
  technology, 28
  transitions of care, 28
physician billing, 22
physicians, 20
resident characteristics, 19–20
suggestions on improving care
  AL transfer/communication forms, 30
  encourage preventive medicine, 32
  ensure communication, 30–31
  families/colleagues guide, 32
  high-risk medications focus, 31
  initiate discussion, advanced directives., 31

medical problems
 focus, 31
 mini-ALWs, 34
 procedures
  adaptation, 29
 provide in-services, 29–30
 regular meeting, facility
  administrator, 29
 urge hiring, 32, 33
Assisted living communities
 (ALC). *See* Assisted
 living (AL)
Assisted living workgroup
 (ALW), 17
Asymptomatic bacteriuria.
 *See* Urinary tract
 infections (UTI)

## B

Beta-blockers, 302
Breast cancer, 155–156
Bronchodilators, 94–95

## C

Cancer screening
 breast, 155–156
 cervical, 155
 colon, 156
 definition, 154
 prostate, 156
Care
 barriers, 24, 26–27
 direct care services, 22
 end-of-life
  comfort-directed
   pharmacologic
   interventions, 185–186
  compounded formulations, 186
  death, 184–185
  nonessential drugs, 185
  physiologic changes, 184
  practical
   interventions, 185
  serious illness, 184
 facility operations, 24
 fracture, 329–330
 hospice, 316

improvement suggestions
 AL transfer/communication
  forms, 30
 encourage preventive
  medicine, 32
 ensure communication,
  30–31
 families/colleagues
  guide, 32
 high-risk medications
  focus, 31
 initiate discussion, advanced
  directives., 31
 medical problems
  focus, 31
 mini-ALWs, 34
 procedures adaptation, 29
 provide in-services, 29–30
 regular meeting, facility
  administrator, 29
 urge hiring, 32, 33
medication management,
 22–24
provider responsibilities,
 24, 26
resident rights, 24–26
staff training, 24
standards, 265
Care plan oversight (CPO), 9
Center for Excellence in Assisted
 Living (CEAL), 17
Centers for Medicare and
 Medicaid Services
 (CMS), 208
Cervical cancer, 155
Chronic obstructive pulmonary
 disease (COPD)
 acute exacerbations,
  96, 98
 algorithm, 95, 96
 bronchodilators, 94–95
 clinical indicators, 93
 criteria, 94
 diagnosis, 93–94
 identification of, 92–93
 management, 94–97
 pharmacological treatments,
  96, 97

Clinical conditions
　anemia
　　acute or chronic immune activation (ACI), 86
　　causes of, 84–86
　　CKD, 86
　　definition, 83
　　impairments, 82–83
　　outcomes, 83
　　signs and symptoms, 83–84
　　treatment, 86, 87
　chronic obstructive pulmonary disease (COPD)
　　acute exacerbations, 96, 98
　　algorithm, 95, 96
　　bronchodilators, 94–95
　　clinical indicators, 93
　　diagnosis, 93–94
　　identification of, 92–93
　　management, 94–97
　　pharmacological treatments, 96, 97
　diabetes, 98
　　challenges, 99, 100
　　complications, 99
　　goals of, 103–105
　　hypoglycemia, 105–106
　　insulin, 101–104
　　monitoring, 106
　　treatment selection, 101, 102
　heart failure (HF)
　　care considerations process, 90–91
　　diastolic dysfunction, 87
　　evaluation, 88–89
　　laboratory testing, 89–90
　　left ventricular ejection fraction (LVEF), 87–88
　　management, 91–92
　　precipitators, 90
　　refractory, 92
　　staging, 88
　　thyroid disease, 89
　　treatment, 91
　hypertension (HTN)
　　evaluation, 79
　　goals of therapy, 79–82
　　LTC implications, 82
　　treatment benefits, 78–79
　hypothyroidism
　　causes of, 110
　　clinical evaluation, 110–111
　　definition, 106–107
　　drugs affections, 108, 109
　　interpretations, 108, 109
　　management, 112–113
　　nonthyroidal illness, 112–113
　　screening, 107–110
　　subclinical, 112
　　thyroid function tests (TSH), 108–110
　　treatment, 111–112
　skin disorders
　　herpes zoster (HZ), 118–119
　　scabies, 115–118
　subclinical hypothyroidism, 120
　vitamin $B_{12}$ deficiency
　　causes, 113–114
　　diagnosis, 114–115
　　food-cobalamin deficiency, 113
　　hematologic, 114
　　neurological consequences, 113
　　neuropsychiatric, 114
　　treatment, 115
Coding
　assisted living facilities, 319, 320
　consultations, 316
　CPT codes, 312
　home visits, 319–320
　hospice care, 316
　"Incident To" services, 317
　multisite same day visits, 317
　nursing/skilled nursing facility (NF/SNF)
　　discharge stage, 313, 315
　　health evaluation, 316
　　initial stage, 312, 313
　　subsequent stage, 313, 314
　physicians in group practice, 317
　prolonged services, 319
　qualified nonphysician practitioners visit, 317–319
Colon cancer, 156
Communication efficiency, 275

Competency, 255–256
Confusion assessment method (CAM), 235
Constipation, 169–171
COPD. *See* Chronic obstructive pulmonary disease
Cross-cultural issues, 273
Cultural barriers, 281–282
Current procedural terminology (CPT) codes
    coding, 312
    documentation, 309

## D

Delirium
    assessment, 235–236
    clinical evaluation, 225, 227
    comparison with depression and dementia, 225, 226
    confusion assessment method (CAM), 235
    importance of, 234–235
    palliative care, 171–172
    prevention interventions, 235, 236
    risk factors, 235
Dementia
    Alzheimer's disease, 227–228
    clinical evaluation, 225, 227
    cognitive impairment, 229–230
    comparison with depression and delirium, 225, 226
    definition of, 225–228
    diagnosis implications, 230
    evaluation of, 228
    medication management, 229
    neuro-imaging, 230
    nursing facility, 229
    progression of, 230
    resident evaluation, 229–230
    screening, 228
    surrogate decision making, 260
    treatments
        Alzheimer's disease (AD), 231
        behaviors, 232–233
        challenging behaviors, 231–232
        pharmacologic, 233
Department of Health and Human Services (DHHS), 50
Depression
    clinical evaluation, 225, 227
    comparison with delirium and dementia, 225, 226
    *vs.* dementia, 237–238
    diagnosis, 238–239
    diagnostic tools, 240–241
    geriatric depression scale, 240
    SIGECAPS mnemonic, 240
    symptoms, 236, 238
    treatment
        antidepressants affect, 242
        medication classes, 241–242
        monoamine oxidase inhibitors, 242
        psychotherapy, 241
        response rate, 242–243
        serotonin/norepinephrine reuptake inhibitors (SNRI's), 241, 242
        serotonin-reuptake inhibitors (SSRIs), 241, 242
        side effects, 242
Diabetes
    analog insulin therapy, 103, 104
    challenges, 99, 100
    complications, 99
    facility management assessment, 106
    glycemic control assessment, 106
    goals of, 103–105
    hypoglycemia, 105–106
    insulin
        adequate glucose control, 103–104
        basal insulin analogs, 101–102
        sliding-scale, 102–103
    monitoring, 106
    risk factors, 105
    standard human insulin therapy, 103
    treatment selection, 101, 102
    wounds, 213–214

Documentation
    CPT codes, 309
    evaluation and management
        (E/M) codes, 309–310
    history, 310–311
    medical decision making,
        311–312
    practitioners, 309, 310
    time, 312
Driving, 254–255
Durable medical equipment
    (DME), 4
Dyspnea, 167–168

### E
Elder abuse, 250, 252
End-of-life (EOL)
    care
        comfort-directed
            pharmacologic
            interventions, 185–186
        compounded
            formulations, 186
        death, 184–185
        nonessential drugs, 185
        physiologic changes, 184
        practical interventions, 185
        serious illness, 184
    issues
        American Medical Directors
            Association (AMDA)
            Policy Statements,
            262–263
        Do Not Resuscitate (DNR),
            260–261
        Living Will, 261–262
Erythropoietin secretion (EPO), 82
Ethical and legal issues
    capacity evaluation, 258–260
    care standards, 265
    Centers for Medicare and
        Medicaid Services State
        Operations Manual,
        253–254
    compilation of rules, 247
    driving, 254–255
    elder abuse, 250, 252
    end-of-life issues
        American Medical Directors
            Association (AMDA)
            Policy Statements,
            262–263
        Do Not Resuscitate (DNR),
            260–261
        Living Will, 261–262
    everyday practice, 266–267
    exploitation, 252–254
    feeding tubes, 202, 203
    health care ethics,
        248–249
    long-term care
        liability, 264–266
        vulnerable population,
            262–264
    medical decisions,
        267–268
    medical malpractice,
        264–266
    neglect, 252
    practitioners, 265–266
    resident rights, 249–252
    surrogate decision making
        capacity evaluation,
            258–260
        competency, 255–256
        dementia, 260
        guardianship,
            257–258
        judgment, 259
        mental capacity, 256
        mental illness, 260
        power of attorney,
            256–257

### F
Fall prevention.
        *See* Physical activity
Family care
    adult children, 271
    attitudes, 272–273
    chronic illness, 274
    communication
        efficiency, 275
    cross-cultural issues, 273
    cultural barriers, 281–282
    health care system, 273

interdisciplinary team
(IDT), 271
knowledge, 273–274
prudence, 274
skills, 274
  family meeting, convening
    and conducting,
    278–279
  genogram, 280–281
  progress note, 280
  responding to a phone call,
    275–277
  spokesperson
    selection, 275
translators, 282
Family meeting, 278–279
Family spokesperson, 275
Feeding tubes
  artificial feeding, 200
  enteral feedings, 201
  ethical and legal issues,
    202, 203
  immune formulas, 202
  nasogastric (NG)
    tubes, 200
Food-cobalamin
  deficiency, 113
Fragility fracture, 150–151
F-Tags, 65–67

## G
Genogram, 280–281
Geriatric depression scale, 240
Gout, 301
Gradual dose reduction
  (GDR), 303

## H
Health care
  ethics, 248–249
  system, 273
Health maintenance and
  prevention
  cancer screening
    breast, 155–156
    cervical, 155
    colon, 156
    definition, 154
    prostate, 156
  osteoporosis, 157
    fragility fracture, 150–151
    treatment of, 151
  physical activity and fall
    prevention, 156
    environmental changes, 149
    exercising, 149
    medicines arrays, 150
    occupational therapy, 149
    recommendations, 148
  preventive care, 147–148
  tuberculosis (TB) screening,
    153–154
  United States Preventive
    Services Task Force
    (USPSTF), 150
  vaccinations, 157
    herpes zoster
      vaccine, 153
    influenza
      vaccine, 153
    pneumococcal vaccine,
      152–153
  vitamin D deficiency,
    151–152, 157
Heart failure (HF)
  care considerations process,
    90–91
  diastolic dysfunction, 87
  evaluation, 88–89
  laboratory testing, 89–90
  left ventricular ejection fraction
    (LVEF), 87–88
  management
    cautions, 91–92
    digoxin, 92
    treatment, 91
  medication
    management, 301
  precipitators, 90
  refractory, 92
  staging, 88
  thyroid disease, 89
  treatment, 91
Herpes zoster (HZ),
  118–119, 153
HF. *See* Heart failure

Home care
  activities of daily living (ADLs), 3, 4
  agency home health care
    future of, 10
    homebound status
      definition, 5, 6
    members of, 5
    physician reimbursement, 9
    requirements, 5–7
  care plan oversight (CPO), 9
  definition, 2
  durable medical equipment (DME), 4
  physician house call
    acute care visit, 2
    doctor's bag, 3
    home assessment, 4
    medicare part B reimbursement, 5
    preparations, 3–4
    services billing, 4–5
  team members
    aide in attendance, 8
    occupational therapist, 8
    physical therapist, 8
    skilled nursing care, 7
    speech therapist, 8
Hospice
  billing, 184
  certification, 183–184
  disease-specific eligibility criteria, 181–183
  practitioner awareness, 181
House call
  acute care visit, 2
  doctor's bag, 3
  home assessment, 4
  medicare part B reimbursement, 5
  preparations, 3–4
  services billing, 4–5
Hypertension (HTN)
  evaluation, 79
  goals of therapy
    antihypertensive medication classes, 80, 81
    factors, 82
    pharmacological treatment, 79–80
  LTC implications, 82
  medication management, 301–302
  treatment benefits, 78–79
Hypertension in the Very Elderly Trial (HyVET), 301
Hypodermoclysis, 204
Hypothyroidism
  causes of, 110
  central, 110
  clinical evaluation, 110–111
  definition, 106–107
  drugs affections, 108, 109
  interpretations, 108, 109
  management, 112–113
  nonthyroidal illness, 112–113
  primary, 110
  screening, 107–110
  subclinical, 112
  thyroid function tests (TSH), 108–110
  treatment, 111–112
HZ. *See* Herpes zoster

# I

Illness trajectories, 162
Infection Disease Society of America (IDSA), 127
Influenza vaccine, 153
Instant nutritional assessment (INA), 195
Institute for Healthcare Improvement (IHI), 214, 215
Interdisciplinary care team, 40
  attending primary care physician, 45
  certified nurses aids, 41
  consultant pharmacists, 46
  dietitian, 43
  DON, 42
  licensed practical nurse, 41
  medical director, 45
  nurse practitioner, 45
  nursing home administers, 46

occupational therapist, 44
physical therapist, 44
recreational therapist, 45
registered nurse, 41
registered nurse assessment coordination (RNAC), 42
social worker, 43
Ischemic wounds, 214

## L

Left ventricular ejection fraction (LVEF), 87–88
Long-term care
liability, 264–266
vulnerable population, 262–264
Lung disease, 301

## M

Medical decision making, 311–312
Medical director
American Medical Director's Association (AMDA), 67–68
characteristics, 64
clinician performance and participation, 73
definition, 64
effective medical direction, 74
facility quality, 72–73
F-Tags, 65–67
Omnibus Budget Reconciliation Act (OBRA) 1987, 64–65
origins of, 64–65
physicians, 73
practitioners
responsibilities, 69–70
surveyor guidance, 69
relationship with the facility, 70–72
responsibilities
professional foundations, 67–68
regulatory foundation, 65–67
Medical malpractice, 264–266
Medicare five star program, 50–51
Medicare Modernization Act, 52–53
Medication errors, 300

Medication management
adverse drug events (ADEs), 285
absorption, 287–288
analgesics, 299–300
antipsychotic medications use, 294, 299–300
diabetic medications, 299
distribution, 288
elimination, 289
medication errors, 300
metabolism, 288–289
pharmacodynamics, 289–298
pharmacokinetics, 286–287
polypharmacy, 286
potentially inappropriate drugs, 290–293
STOPP criteria, 294–298
transition of Care, 300
angina, 301
comorbid medical conditions, 288
diabetes, 301
gout, 301
heart failure, 301
Hypertension in the Very Elderly Trial (HyVET), 301
lung disease, 301
medication selection, elderly
beta-blockers
postmyocardial infarction, 302
gradual dose reduction (GDR), 303
hypertension, 301–302
nonvalvular atrial fibrillation, anticoagulants, 302
Screening Tool to Alert Doctors to Right Treatment (START), 300
subclinical hypothyroidism, 302–303
venous thromboembolism (VTE), 300
pharmacologic treatment, 304
postmyocardial infarction, 301

Medication selection
   beta-blockers postmyocardial infarction, 302
   gradual dose reduction (GDR), 303
   hypertension, 301–302
   nonvalvular atrial fibrillation, anticoagulants, 302
   Screening Tool to Alert Doctors to Right Treatment (START), 300
   subclinical hypothyroidism, 302–303
   venous thromboembolism (VTE), 300
Mental capacity, 256
Mental illness, 260

## N

Nasogastric (NG) tubes, 200
National Pressure Ulcer Advisory Panel (NPUAP) staging system, 211, 212
Nausea, 168–169
Neuro-imaging, 230
Nonvalvular atrial fibrillation, 302
Nursing facilities (NF)
   activities of daily living (ADLs), 48
   Centers for Medicare and Medicaid Services State Operations Manual, 253–254
   dementia, 229
   Department of Health and Human Services (DHHS), 50
   discharge stage, 313, 315
   driving, 254–255
   financing
      medicaid, 53
      medicare benefit coverage, 51
      medicare part A, 52
      medicare part B, 52
      medicare part C, 52–53
      medicare part D, 53
      skilled *vs.* nonskilled nursing facility care, 51
   future changes, 54
   health evaluation, 316
   initial stage, 312, 313
   interdisciplinary care team, 40
      attending primary care physician, 45
      certified nurses aids, 41
      consultant pharmacists, 46
      dietitian, 43
      DON, 42
      licensed practical nurse, 41
      medical director, 45
      nurse practitioner, 45
      nursing home administers, 46
      occupational therapist, 44
      physical therapist, 44
      recreational therapist, 45
      registered nurse, 41
      registered nurse assessment coordination (RNAC), 42
      social worker, 43
   long-term care, 39
   medicare daily base rates, 52
   medicare five star program, 50–51
   Medicare Modernization Act, 52–53
   minimum data set (MDS), 48
   nursing facility regulations, 47–49
   nursing home-acquired pneumonia, 136–138
   Omnibus Reconciliation Act (OBRA), 40, 47, 55
   practitioners, 59–60
   rehabilitation
      deconditioned state, 332
      fracture care, 329–330
      maximizing function, 332
      therapy, 325
      venous thromboembolism, 326
   resident assessment instrument (RAI), 47–48

resident assessment protocols (RAPs), 48
short-term skilled care, 52
special needs plans (SNPs), 52–53
state operations manual (SOM), 48–49
subsequent stage, 313, 314
transitions of care, 39, 53
weight and nutrition, 196
wound development, 211
Nursing home-acquired pneumonia
acid-suppressing medications, 136
causes of, 136
criteria of, 137
nursing facility, 138
risk factors, 136
treatment guidelines, 137–138
Nutritional intervention
appetite stimulating medicines, 199–200
fluids, 198
supplements, 198–199
Nutritional status
assessment, 194–195
wound development, 210

## O

OBRA 1987. *See* Omnibus Budget Reconciliation Act 1987
Occupational therapist
home care, 8
interdisciplinary care team, 44
Occupational therapy, 325
physical activity, 149
rehabilitation and maximizing function, 325
Omnibus Budget Reconciliation Act (OBRA) 1987
federal requirements, 202, 203
medical director, 64–65
nursing facilities (NF), 40, 47, 55
practitioners, 60, 61

Opioid analgesics
acute pain, 177
cautions, 180
chronic pain, 177
dose reduction, 176
equianalgesic starting doses, 177
immediate-release morphine pharmacodynamics, 178
methadone, 180–181
oral morphine equivalents, 179, 180
side effects, 179
sustained-release oral opioids, 177, 178
Optimal medical care
physician practice, 27–28
technology, 28
transitions of care, 28
Orthotics, 331
Osteoporosis, 150–151

## P

Pain management, 332–333
caveats, 175–176
classification of, 173
end-of-life care
comfort-directed pharmacologic interventions, 185–186
compounded formulations, 186
death, 184–185
nonessential drugs, 185
physiologic changes, 184
practical interventions, 185
serious illness, 184
evaluation of, 172–173
goals of, 172
hospice
billing, 184
certification, 183–184
disease-specific eligibility criteria, 181–183
practitioner awareness, 181

Pain management (*cont.*)
  opioid analgesics
    acute pain, 177
    cautions, 180
    chronic pain, 177
    dose reduction, 176
    equianalgesic starting doses, 177
    immediate-release morphine pharmacodynamics, 178
    methadone, 180–181
    oral morphine equivalents, 179, 180
    side effects, 179
    sustained-release oral opioids, 177, 178
  partial opioid agents, 176
  treatment, 174
  WHO recommendations, 174–175
Palliative care
  combination therapy, 170
  illness trajectories, 162
  long-term care (LTC), 161
  pain management
    caveats, 175–176
    classification of, 173
    end-of-life care, 184–186
    evaluation of, 172–173
    goals of, 172
    hospice, 181–184
    opioid analgesics, 176–181
    partial opioid agents, 176
    treatment, 174
    WHO recommendations, 174–175
  principles of, 162–163
  symptom assessment and management
    advanced illness, 163, 164
    anorexia, 166–167
    assessment scales, 165
    constipation, 169–171
    delirium, 171–172
    distressful symptoms, 165
    dyspnea, 167–168
    nausea and vomiting, 168–169

Pharmacodynamics, 289–298
Pharmacokinetics, 286–287
Physical activity
  environmental changes, 149
  exercising, 149
  medicines arrays, 150
  occupational therapy, 149
  recommendations, 148
Physical therapist
  home care, 8
  interdisciplinary care team, 44
Physical therapy, 325
Physiologic stress, 193
Pneumococcal vaccine, 152–153
Pneumonia
  diagnosing, 133–134
  lower respiratory infections, 132–133
  nursing home-acquired pneumonia
    acid-suppressing medications, 136
    causes of, 136
    criteria of, 137
    nursing facility, 138
    risk factors, 136
    treatment guidelines, 137–138
  pneumonia *vs.* pneumonitis, 135
  treatment, 134–135
Polypharmacy, 286
Postherpetic neuralgia (PHN), 118
Postmyocardial infarction, 301
Practitioners
  acute change of condition, 143–144
  assisted living communities, 34–35
  caring for families, 282
  clinician performance and participation, 73
  common clinical conditions, 119–120
  delirium, dementia and depression, 243
  documentation, 309, 310

documentation and coding, 320–321
effective medical direction, 74
ethical and legal issues, 267–268
health maintenance and prevention, 156–157
home care, 10–11
medical director
  responsibilities, 69–70
  surveyor guidance, 69
medication management, 304–305
nursing facilities, 55, 59–60
Omnibus Budget Reconciliation Act (OBRA) 1987, 60, 61
palliative care, 186
physicians, 73
physician's functions and task, 60, 61
rehabilitation and maximizing function, 334
responsibilities, 60, 62–63
role of, 60–63
weight and nutrition, 203–204
wound care, 221–222
Pressure ulcers
  prevention, 214–215
  rehabilitation and maximizing function, 326
  wounds, 213
Preventive care, 147–148
Prostate cancer, 156
Psychotherapy, 241

## R

Recreational therapist, 45
Red cell morphology, 85
Rehabilitation and maximizing function
  acute illness factors, 323–324
  approaches
    amputation, 331
    deconditioned state, 332
    fracture care, 329–330
    joint replacement, 330
    orthotics, 331
    stroke, 327–329
  guiding principles
    depression, 333
    maximizing function, 332
    pain management, 332–333
  health care delivery, 333–334
  occupational therapy, 325
  physical therapy, 325
  pressure ulcer, 326
  prevention, 326–327
  speech and language therapy, 325
  therapeutic interventions, 324
  therapy services
    frailty, 325–326
    medical comorbidities, 325–326
    payment, 325
    types of, 324–325
  venous thromboembolism (VTE), 326–327
Reimbursement
  agency home health care, 9
  house call, 5
  physician house call, 5
Resident assessment instrument (RAI), 47–48
Resident assessment protocols (RAPs), 48
Residential care. *See* Assisted living (AL)
Resident rights, 249–252

## S

Scabies
  definition, 115–116
  diagnosis, 116
  outbreak controlling, 117
  transmission, 116
  treatment, 117–118
Screening Tool of Older Person's Prescriptions (STOPP) criteria, 294–298
Screening Tool to Alert Doctors to Right Treatment (START), 300
Serotonin/norepinephrine reuptake inhibitors (SNRIs), 241, 242

Serotonin-reuptake inhibitors (SSRIs), 241, 242
Short-term skilled care, 52
SIGECAPS mnemonic, 240
Skilled nursing care, 7
Skilled *vs.* nonskilled nursing facility care, 51
Skills, family
 family meeting, convening and conducting, 278–279
 genogram, 280–281
 progress note, 280
 responding to a phone call, 275–277
 spokesperson selection, 275
Skin disorders
 herpes zoster (HZ)
  measures, 118
  postherpetic neuralgia (PHN), 118
  treatment, 119
  vaccination, 119
 scabies
  definition, 115–116
  diagnosis, 116
  outbreak controlling, 117
  transmission, 116
  treatment, 117–118
SNRIs. *See* Serotonin/norepinephrine reuptake inhibitors
SOM. *See* State operations manual
Speech and language therapy, 325
Speech therapist, 8
SSRIs. *See* Serotonin-reuptake inhibitors
Staging, 215–216
Standard human insulin therapy, 103
State operations manual (SOM), 48–49
Stroke, 327–329
Subclinical hypothyroidism, 302–303
Surrogate decision making
 capacity evaluation, 258–260
 competency, 255–256
 dementia, 260
 Do Not Resuscitate (DNR), 261
 guardianship, 257–258
 judgment, 259
 mental capacity, 256
 mental illness, 260
 power of attorney, 256–257

## T
TB. *See* Tuberculosis
Thyroid dysfunction. *See* Hypothyroidism
Transitions of care
 acute care interface, 141, 142
 adverse drug events (ADEs), 300
 nursing facilities (NF), 39, 53
 optimal medical care, 28
Tuberculosis (TB), 153–154

## U
United States Preventive Services Task Force (USPSTF), 150
Urinary tract infections (UTI)
 diagnosing guidelines
  abnormal urinalysis, 126–127
  fever, 129–130
  *indwelling catheter,* 128
  public health service grading system, 127
  symptoms, 127–128
  urinalysis and urine culture, 129
 residents percentage, 132
 treatment, 131–132

## V
Vaccinations
 herpes zoster vaccine, 153
 influenza vaccine, 153
 pneumococcal vaccine, 152–153
Vacuum-assisted closure (VAC), 218
Venous thromboembolism (VTE), 300, 326–327
Venous wounds, 214
Vitamin $B_{12}$ deficiency
 causes, 113–114

diagnosis, 114–115
food-cobalamin deficiency, 113
hematologic, 114
neurological consequences, 113
neuropsychiatric, 114
treatment, 115
Vitamin D deficiency, 151–152, 157
Vomiting, 168–169

# W

Weight and nutrition
  aging, diseases and medications impacts
    anticholinergic drugs, 192–193
    community dwelling, 193–194
    disorders, 193
    drugs, 193
    laboratory assessment and monitoring, 195–196
    normal aging, 190
    nutritional status assessment, 194–195
    physiologic stress, 193
    risk factors, 192
  feeding tubes, 204
    artificial feeding, 200
    enteral feedings, 201
    ethical and legal issues, 202, 203
    immune formulas, 202
    nasogastric (NG) tubes, 200
  hypodermoclysis, 204
  instant nutritional assessment (INA), 195
  nursing facility, 196
  nutrients recommendations, 190, 191
  nutritional intervention
    appetite stimulating medicines, 199–200
    fluids, 198
    supplements, 198–199
  nutritional needs, 189
  OBRA federal requirements, 202, 203
  optimal health and longevity, 203
  weight management, 196–198
Weight management, 196–198
Wound care
  American Medical Directors Association (AMDA), 215–216, 220
  Centers for Medicare and Medicaid Services (CMS), 208
  complications, 219
  documentation, 220–221
  Institute for Healthcare Improvement (IHI), 214, 215
  long-term care (LTC), 207–208
  management, 216
  pressure ulcer prevention, 214–215
  prevalence of, 221
  prevention, 214–215
  staging, 215–216
  treatment
    challenges, 216, 217
    dressing, 218
    enzymatic debridement, 217–218
    saline, 217
    vacuum-assisted closure (VAC), 218
  types of
    diabetic wounds, 213–214
    ischemic wounds, 214
    pressure ulcers, 213
    venous wounds, 214
  ulcers, 221, 222
  wound development
    blood loss, 209–210
    Braden scale, 211
    cognitive impairment, 210
    comorbid medical conditions, 210
    National Pressure Ulcer Advisory Panel (NPUAP) staging system, 211, 212
    nursing facilities, 211
    nutritional status, 210
    risk factors, 208, 209

Printed by Publishers' Graphics LLC
SO20120926-3530-024